Dr. J. Jansen
*internist*

# The Pathology of Bone Marrow Transplantation

Edited by

## GEORGE E. SALE, M.D.

Associate Professor of Pathology
University of Washington

Associate Member
Fred Hutchinson Cancer Research Center
Seattle, Washington

and

## HOWARD M. SHULMAN, M.D.

Associate Professor of Pathology
University of Washington

Associate Member
Fred Hutchinson Cancer Research Center
Seattle, Washington

*Distributed by*
YEAR BOOK MEDICAL PUBLISHERS • INC.
35 EAST WACKER DRIVE, CHICAGO

**Library of Congress Cataloging in Publication Data**
Main entry under title:

The Pathology of bone marrow transplantation.

(Masson monographs in diagnostic pathology ; 9)
Bibliography; p.
Includes index.
   2. Marrow—Transplantation—Complications and sequelae.
2. Graft versus host reaction. I. Sale, George E.
II. Shulman, Howard M. III. Series. [DNLM: 1. Bone
Marrow—Transplantation. 2. Graft vs host disease—
Etiology. 3. Graft vs host disease—Pathology.
4. Postoperative complications. 5. Transplantation—
Adverse effects. W1 MA9309S v.9 / WH 380 P297]
RD123.5.P38 1984        617'.44        84-3890
ISBN 0-89352-220-1

ISBN 0-89352-220-1

*Library of Congress Catalog Card Number:*  *84-3890*

Printed in the United States of America

# Masson Monographs in Diagnostic Pathology

*Series Editor:* **Stephen S. Sternberg, M.D.**

1. *Tumors and Proliferation of Adipose Tissue:*
   *A Clinicopathologic Approach*

   By Philip W. Allen (1981)

2. *Diagnostic Immunohistochemistry*

   Edited by Ronald A. DeLellis (1981)

3. *Diagnostic Transmission Electron Microscopy*
   *of Human Tumors*

   By Robert A. Erlandson (1981)

4. *Meningiomas: Biology, Pathology,*
   *and Differential Diagnosis*

   By John J. Kepes (1982)

5. *Pathology and Clinical Features of Parasitic Diseases*

   By Tsieh Sun (1982)

6. *Pathology of Radiation Injury*

   By Luis F. Fajardo (1982)

7. *Advances in Immunohistochemistry*

   Edited by Ronald A. DeLellis (1984)

8. *Pathology of the Gallbladder*

   By David Weedon (1984)

9. *The Pathology of Bone Marrow Transplantation*

   Edited by George E. Sale and Howard M. Shulman (1984)

To three other generations of George Sales.

My grandfather, the Reverend George Sale,
   President, Morehouse College, 1896–1905
My father, George Goble Sale, b. 1909
My son, George Gregory Sale (Colby), b. 1962

And to my wife Nancy.

**George E. Sale, M.D.**

To my parents Albert and Della Shulman,
   and to my wife Barbara.

**Howard M. Shulman, M.D.**

# Introduction

**B**one marrow transplantation has become an important new form of therapy the full potential of which has yet to be realized. Currently, there are clear indications in patients with acute nonlymphoblastic leukemia, aplastic anemia, immunodeficiency disorders, and some inborn errors when an identical twin or matched sibling donor is available. Autografting and matched unrelated transplants also show promise. New marrow transplantation programs have sprung up all over the world following these substantial successes. Any new therapy, particularly for malignant diseases, carries with it toxicity and complications, many of which are iatrogenic. Marrow transplantation ushers in a whole spectrum of new diseases or new combinations of previously known complications.

It has been ten years since the last review of the pathology of marrow transplantation.[592] Since that time much new data about graft-versus-host disease (GVHD), chemoradiation toxicity, and interstitial pneumonia have been published. Weiden et al. begin this volume with an overview of marrow transplantation. Dr. Tsoi summarizes nearly a decade's work on immunological mechanisms of GVHD in humans based on several types of *in vitro* tests, as well as immunofluorescent studies of biopsy material. This is a particularly useful background for the pathologist attempting to understand the disease processes that afflict marrow transplant recipients. Drs. Shulman, McDonald, Hackman, and I review the animal and human pathology and differential diagnosis of skin, liver, and gut in GVHD, as well as the pulmonary and infectious problems facing the pathologist who may be required to help care for such patients. Multiple knotty problems remain both for pathologists and others in this fascinating new field.

GEORGE E. SALE, M.D.

# Acknowledgments

It was a rare privilege to be invited by Dr. Sternberg for Masson to make this review for their Diagnostic Pathology Series. Little of the field would exist today were it not for the pioneering research and leadership of our esteemed senior faculty: Drs. E.D. Thomas, Rainer Storb, Dean Buckner, Alex Fefer, and Mr. Clift. We received helpful comments, encouragement, and suggestions from Drs. Thomas, Storb, Joel Meyers, H. Joachim Deeg, Jan Wulff, Keith Sullivan, Konrad Muller-Hermelink and Mr. Reginald Clift. Charles Mahan has been invaluable in histologic and photographic work, and Dorothy Hansen and Audrey Kupfer in the secretarial arts. Considerable assistance has come from many other staff members, including Mary Rastetter, Kathleen Schaefers, Betty Pannunzio, Roderick Browne, and Larry and Rudy Lizama.

The Seattle Marrow Transplant Team has been supported by a large number of research and training grants. American Cancer Society Junior Faculty Fellowships have assisted Drs. Sale, Shulman, and Hackman. Additional grants directly or indirectly helpful have included NCI Grants No. CA18221, CA30-924, CA18029, CA15704, CA31787, and CA18105, and ACS Grant NO. CH137.

# Contributors

**ROBERT C. HACKMAN, M.D.**, *Instructor in Pathology, University of Washington; Associate in Medical Oncology, Fred Hutchinson Cancer Research Center, Seattle, Washington 98104*

**GEORGE McDONALD, M.D.**, *Associate Professor of Medicine, University of Washington; Division of Gastroenterology and Consultant, Fred Hutchinson Cancer Research Center; Attending Gastroenterologist, Veterans Administration Medical Center, Seattle, Washington 98104*

**GEORGE E. SALE, M.D.**, *Associate Professor of Pathology, University of Washington; Associate Member, Fred Hutchinson Cancer Research Center; Director of Bone Marrow Transplant Pathology, Fred Hutchinson Cancer Research Center, Seattle, Washington 98104*

**HOWARD M. SHULMAN, M.D.**, *Associate Professor of Pathology, University of Washington; Associate Member, Fred Hutchinson Cancer Research Center, Seattle, Washington 98104*

**MANG-SO TSOI, Ph.D.**, *Associate Professor in Microbiology and Immunology, University of Washington; Associate Member, Fred Hutchinson Cancer Research Center, Seattle, Washington 98104*

**PAUL WEIDEN, M.D.**, *Associate Professor of Medicine, University of Washington; Attending Physician, Virginia Mason Clinic and Hospital, Seattle, Washington*

# Contents

# Chapter 1

# Human marrow transplantation: An overview

Paul Weiden, M.D.
George E. Sale, M.D.
Howard M. Shulman, M.D.

## Introduction

In the early 1950s, infusions of marrow or spleen cells were shown to be capable of saving mice exposed to superlethal doses of total body irradiation (TBI). Subsequent studies established that this protection was due to repopulation of the host's marrow and lymphoid organs by cells of donor type, raising the possibility of replacement of diseased or inadequate marrow or lymphoid tissue in man. Clinical marrow grafting was, in fact, attempted in the late 1950s, primarily in patients with leukemia, but results were poor. Failures were principally related to lack of engraftment or fatal graft-vs.-host disease (GVHD), and to early deaths in patients who were already terminally ill at the time marrow transplantation was attempted.

During the 1960s, studies in a variety of animal systems laid the groundwork for improved clinical results. Studies in inbred rodents established the immunological principles involved in marrow grafting, especially the need for adequate immunosuppression and the importance of the major histocompatibility complex (MHC). Studies in the dog demonstrated that it was possible to achieve long-term stable chimerism by TBI and allogenic marrow transplantation in a large outbred animal. Rapid progress was achieved in defining the human MHC by serological and cellular techniques. Supportive care for pancytopenic patients also advanced dramatically with the development of antibiotics effective against staphylococci and *Pseudomonas* and the development of practical methods and principles for platelet and granulocyte support.

The 1970s saw clinical marrow transplantation emerge from a "last ditch" attempt to save a terminally ill patient to an established treatment modality for some patients with acute leukemia, severe aplastic anemia, severe combined immunodeficiency disease (SCID), and a variety of other miscellaneous disorders. In this overview, we shall review aspects of the technique, histocompatibility considerations, and supportive care common to all marrow transplants, and then aspects of patient selection, conditioning regimen, and results for each of the disease categories mentioned. A final section of this chapter will review acute and chronic GVHD briefly.

### TECHNIQUE

The technique of marrow aspiration, processing and infusion is actually quite simple.[668] Sufficient quantities of marrow can be obtained by multiple aspiration from the anterior and posterior iliac crests of living donors. The aspirations

1

are generally done in an operating room, utilizing spinal, or occasionally general, anesthesia. The marrow is anticoagulated and screened to break up clots and remove any particulate material. Usually 400–700 ml of marrow containing 5–30 billion nucleated marrow cells are obtained and infused intravenously without manipulation. By some unknown mechanism, the marrow cells find their way to the marrow spaces and in 10–20 days, islands of hematopoietic activity can be detected by marrow aspiration. Engraftment of donor cells can be confirmed by karyotyping (if donor and recipient are of opposite sex or differ for some other detectable chromosomal marker), or by detection of donor red or white cell enzymes or membrane antigens.

### HISTOCOMPATIBILITY

The genetically determined human leukocyte antigens (HLA) pose a "double" barrier to successful marrow transplantation. First, a marrow transplant, like any other organ transplant, contains histocompatibility antigens which may stimulate a rejection reaction. Second, transplanted marrow cells, unlike other organ transplants, are immunologically competent and thus able to react against histocompatibility antigens of the host, resulting in a syndrome of signs and symptoms we call GVHD. Thus tissue typing designed to select a compatible donor and recipient is of paramount importance, as has been extensively demonstrated in animal studies involving rodents, dogs, and primates (Chapter 3).

An ideally suitable, albeit infrequently available, marrow donor is an identical twin. Transplants between genetically identical individuals, referred to as syngeneic transplants, can be performed without concern that histocompatibility differences will result in either graft rejection or GVHD. These transplants, therefore, provide the opportunity of determining the influence on marrow graft results of either GVHD or attempts to prevent GVHD by providing a group of marrow transplant recipients in whom no alloimmune reaction can occur and who, therefore, do not receive postgrafting immunosuppression designed to ameliorate GVHD.

The major transplantation antigens in all species studied are determined by a complex of genetic loci on one autosomal chromosome pair and

designated the MHC. The antigens of the MHC in man are known as human leukocyte antigen (HLA) and occur in several segregant series known as HLA-A, HLA-B, HLA-C, HLA-D, and HLA-DR. Antigens of each series, except HLA-D, can be recognized by the use of appropriate antisera in cytotoxicity assays, while those of HLA-D are recognized by reactivity in mixed leukocyte culture. Almost all allogeneic marrow transplants in man have been between HLA-matched sibling pairs. In such a pair, each individual has inherited the same two MHC-bearing chromosomes, one from each parent. Any sibling of a patient has a 25% chance of being HLA-identical with the patient. It is important to emphasize that HLA-identical siblings do differ for other transplantation antigens whose genetic loci are on other chromosome pairs and that cannot generally be detected *in vitro*. Although designated "minor," these transplantation antigens can result in marrow graft rejection or fatal GVHD.

Recently, attempts have been made to expand the potential of marrow transplantation by finding acceptable alternatives to the use of HLA-matched sibling donor-recipient combinations. The general approach has been to utilize donors and recipients who are HLA-phenotypically identical for one haplotype (i.e., chromosome) and have well-defined similarity for the other.[113,114] Examples include parent-child, unrelated HLA-phenotypically identical pairs, or pairs who differ by only a portion of the dissimilar haplotype. An exemplary pair would be HLA-A- and HLA-B-identical, but dissimilar for one HLA-D antigen. Although the number of patients is limited, successful grafts have been achieved even in the absence of genotypic HLA identity, especially in HLA-phenotypically identical combinations.

ABO incompatibility does not preclude successful marrow transplantation. Type O marrow can be transplanted into individuals of any ABO type, and AB recipients can receive marrow from any individual. In either circumstance, the transplanted marrow and immune system will make antibodies against recipient-type red cells, resulting in accelerated destruction. Thus, red cell support should be of donor ABO type. If the donor red cells represent a "major" mismatch (type A into type B or O), two approaches have been used: 1) recipient isohemagglutins have been removed by plasmapheresis and absorption of remaining antibody by donor type red cells;[86] or 2) donor red cells have been removed from the marrow graft by differential centrifugation.[79] Either technique has avoided major hemolytic transfusion reactions and permitted successful engraftment. It is interesting that neither ABO nor Rh antigens are histocompatibility antigens; that is, graft rejection and GVHD are not influenced by ABO/Rh incompatibility.

## SUPPORTIVE CARE

Marrow transplant candidates will often have severely compromised marrow and immune function as a consequence of their underlying disease and/or previous therapy. The conditioning regimen given before marrow transplantation will destroy the remaining function. The newly transplanted marrow does not function usefully for at least 2–3 weeks and immune function remains compromised for 3–4 months. Therefore, all patients will require blood product support and intensive efforts to prevent and treat infectious complications.[643] Platelet transfusions are given to maintain a platelet count of 20,000/$\mu$l whether or not the patient shows evidence of bleeding. Platelet requirements increase in the face of infection, GVHD, or immunization.

During the early post-transplant period all patients are profoundly granulocytopenic and the risk of bacterial and fungal infection is high. Most patients become febrile and are started empirically on broad-spectrum, intravenous antibiotics, generally an aminoglycoside and broadspectrum penicillin. Patients with persistent fever after 2 or 3 days are started on antifungal therapy, generally with amphotericin. Vigorous bacterial and fungal surveillance is maintained to make certain that any pathogen is identified rapidly and treated appropriately.

Granulocyte transfusions are used empirically to treat pyogenic infections not controlled by antibiotic/antifungal drugs. The value of therapeutic granulocyte transfusions has been established in granulocytopenic dogs with experimental bacteremia and in leukemic patients with Gram-negative septicemia and is assumed to extend also to granulocytopenic marrow transplant recipients.[111] The most suitable donor is a family member (occasionally the marrow donor) whose platelets survive normally in the recipient. Daily continuous-flow centrifugation using arteriovenous shunts has proven to be the most effective method for procuring adequate numbers of granulocytes from a single donor.

Two approaches to the prevention of infection in marrow graft recipients have been explored. Ultraisolation consisting of a protective environment with laminar airflow isolation, skin and intestinal decontamination, and sterile diet resulted in significantly fewer episodes of systemic and major local infections than those observed in marrow transplant recipients nursed in standard rooms without oral antibiotics.[85] Similarly, the prophylactic transfusion of granulocytes from a compatible single donor during the period of profound granulocytopenia was shown to be effective in decreasing both local infections and septicemia during the first 21 days post-transplant, compared to a randomized control group.[112] Neither method of infection prophylaxis affected patient survival, however, primarily because pyogenic infection had become a rare cause of patient mortality following marrow transplantation.

### ACUTE LEUKEMIA

### Transplantation in relapse

As is appropriate for any new therapeutic modality, initial studies of marrow transplantation were undertaken in end-stage patients who had acute leukemia in relapse. Syngeneic transplantation in this setting in patients conditioned with 1000 rad TBI demonstrated. marrow reconstitution but early relapse of leukemia.[669] Addition of cyclophosphamide (CY), 60 mg/kg, on each of 2 consecutive days before TBI, improved results. In Seattle, 34 patients with leukemia in relapse were treated with CY, TBI, and syngeneic marrow transplantation.[200] Of these, 23 died of persistent or recurrent leukemia, and three of nonleukemic causes. Eight remain alive in complete remission without any maintenance therapy at 37–111 (median 88) months after grafting. These figures demonstrate that syngeneic marrow transplantation after CY and TBI results in tolerable morbidity, rare nonleukemic fatality, frequent remissions, and occasional long-term, disease-free survival (cures), even when applied to end-stage patients.

Allogeneic marrow transplantation using HLA-identical sibling donors was also undertaken initially with end-stage patients in relapse. The first 10 patients were conditioned with TBI alone, but because of the results in syngeneic recipients described above and the observation of recurrent leukemia in cells of donor origin, CY was added to the conditioning regimen.[669] Of the next 100 patients, all treated with CY, TBI, and HLA-matched sibling marrow, 12 remain alive 6–11 years after grafting with functioning marrow of donor origin, without leukemia and without maintenance chemotherapy. Among those who died, major causes of death included recurrent (or persistent) leukemia, GVHD, interstitial pneumonia, and early pyogenic infection.[671] An important observation was that patients in better clinical condition at the time of transplantation fared better. Results of over 300 transplants reported in the literature and evaluated by Gale[227] indicate an actuarial survival rate of approximately 10%. As in the Seattle series, recurrent or resistant leukemia was the most important cause of treatment failure, followed by GVHD and interstitial pneumonia. Attempts to condition patients without TBI have generally been followed by recurrent leukemia, while a more intensive chemoradiotherapy conditioning regimen (known as the SCARI regimen), did result in fewer leukemic deaths but in more nonleukemic deaths.[701] Despite poor survival for these end-stage patients, the results have demonstrated that "cure" is achievable by marrow transplantation in acute leukemia.

### Transplantation in remission

Based on the "cure" achieved in end-stage patients, it was logical to attempt to improve the results by performing marrow transplantation earlier in the course of acute leukemia. Such patients are in optimal clinical condition, have a lesser burden of leukemic cells, and should be less likely to have leukemic cells refractory to chemoradiotherapy. Patients with acute lymphoblastic leukemia (ALL) and acute nonlymphoblastic leukemia (ANL) present somewhat different problems and will be considered separately.

Although as many as 50% of children with ALL can be cured with optimal combination chemotherapy, once relapse has occurred the prognosis is grim. Adults with ALL have little likelihood of long-term survival with conventional therapy. Accordingly, the Seattle transplant group compared the results of transplantation of patients with ALL in second or subsequent remission to those obtained in concurrently treated patients with ALL in relapse.[673] Patients transplanted in remission had a lower likelihood of death from nonleukemic causes and were less likely to develop recurrent leukemia, resulting in a significant improvement in survival. Even among the patients transplanted in remission, however, recurrence of leukemia was the major cause of treatment failure. Nevertheless, for children with ALL in second remission (reinduced with chemotherapy after an initial treatment failure), marrow transplantation has been shown to result in improved survival as compared to conventional chemotherapy, and to offer the best chance of long-term remission and potential cure.[320]

Although an initial complete remission can now be induced with combination chemotherapy in 60–80% of patients with ANL, median duration of first remissions is only 10–14 months, and only 10–25% of patients who achieve a complete remission will remain free of recurrent leukemia after 3–5 years.[228,246,343,517] Because of this still dismal long-term prognosis, the results of marrow transplantation in end-stage patients, and the considerations summarized above, several groups have transplanted patients with ANL in first remission after intensive chemotherapy (generally CY and 920–1200 rad TBI) using HLA-identical sibling marrow donors.[65,66,512,672] In Seattle, 12 of the first 22 ANL patients transplanted in first remission are living in remission, well out on a plateau and probably cured of their disease. In a subsequent series of 53 such patients, randomized between two different radiation schedules, 26 patients were alive in remission 1–3 years after treatment.[675] Recurrent leukemia has been an unusual cause of failure, observed in only seven of the 75 patients, while transplantation-related problems, such as interstitial pneumonia and GVHD, have been the principal cause of morbidity and mortality. Similar results have been obtained by transplant centers in England[512] and California.[65,66]

One of the early theoretical indicators for attempting allogeneic marrow transplantation in patients with leukemia was the possibility that the marrow graft would exert an antileukemia effect. Recent statistical analyses, in fact, have shown the recurrence rate of leukemia is less in patients who develop significant acute or chronic GVHD, compared to allogeneic marrow graft recipients without GVHD, or to syngeneic marrow graft recipients.[737]

## CHRONIC MYELOGENOUS LEUKEMIA

Although the median survival of patients with chronic myelogenous leukemia (CML) is longer than that of patients with acute leukemia, there is no suggestion of a plateau in the survival curve and little evidence that currently available chemotherapy is of any value in prolonging survival. Myeloblastic transformation of "blast crisis" terminates the "chronic phase" of the disease and is the major cause of death.

Initially, marrow transplantation was attempted in patients in blast crises using a variety of chemoradiotherapeutic regimens. Morbidity and early mortality were high, both among syngeneic and allogeneic marrow graft recipients. Of 10 patients treated with identical twin marrow, two are alive, 2 and 6 years after grafting (one after a second transplant).[675] Of the initial 10 patients to receive allogeneic marrow, the only long-term survivor relapsed at 16 months (Doney, 1978). Five of the 14 patients studied recently are alive 5–43 months after grafting. Overall, these results are comparable to those achieved in patients with end-stage acute leukemia, though a "clinical impression" exists that these patients have particularly difficult posttransplant courses.

Transplantation while still in the chronic phase of CML has recently been reported in 12 patients with syngeneic donors.[201] Morbidity was low, and eight patients remain in cytogenically complete remission without the Philadelphia chromosome 21–65 (median 30) months post grafting, results clearly superior to those achieved in blast crisis. Nine patients with HLA-identical sibling donors have been transplanted while still in chronic phase. Although five are alive with the Philadelphia chromosome 5–29 months post grafting, four died of transplant-related complications.[115] These results do not yet define the role of marrow transplantation in the treatment of patients without identical twins, but do justify continued investigation of this treatment approach.

## APLASTIC ANEMIA

Aplastic anemia is characterized by marrow hypoplasia with pancytopenia secondary to any of a variety of possible etiologic agents or often of unknown etiology ("idiopathic"). A wide range of therapeutic modalities has been employed in the treatment of aplastic anemia, including corticosteroids, androgens, splenectomy, and, more recently, antithymocyte globulin (ATG), and marrow transplantation. Interpretation of the effectiveness of these approaches has been difficult, in part because of differences in definition (i.e., severity) of disease, supportive care, and onset of therapy in relation to onset of disease, and because of the innate variability and unpredictability of this disease. The emergence of marrow transplantation as a realistic therapeutic alternative has played a significant role in encouraging agreement on definition of criteria for severe aplastic anemia and in the design of prospective, controlled therapy trials.

Criteria for severe aplastic anemia, defined by the International Aplastic Anemia Study Group, are indicated in Table 1. Survival of patients meeting these criteria was approximately 50% at 4 months and 25% at 2 years, with no difference observed in patients treated or not treated with oral or parenteral androgens.[91]

Patients with aplastic anemia who have identical twins provide a special opportunity to determine the pathophysiology of this disease, since any mechanism that would prevent the growth of syngeneic marrow infused without preconditioning the patient would, by definition, be nongenetic. In 6/8 patients treated in Seattle, beginning marrow regeneration was observed 1–2 weeks after marrow infusion with subsequent restoration of normal hematopoietic function. Similar results have been obtained elsewhere, indicating that in the majority of cases, aplastic anemia is due to

**TABLE 1**
Criteria for Severe Aplastic Anemia[91]

---

Peripheral blood (two or more of the following):
  1. Granulocytes: fewer than 500/$\mu$l
  2. Platelets: fewer than 20,000/$\mu$l
  3. Anemia with reticulocytes: less than 1% (corrected for hematocrit)
Bone marrow (one of the following):
  1. Cellularity: less than 25% of normal
  2. Cellularity: less than 50% of normal with over 70% of remaining cells being nonhematopoietic

---

failure of the marrow stem cell population rather than to the lack of a nutrient or hormone or defect in the marrow "microenvironment." In a minority of patients, however, simple infusion of syngeneic marrow did not result in restoration of marrow function, while a second infusion after preparation of the patient with high-dose CY was successful.[10] Thus, in a minority of patients, some host factor which can be eliminated by CY, possibly an immunologic mechanism, appears to be responsible for the development of aplastic anemia.

Initially, HLA-identical sibling marrow transplants were performed for patients with aplastic anemia only after many transfusions and failure of conventional therapy. Patients were frequently infected and sensitized to random platelet transfusions at the time of transplantation. Immunosuppression to permit engraftment most commonly employed CY, 50 mg/kg, on each of 4 successive days. Between 1971 and 1975, 73 patients were transplanted in Seattle and 42% survived more than 5 years with normal marrow function.[634,637] Major causes of failure were graft rejection (failure to achieve sustained engraftment) in 17 patients, GVHD in 16 patients, and infection not associated with rejection or GVHD in four patients. Similar results were obtained in other centers and by the International Aplastic Anemia Study Group.[91] In their study, patients with newly diagnosed severe aplastic anemia and an HLA-identical sibling who could serve as a marrow donor underwent allogeneic marrow transplantation. Twenty-seven of 48 patients treated (56%) were alive at 3 years, compared with 25% in the nontransplant arms ($p$ was less than 0.001 for all patients, but not significant when only patients older than 25 years were analyzed).

Several efforts have been made to decrease the incidence of graft rejection following allogeneic transplantation for aplastic anemia. Animal studies, primarily in the dog, suggested that graft rejection was due to sensitization to minor histocompatibility antigens from transfused blood products and could be overcome by more intensive immunosuppressive conditioning regimens or by infusion of a larger number of donor cells.[734] Procarbazine and ATG were added to the CY conditioning regimen based on impressive results in sensitized dogs, but failed to alter

the incidence of graft rejection in a randomized study in humans.[637] Addition of TBI was successful in preventing rejection but failed to improve survival because of increased mortality from GVHD and interstitial pneumonia.[642,702] Other groups, however, have used lower doses of TBI and/or shielding of the lungs or total lymphoid irradiation in combination with CY in order to decrease the incidence of rejection without excessive short-term morbidity.

Infusion of additional donor cells (peripheral blood buffy coat cells for the first 5 days after grafting) has resulted in a decrease in marrow graft rejection among sensitized patients transplanted in Seattle.[640] Thirteen of 16 such patients given marrow only rejected their graft, compared to only three of 23 subsequent patients given marrow plus peripheral blood leukocytes. The precise mechanism by which these cells decrease the likelihood of graft rejection is not fully elucidated.

Another approach to decrease the incidence of rejection is to transplant patients before they have an opportunity to become sensitized, that is, before they are transfused. Only 3/30 nontransfused patients conditioned with CY alone failed to achieve a sustained graft, and 75% are alive 2–6 years after grafting.[642] These results show that in the vast majority of patients, rejection is related to transfusion-induced sensitization against minor HLA antigens and can be avoided by early transplantation before transfusions are given.

## TRANSPLANTATION FOR CONGENITAL ABNORMALITIES

Marrow transplantation has been used in the treatment of a wide range of hematologic and immunologic congenital disorders, many of which present special opportunities or problems. SCID is a rare congenital disorder characterized by profound immunodeficiency involving both T- and B-lymphocytes and is generally fatal within the first year of life. This profound immunodeficiency permits the engraftment of viable donor hematopoietic/lymphoid cells without any immunosuppressive conditioning of the recipient. This has led to fatal GVHD when unintended engraftment has occurred following transfusion of blood products. In a series of 69 SCID patients reported by the International Bone Marrow Transplant Registry, transplantation of HLA-genotypically identical marrow resulted in 63% 6-month survival, transplantation of fetal tissues in 43% 6-month survival, marrow from HLA-D-matched donors in 38%, and marrow from HLA-D-mismatched donors in 5%. Infection was the most frequent cause of death, followed by GVHD, and then by multiple other causes.[73] Nine of 12 SCID patients transplanted by Good and colleagues using matched sibling donors are alive and healthy as late as 11 years after transplantation.[280] It is of interest that, even though no postgrafting immunosuppression was used to ameliorate GVHD, this complication was observed in only five patients and was usually mild to moderate and transient.

Marrow transplantation has also been used in other congenital immunodeficiencies and in phagocytic disorders, such as Wiskott-Aldrich syndrome,[490] chronic granulomatous disease, infantile agranulocytosis, Chediak–Higashi syndrome, etc., summarized in Hobbs.[293] These disorders seem to have in common: first, the need to immunosuppress the marrow graft recipient adequately to permit engraftment (since, otherwise, immune function in these disorders is intact enough to result in graft rejection); and, second, the need to "make space" in the recipient marrow by administration of radiation or myleran in addition to CY.[490] It appears that CY alone does not reduce the recipient's hematopoietic stem cell population enough to prevent overgrowth of the infused normal-donor (allogeneic) stem cells.

Marrow transplantation may also have a role in the treatment of inborn metabolic diseases, including, to date, Hurler-Scheie disease (a mucopolysaccharidosis) and Fabry disease (a lipidosis), reviewed in Hobbs.[293] Infantile osteopetrosis, an otherwise fatal disorder of marrow osteoclasts, also has been successfully treated by marrow transplantation.[115a] The marrow aplasia of patients with Fanconi's anemia has been reversed by marrow transplantation, just as in patients with acquired aplastic anemia.[139] Congenital hemolytic anemia has been treated successfully in the mouse[617] and the dog.[735a] Two patients with thalassemia major have been transplanted successfully (unpublished data).[675a]

## AUTOLOGOUS MARROW TRANSPLANTATION

Autologous marrow transplantation is a special case in which some of a patient's marrow is removed, preserved, and stored. Tumor therapy with large doses of radiation or drugs is then followed by autologous marrow rescue to prevent aplasia. The value of this technique is still under active study. The topic is reviewed elsewhere.[87] Of interest to the study of GVHD is the fact that these patients are by definition incapable of a true GVHR.

## ACUTE GRAFT-vs.-HOST DISEASE

The GVHD syndrome refers to the clinical features caused by the attack of immunocompetent donor lymphoid cells against certain target organs. In man, GVHD has been separated into an early acute form occurring in the first 3 months post transplantation and a later chronic form. Although the distinction between acute and chronic GVHD is partially an arbitrary and temporal one, there are also definite histologic and immunologic differences.

The most common onset of acute GVHD occurs in the third to fourth week post transplant. However, the range extends from the first week to infrequent cases starting after day 60. The cases of GVHD which occur during the early period pose the greatest diagnostic difficulty because of toxicity reactions from chemotherapy and radiation that mimic the signs of GVHD in the skin, liver, and gut. Fortunately, in most patients, GVHD can be separated from these other events by combining clinical judgment, histologic findings, and, sometimes, radiographic studies. The pathologist's role is to determine if the histological findings are consistent with GVHD.

Typical features of acute GVHD are skin rashes, enterocolitis with diarrhea, jaundice with hepatic dysfunction, and fever. The initial target organ and the severity of involvement vary. In the initial report of 61 patients transplanted in Seattle before May 1973, 43 (70%) developed GVHD.[245] This early incidence seemed higher than that of ensuing years. The frequency inexplicably fluctuated between 70–40% from 1974 to 1979. The overall incidence is approximately 55% among HLA-matched recipients who received standard post-transplant, intermittent methotrexate (MTX) until day 100. The clinical severity of GVHD is graded as in Table 2. Grades II–IV have prognostic significance, where grade I is similar to grade 0 in prognosis. Severe acute GVHD may result in fatal infection via denudation of the gut mucosa or through general immunodeficiency producing a greater susceptibility to pneumonia or deep fungal infections. Early liver disease with ascites is usually veno-occlusive disease rather than GVHD and is treated differently. Treatment of acute GVHD employs steroids, ATG, or cyclosporin (CYA). Optimal treatment is still under active study.

### CHRONIC GRAFT-vs.-HOST DISEASE

Chronic GVHD, a later sequela of allogeneic marrow transplantation, is a multisystem disorder with features of autoimmunity and immunodeficiency that has an unfavorable natural history. Even in the earliest reports of clinical marrow transplantation, a few of the longer-lived patients developed what now would be diagnosed as chronic GVHD. Mathe reported a patient surviving 75 days with a dry, scaly, erythematous rash.[413] Early reports by transplant groups from NIH[365] and Minnesota[432] described a few patients with scleroderma-like skin changes with epidermal atrophy and dermal fibrosis. Speilvogel's case report[609] provided the first chronological demonstration of gross and histological progression from acute to chronic cutaneous GVHD. In separate short reports in 1975, Touraine[680] and Saurat[557] described features of early chronic cutaneous GVHD. When larger series of patients with chronic GVHD were eventually reported from other marrow transplantation centers,[263,584] a more complete picture of chronic GVHD emerged.

### Onset of chronic GVHD

Chronic GVHD may present in one of three modes of onset: *progressive*, if it follows as a direct extension of acute GVHD; *quiescent*, if it is preceded by a resolution of acute GVHD; or *de novo*, if it occurs without any preceding acute GVHD. The type of onset also influences the morbidity, which is highest in progressive and lowest in *de novo*. The progressive onset was slightly more common (37%) than either the quiescent (33%) or the *de novo* (31%) presentations. In the absence of specific therapy directed at chronic GVHD, clinical signs usually develop between days 70–250, and occasionally as late as day 500. The most frequent onset is between days 120–150, perhaps corresponding to the usual cessation of intermittent prophylactic MTX at day 100, or to the more competent state of immunological reconstitution. In many patients, the onset of chronic GVHD may be immediately preceded by sun exposure or a febrile illness. The initial sites involved with chronic GVHD may correspond to photoexposure, trauma, venous stasis, a viral exanthem (measles or varicella zoster), or previous local radiation. Once chronic GVHD begins, the manifestations usually become more widespread.

### Clinical Manifestations

Chronic GVHD has typical manifestations which are variable in frequency and may occur together. These include the following (in order of decreasing frequency): either of two scleroderma-like skin disorders (98%); chronic liver disease (89%); Sjogren's syndrome with xerophthalmia (89–90%); xerostomia and oral stomatitis (60%); and/or dryness of upper respiratory tract and a desquamative esophagitis (36%). Less frequent manifestations are musculoskeletal serositis (approximately 20%), including arthralgias, sterile effusions, arthritis, and polymyositis (8%), and dryness and stenosis of vaginal vault (stenosing vaginitis).[129] Circulating autoantibodies, usually in low titer, were found in approximately two-thirds of untreated patients with chronic GVHD, as follows (in order of decreasing frequency): ANA, rheumatoid factor, antimitochrondrial antibody, and direct Coombs' test.

**TABLE 2**
Overall Clinical Grading of Severity of GVHD[669]

| Grade | Degree of Organ Involvement |
|---|---|
| I | + to ++ skin rash; no gut involvement; no liver involvement; no decrease in clinical performance. |
| II | + to +++ skin rash; + gut involvement or + liver involvement (or both); mild decrease in clinical performance. |
| III | ++ to +++ skin rash; ++ to +++ gut involvement or ++ to ++++ liver involvement for (or both); marked decrease in clinical performance. |
| IV | Similar to grade III with ++ to ++++ organ involvement and extreme decrease in clinical performance. |

With the advent of immunosuppressive therapy, autoantibodies, other than rheumatoid factor, are infrequent. Increasing circulating eosinophils (greater than 7500/$\mu$l) were found in 75% of patients with chronic GVHD. Approximately 20% of patients with chronic GVHD fulfill the criteria of the American Rheumatological Association for the diagnosis of systemic lupus erythematosus in spite of the more obvious dermatopathologic similarities to scleroderma.

The manifestations of chronic GVHD have been classified as *limited* or *extensive*, depending on the type of cutaneous histopathology and the extent of systemic involvement (Table 3). In *limited* chronic GVHD, skin histopathology was exclusively of the localized type and resembled localized scleroderma; no other organs were involved, except occasionally the liver. Patients with limited chronic GVHD had an indolent clinical course and usually did not require therapy, or they improved spontaneously. In *extensive* chronic GVHD, the patients had a more inflammatory and *generalized* type of skin involvement, and/or sicca syndrome, and involvement of other viscera. In contrast to limited chronic GVHD, extensive chronic GVHD has a high morbidity and mortality rate. The morbidity results from cosmetic deformities, immobility from skin contractures, ulcerations, xerophthalmia, failure to thrive with weight loss, and frequent infections. The weight loss in these patients is multifactorial, stemming from debility, poor caloric intake from xerostomia, painful swallowing or esophageal strictures, and, occasionally, from malabsorption of fats. Patients dying with chronic GVHD usually succumb to infections by Gram-positive organisms. Although these patients are at increased risk for varicella zoster,[20] they do not appear at a markedly increased risk for other viral infections, as was initially suggested by Graze and Gale.[263] As discussed elsewhere, tests of *in vivo* and *in vitro* cellular immunity remain impaired in such patients. The unfavorable natural course of chronic GVHD has stimulated efforts at developing predictive tests for early diagnosis[305,548] and various treatment regimens.[653] The apparent initial success with prednisone and azothioprine is being further tested by randomized clinical trials to compare the regimen with prednisone alone.

### CONCLUSION

During the 1980s, we can expect further refinement in both the indications for and management of allogeneic marrow transplantation. Indications for marrow transplantation are relative, influenced, that is, not only by the results of transplantation, but also by the results of alternative therapy. For example, if idiopathic aplastic anemia could be treated with an alternative, less toxic, equally or more effective therapeutic approach, the indications for early marrow transplantation would be decreased. Similarly, if the percentage of patients with ANL cured by conventional combination chemotherapy were to increase, indications for transplantation in first remission would be less clear. Further, as risk factors which identify patients with poor prognosis are more clearly delineated (in ALL: age, sex, initial white cell count, T-cell versus non-T-cell disease), certain subpopulations of patients may be identified in whom early marrow transplantation is justified.

Improvement in results of marrow transplantation itself can also be anticipated. For example, eradication of leukemia cells might be facilitated and toxicity decreased by fractionation of the TBI, an approach under active investigation in several centers. New immunosuppressive agents will be developed and employed; at present, CYA is such an agent—one that has initially shown great promise and is being actively studied in many centers. Monoclonal antibodies will also undoubtedly be used in marrow transplantation in at least two ways: first, specific anti-T-cell

**TABLE 3**
Classification Scheme for Patients with Chronic GVHD[584]

Limited chronic GVHD
  Either or both:
    1. Localized skin involvement
    2. Hepatic dysfunction due to chronic GVHD
Extensive Chronic GVHD
  Either:
    1. Generalized skin involvement; or
    2. Localized skin involvement and/or hepatic dysfunction due to chronic GVHD, plus:
    3. a. Liver histology showing chronic aggressive hepatitis, bridging necrosis or cirrhosis; or
       b. Involvement of eye: Schirmer's test with less than 5-mm wetting; or
       c. Involvement of minor salivary glands or oral mucosa demonstrated on labial biopsy; or
       d. Involvement of any other recognized target organ

antibodies may be used *in vitro* or *in vivo* to suppress GVHD; and second, antibodies directed against leukemia-associated antigens may be used to help eradicate residual leukemia cells.

Thus, marrow transplantation in the future is likely to remain both an area of active clinical investigation and a treatment approach of increasing clinical value.

# Chapter 2

# Introduction to the experimental pathogenesis of GVHR

George E. Sale, M.D.

## Introduction

The phenomenon of the graft-vs.-host reaction (GVHR) has been studied in a bewildering variety of experimental settings, and has been operationally defined in several ways.[178-180,264,587,713] This chapter attempts only a skeletal introduction of some of the ideas in this field. Special cases summarizing various *in vitro* and *in vivo* models are described in Chapter 3.

### Generic definition

The fundamental requirements for a *true* GVHR are:

1. A donor with one or more *genetically* determined differences from the host
2. The introduction of living, "immunocompetent" cells (e.g., lymphocytes or stem cells) from the donor into the host
3. The survival of the donor cells in the host at least long enough to subserve an immunological reaction
4. Assessable evidence of an immunological reaction by the donor cells against host tissues or cells (e.g., target cell damage)

There is a wide range of special cases and models for GVHR, the diversity of which has been responsible for occasional confusion.

### Pseudo-GVHRs: GVHD-like reactions

Classified here for purposes of this discussion are all GVHR-*like* reactions arising in autologous (self-donor, self-host) and syngeneic (identical twin donor or congenic animal strain donor) situations. These include all the skin reactions reported in human identical-twin and autologous bone marrow graft recipients[78,520,545,664] as well as the *in vitro* autocytotoxicity and autostimulation reactions.[241,619-621] These reactions have been variously called GVHR or GVHR-like but, by definition, are *not* initiated by GVHR.[180] Also numbered among these might be the so-called "autoimmune" diseases such as systemic lupus erythematosus, rheumatoid arthritis, systemic scleroderma, mixed connective tissue disease, primary biliary cirrhosis, and those viral diseases which may mimic alloimmune disease or GVHR/GVHD, such as infectious mononucleosis.

### BASIC LAW OF TRANSPLANTATION

This basic law derives from classical studies of Burnet, Medawar, Snell, and others. It states that the degree of genetic disparity between donor and host controls rejection. Succinctly stated by Snell, it is that "isografts and autografts succeed, and allografts fail."[601] Grafts between genetically identical host and donor are accepted readily; grafts between nonidentical host and donor are rejected. A "syngeneic" donor–host combination (isograft) is genetically identical; i.e., identical twins or inbred strains with the same genes. Individuals of the same species who are not genetically identical define an "allogeneic" combination; such a graft is an "allograft;" a graft between species is "xenogenic," and is a "xenograft." Graft rejection occurs when a relatively vigorous immunologic reaction develops in an allograft situation. The GVHR is an allograft rejection in reverse, in which the graft is lymphoid cells from the donor that recognize host tissues as foreign and attempt to eliminate ("reject") them. This is usually manifested as a syndrome of wasting with dermatitis, enteritis, and hepatitis.

## MAJOR HISTOCOMPATIBILITY COMPLEX

There is considerable evidence in mice, humans, dogs, horses, rats, hamsters, and monkeys that genetic control over the most vigorous component of graft rejection is localized to a relatively short segment of genetic (chromosomal) material. The general biological term for this is the "major histocompatibility complex" (MHC), which is given the designation "H2" in mice, "HLA" in humans, and "DLA" in dogs. The MHC of humans is a group of genetic loci on the short arm of the sixth chromosome. The major loci are called A,B,C, and D. A,B, and C are serologically defined; D is defined either by mixed lymphocyte culture (MLC) methods or by serology. Gene products of A, B, and C are widely distributed and are found on nucleated cell surfaces and platelets. Gene products of the D locus are found on the monocytic series, B-lymphocytes, activated T-lymphocytes, and certain epithelial tissues such as endothelial cells.

Much research has been devoted to finding the natural and evolutionary role of the MHC, since allografting or rejection is obviously an unnatural event. A vigorously debated hypothesis is that of Doherty and Zinkernagel[156] which states that a major function of the MHC may be to signal changes in "self" to the immune system. This is based on evidence showing that the ability of T-cells to lyse virus-infected cells is dependent on the histocompatibility of the infected cells with the T-cell source. In other words, T-cells

from a mouse must have the same histocompatibility type as virally infected mouse target cells in order to be able to kill the target cells. The virus is thought to produce a chemical change on the target cell surface which is recognized as a combination of foreign *and* self by the T-cell. Cells from a histo*in*compatible animal will *not* become targets for viral antigen-induced, T-cell killing by this mechanism (although they may, of course, still be recognized as allogeneic). The evolutionary role of this phenomenon, often called $H_2$ restriction, is thought to be two-fold:

1. It provides a way to attack a virus which hides within the host's very cell machinery.

2. It may explain the polymorphism of the histocompatibility loci which have been discovered so far. Such a polymorphism, it is argued teleologically, would render a virus unable to eradicate entire populations because the genetic diversity generates a similar diversity in the range of viral susceptibility.

Naturally occurring viral diseases of mice, such as lymphocytic choriomeningitis, ectromelia (mouse pox), and paramyxovirus (Sendai) infection, have shown evidence of sensitization to altered self-antigens, which tends to support this hypothesis. Similar reactions have been demonstrated in chemically altered target cell surfaces by Shearer and others[579] using such chemical modifiers as trinitrophenol. The potential importance of such a mechanism induced by viruses in GVHD is discussed below under the superinfection theory. New knowledge on the MHC in rats, guinea pigs, dogs, Arabian horses, chickens, and other species promises to strengthen this backbone of transplant research and to elucidate its biological role.

## PATHOGENESIS OF GVHD

Initial research indicated that graft rejection and GVHR are cell-mediated or humorally mediated immunological reactions. Graft rejection is specifically related to antigens present in the donor tissue and expressed on its cell surfaces. Rejections can be primary or "second set." Second-set rejections, which are much more vigorous, are due to hypersensitive recipients previously immunized to donor antigens by earlier grafts or other exposure routes.

There is much evidence that graft rejection (or GVHD, its converse) is mediated by T-lymphocytes. To deal with this subject, we consider three stages of the pathogenetic process, using the conceptual framework employed by immunologists to describe the immune response. These are:

1. Afferent phase (stimulation: exposure to and recognition of specific antigens)
2. Central phase (information processing, recruitment of effector mechanisms)
3. Efferent phase (target cell destruction)

At some point during phase 3, possibly even during phase 2, mechanisms less specific for the stimulating antigen, and perhaps even independent of the stimulating process, come into play. Much of the debate about GVHD and autoimmune disease centers around the problem of distinguishing the steps which are "specific" in one sense or another from those which constitute the nonspecific, final common pathways of inflammation.

The immunological network theory of Jerne has significantly influenced the thinking of workers in transplantation immunology.[290] Proposed is a network of immunoregulatory lymphocyte subsets, particularly T-lymphocytes which, under the influence of immune response genes, regulate the organism's immune function. Inducer/helper cells assist the B-lymphocyte compartments to proliferate and to produce antibody. Suppressor/cytotoxic subsets inhibit such activity or kill target cells.

A complex network of feedback loops is a necessary feature of this hypothesis. Investigation is directed at understanding how such a system might function both in autoimmune disease and graft rejection. One general hypothesis is that the GVHR may be controlled by such a network. Parkman et al. have constructed a paradigm by which this potential interaction may be described in humans and by which some of the hypothesis may be tested.[491,520]

Another hypothetical framework involves the destructive capabilities of natural killer (NK) cells. The recognition mechanisms of these cells are less clear than those of T-killer cells, although they may be related to the $H_2$ restriction phenomenon mentioned above and seem to be MHC-linked. It is hypothesized, furthermore, that NK cells may be under the influence of an immunoregulatory network composed of subsets of T-helper and T-suppressor lymphocytes, and that imbalances in these regulatory cell populations may be important determinants of the effector cell reactions.

Such a network imbalance could be caused by severe thymic damage, as hypothesized by Seemayer and colleagues,[572–575] particularly in young or developing animals. Recent studies by cellular immunologists have suggested that helper and suppressor T-cells may fail to differentiate normally in human marrow recipients who get chronic GVHD.[397,398] If this is an effect rather than a cause of GVHD, the thymic damage hypothesis might gain further support as a prior cause. Figure 1 is a flow diagram illustrating several hypothetical afferent, recruitment, and efferent mechanisms in GVHD.

The possible interactions among these immunoregulatory cells are further discussed in Chapter 4. Several specific mechanisms have been prosposed which may contribute to the organ damage in GVHD. These include the "innocent bystander," the "aggressor lymphocyte," and variations on a superinfection theory.

### "Innocent bystander" theory

Steinmuller tested the concept of the "passenger leukocyte."[618] His studies manipulated the genetic composition of the blood cells in skin grafts. A skin graft from animal $B_1$ containing blood cells from animal A was placed on another animal $B_2$ with the same genetic composition as animal $B_1$. This graft was rejected. Since the only foreign cells present were blood cells, the result suggests that the antigenic differences on the blood cells were enough to excite rejection. This was called the "passenger leukocyte phenomenon." The damage to the graft has become known as an "innocent bystander" effect. Lymphokine or other toxins released in the interaction between donor and host lymphoid cells are postulated by some as mediators of this damage. The animal $B_1$ (donor of the skin graft) is known as a radiation chimera (pronounced ki-me'rah) and is produced by irradiating the animal and giving it a bone marrow transplantation from animal A. A certain percentage of such animals will be stable chimeras (without rejection or GVHR). These can then be used as sources of the skin grafts to

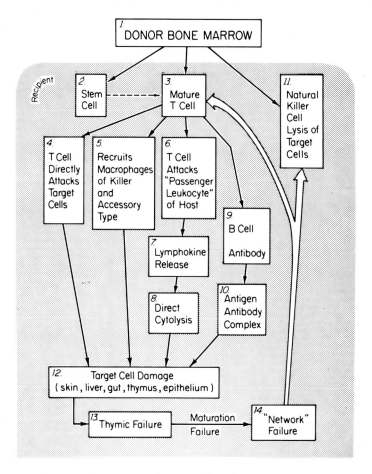

**Figure 1.** Pathogenesis of GVHD: some hypothetical mechanisms:

1. The donor bone marrow is infused into the recipient.

2. Stem cells, present in the graft, may mature in time to T-cells, as well as to other cell types.

3. Mature T-cells, also in the graft, may mediate several reactions.

4. T-cells may directly attack epithelial cells bearing nonself antigens or infected with viruses (altered self). Presentation of these antigens probably requires macrophages (5.) which may recruit or be recruited by T-cells. Macrophages of killer type may be recruited also at this stage.

6. Mature T-cells attacks lymphoid cells of host (passenger leukocyte). The reaction may release toxic lymphokines (Step 7).

8. Lymphokines may be capable of causing direct lysis of target cells.

9. T-cells may recruit B-cells to produce antibody against several antigens. Control of this process may be poor, so that polyclonal hypergammaglobulinemia results from B-cell hyperplasia in nodes and spleen.

10. Antigen–antibody complexes may form and deposit in skin or kidneys of some recipients (human skin; mouse $F_1$ hybrid glomerulonephritis).

11. Graft (or host) may contain natural killer cells capable of mediating autologous reactions ("pseudo-GVHR") or of amplifying or aggravating *true* alloimmune reactions. This has been proposed for both acute and chronic GVHD-like syndromes by Parkman et al. and may explain the unusual "pseudo-GVHR" in twins and autografts.[491]

12. End-organ damage of a certain spectrum is the observation made by the histopathologist. Obviously, very limited deductions about *either* etiology *or* relationship to the *alloantigenic* (nonself) difference between donor and host can be made solely on the basis of observing this end-organ damage. This spectrum is sensitive to species differences, strain differences within species, and is also sensitive to minor or major histocompatibility antigen differences, rendering generalizations risky. It also varies within the same recipient over time (waxing and waning acute GVHD, quiescence, chronic GVHD, photoactivation, and other triggering events).

13. A fundamental hypothesis suggests that thymic epithelial cell damage produces thymic failure and profoundly delays maturation or function of the normal immunoregulatory cell network.

14. This might feed back, as illustrated, into a *failure to regulate* B-cells, T-cells, or even NK-cells. The immunodeficiency is a well-supported fact. Secondary theories of GVHD ascribe the majority of the end-organ damage of GVHD to this immunodeficiency. Viral and bacterial infection with antigenic cross-reactivity between self and microorganisms are postulated by two such ideas,[156,710] and simple endotoxin-induced damage is proposed by a third.[133]

the second animal $B_2$, syngeneic to $B_1$. Figure 2 illustrates this experiment schematically. Similar experiments in the model of local skin GVHR in the hamster[647,648] support a passenger leukocyte mechanism for that local GVHR. Studies of similar design by Elson[181] have shown that an innocent bystander effect may account for intestinal crypt epithelial injury in the mouse. In those studies, sterile gut grafts were used rather than skin grafts. Otherwise, the principles were identical (see Chapter 6).

These passenger leukocyte experiments are elegant and instructive. However, the phenomenon can only be demonstrated under highly artificial circumstances and its contribution to systemic GVHR or GVHD in whole animals has never been demonstrated. Furthermore, it may be a vast oversimplification to invoke it as a sole mechanism by which most grafts are rejected or most GVHRs are mediated, because in

allografted animals there is no shortage of foreign antigens. To use Steinmuller's own simile, the passenger leukocyte is like a "lawn sprinkler in a rainstorm" when most alloreactions are considered.

A particularly informative example in this regard is thymic transplantation, in which incubation of unrelated donor thymic fragments has been attempted in order to allow the "passenger leukocytes" to die prior to grafting. This procedure has been thought capable of increasing the likelihood of an engraftment by removing the critical MHC antigens[296,367] expressed by the lymphocytes and macrophages in the graft. Recent data from Rouse et al.[540] and Janossy et al.[314] have shown, however, that in both mice and humans, antigens of *all* major histocompatibility loci are expressed on the surfaces of most, if not all, of the thymic epithelial cells of the medulla, including those of Hassal's corpus-

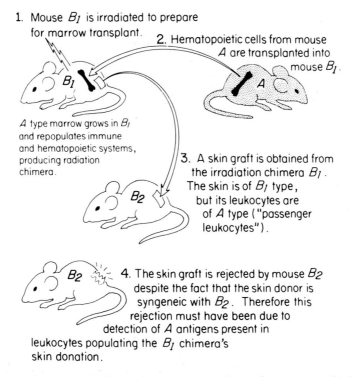

1. Mouse $B_1$ is irradiated to prepare for marrow transplant.

2. Hematopoietic cells from mouse $A$ are transplanted into mouse $B_1$.

$A$ type marrow grows in $B_1$ and repopulates immune and hematopoietic systems, producing radiation chimera.

3. A skin graft is obtained from the irradiation chimera $B_1$. The skin is of $B_1$ type, but its leukocytes are of $A$ type ("passenger leukocytes").

4. The skin graft is rejected by mouse $B_2$ despite the fact that the skin donor is syngeneic with $B_2$. Therefore this rejection must have been due to detection of $A$ antigens present in leukocytes populating the $B_1$ chimera's skin donation.

**Figure 2.** The passenger leukocyte phenomenon: Animals $B_1$ and $B_2$ are genetically identical. Animal A differs from them both. We use animal A as the donor of bone marrow (and, therefore, blood and lymphoid cells). We transplant this marrow into irradiated animal $B_1$. This accepted graft replaces $B_1$'s native marrow and makes $B_1$ a "radiation chimera." Then, $B_1$'s skin is grafted onto animal $B_2$. This skin graft is now populated by A's blood cells, and is rejected by $B_2$. **Interpretation:** $B_2$ was able to recognize the A blood cells in the $B_1$ skin graft and was therefore able to reject the skin graft because it contained foreign A "passenger leukocytes." This demonstrates that under carefully contrived conditions, "passenger leukocytes" can serve as a *sufficient* source of foreign antigenic stimulus to incite rejection.

cles as well as those in the thymic cortex. Therefore, the removal of a few macrophages should
have no significant effect on the total number of
major histocompatibility antigens expressed on
cells of the thymic graft—no more significant,
again, than turning off a lawn sprinkler in a rainstorm would be. The difficulties encountered by
some workers in achieving long-term histoincompatible thymic fragment engraftment in man[24]
may be explained by these histocompatibility
antigen-bearing thymic epithelial cells.

**Direct attack or "aggressor lymphocyte"**
This straightforward theory states that direct attack upon the target epithelial cell (whether
epidermal, hepatic, biliary ductular, or enterocy-
tic) is mediated by a cytotoxic lymphocyte. Support for this idea comes from two directions. The
first is careful morphology of the cytotoxic T-cell
reactions against target cells *in vitro*. These include studies of the MLC reaction coupled to
chromium release assays as well as studies of
morphologically definable events attending the
killing of such targets as mastocytoma cells by
cytotoxic lymphocytes.[58,554,555] These studies
show intimate contact between the membranes
of lymphocytes and target cells. "Point contact"
occurs, in which a sharply pointed projection of a
lymphocyte indents the target cell cytoplasm. No
breach of either cell membrane, however, has
been detected in such reactions. The earliest evidence of damage to the target cell appears to be
local swelling of mitochondria, according to
Leipins et al.[383]

The second line of evidence is direct *in vivo*
observation. Woodruff et al.[760] illustrated close
contact of lymphocytes to epithelial cells of the
lip in monkeys and coined the term "aggressor
lymphocytes" for these cells. Similar lesions have
been seen in skin,[143,229] liver,[46,575] and rectal
mucosa.[230] We have studied these lesions particularly carefully in the human epidermis and
rectum, where both point contact and broad-
zone contact were observed between lymphocytes and four types of target cells: basal keratinocytes, melanocytes, Langerhans' cells, and
rectal enterocytes.[229,230]

Serious problems exist with both lines of evidence, much of which is circumstantial. Ware
and Granger[731] proposed that lymphokines,
such as lymphotoxin, are produced by the attack-

ing cytotoxic T-cells, and that these mediate target cell lysis. A multimolecular model analogous
to that of the complement system is proposed for
this. Unexplained by this hypothesis, and a major
flaw, is the escape of the cytotoxic cell itself from
that lysis. Similarly, our understanding suffers
from ignorance of the type of lymphocyte invad-
ing the epithelium *in vivo*. Is it a donor or host
cell, a B- or T-lymphocyte, an NK cell or a macrophage? If T-cells are present, which subtypes
predominate? Edelson et al.[167] found that macrophages predominated in human skin lesions of
GVHD, but their method was to perform
erythrocyte rosettes on frozen sections, which
has not been deemed very reliable. Immu-
nolabeling and cytochemical methods will contribute answers to some of these questions.

Focal acid naphthylacetate esterase (ANAE)
has been proposed as a T-cell marker in humans,
dogs, and mice.[350,454,763] Formol sucrose-fixed
frozen sections can be used for this technique, so
we examined biopsy and autopsy tissue from patients with and without GVHD. We found focally
ANAE-positive cells with ease in GVHD (Fig. 3),
but also in nonspecific skin reactions.[550] In fact,
T-cells have been found to predominate in studies of a variety of forms of dermatitis by other
investigators.[57,60] Therefore, no disease specificity can be assigned to the demonstration of T-
cells in such lesions. Furthermore, some of the
evidence in man[292] and the rat, and some of our
unpublished data subsequent to our recent canine studies,[763] suggest that ANAE may not be a
completely specific or stable T-cell marker. Preliminary evidence in humans suggests that it cor-
relates with the OKT4 antigen which marks
helper T-cells, but not with OKT8 antigen which
marks suppressor/cytotoxic T-cells.[409]

Although the presence of T-cells in skin lesions
is probably not disease-specific, analysis of subsets of T-cells using newly available methods,
such as monoclonal antibodies, may shed further
light on this subject. Some evidence is available
from solid tissue grafts. Platt et al.[505] recently
reported high OKT8/OKT4 (killer cell–helper
cell) ratios in the interstitial infiltrates of renal
allografts undergoing rejection. These ratios
were significantly higher than those observed in
forms of interstitial nephritis other than graft rejection. Recent immunofluorescence data from
England in patients with GVHD showed a pre-

ponderance of OKT8 (suppressor–killer cells) in frozen sections of the skin lesions. However, since most marrow transplant recipients have high peripheral blood OKT8/OKT4 ratios after transplant,[22] this may simply be a passive reflection of the peripheral blood ratio.[368] The ratio may be secondary to the lymphocyte maturation or distribution defects of GVHD, as hypothesized by Lum et al.,[398] rather than directly indicating the actual mechanisms of GVHD at the target tissue level. Such tissue studies, to be interpretable, should probably analyze blood and tissue ratios simultaneously. A recent study by Vosak et al.,[719] in fact, very strongly suggests that these ratios are passive reflections of those in the peripheral blood and therefore may have no direct implications for the pathogenesis of these lesions. This is the only study which has so far done the appropriate detailed comparisons between blood and tissue in the same patient. Furthermore, the presence of helper T-cells in rejected tissues in various studies of mice, rats, and humans has stimulated a reevaluation not only of the dogma that humoral immunity is relatively unimportant in rejection, but also the dogma that cytotoxic T-cells mediate rejection.[392] The conflicting data and interpretations indicate a dynamic field in which unexpected findings challenge present thinking.

## Cross reaction between epithelial cell and bacterial antigens

van Bekkum[711] suggested that cross reaction between bacterial and epithelial cells may be a route for pathogenesis of gut GVHD. This hypothesis was based on observations in fetal gut

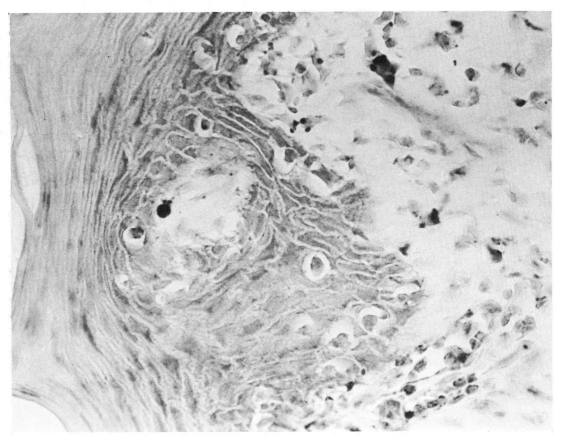

**Figure 3.** Photomicrograph of squamous epithelium in frozen section of lip of patient with chronic GVHD shows multiple infiltrating lymphoid cells staining with focal acid naphthylacetate esterase reaction product. This focal reaction is thought to occur primarily in a T-cell subset, possibly the helper subset identified by the OKT4 monoclonal antibody. Several lymphocytes with focal pattern hug the dermal vessel at the lower right. One focally positive cell invades the epidermis at the upper midleft of the photograph. The large and strongly positive cells are macrophages with some residual positivity incompletely inhibited by fluoride.[763]

transplant experiments. Two sets of experiments were done. In the first, conventional (not germ-free) animals were given lymphoid cell transplants from both allogeneic and syngeneic donors. Each group was also implanted with sterile syngeneic and allogeneic fetal gut. Fetal gut implant damage was quantified histologically. The gut implants allogeneic to the lymphoid cells were damaged markedly (about 50% of crypts degenerated). Gut implants *syngeneic* to the lymphoid cells were also damaged (about 22% of crypts degenerated). Controls consisted of animals given syngeneic lymphoid grafts and syngeneic gut implants. These implants were normal histologically. However, when the same experiments were done with germ-free mice, the damage to syngeneic gut implants seen in conventional animals disappeared. This suggests that bacteria sensitized the lymphocytes against syngeneic gut epithelial cells (at least when the gut and lymphocytes are being carried in an allogeneic host).

**Superinfection theory**

This theory states that the GVH*R* occurs only between lymphoid cell types (as in the passenger leukocyte phenomenon) and that immune suppression resulting from the GVHR (and from additional factors such as irradiation, if present) is the primary event. Subsequent events are explained purely as superinfection by viruses, bacteria, or fungi (the GVH*D*). Often overlooked are the effects of endotoxin alone, which, as emphasized by Cudkowicz et al. (pp. 265–266),[133] mimic facets of GVHD. A variation on the superinfection theme is that viral infection alters the surfaces of infected host cells, such that these cells are recognized as foreign by donor, or even recipient T- or null (NK) lymphocytes (induced autoimmune reaction). This theory has become more attractive recently because of the observation of $H_2$ restriction in mice and autoimmune-like phenomena in human identical twin marrow graft recipients. Some of these cases were simultaneously infected with cytomegalovirus.[243]

These diverse mechanisms, in summary, are difficult or impossible to sort out in clinical settings. Experimentally, many have been demonstrated, and it is unlikely that they are mutually exclusive. Any comprehensive pathogenetic theory of GVHR must take into account the known effects of preconditioning regimens used, and also must admit the existence of not only a whole family of potential recruitment and effector mechanisms derived from the donor, but also a broad spectrum of target tissues, target *or* effector cells, and antigens derived from the host.

# Chapter 3

# *In vitro* and *in vivo* animal models of GVHR and GVHD

George E. Sale, M.D.

## *IN VITRO* MODELS OF THE GVHR

Elkins[178] lists three reactions which constitute an *in vitro* GVHR: 1) the mixed leukocyte culture (MLC) reaction; 2) the rat cytotoxic lymphocyte versus mouse embryo monolayer target system of Berke et al.;[42] and 3) the splenic fragment technique in which fragments of F₁ hybrid mouse spleen are exposed to parental lymphocytes in culture. The MLC reaction is the most important of these assays clinically, as it is now used routinely to test for two-way reactivity between donor and host at the DR locus in matching procedures. Reduced to its principles, it consists of mixing donor and host lymphocytes together and testing their ability to stimulate each other in a tritiated thymidine incorporation assay. Radiation is used to inactivate host and donor cells, in turn, as responders. Reactivity of host against donor theoretically suggests the likelihood of graft rejection, whereas that of donor against host predicts GVHD. Quantitation of these reactions in the form of a relative response index[441] has led to predictive tests for graft rejection, which may be useful in certain transfused aplastic anemia patients who ordinarily receive less ablative preparation for transplantation than do patients with hematologic malignancies. A variety of such *in vitro* studies in man are reviewed in Chapter 4.

## *IN VIVO* MODELS

The several *in vivo* models have to be differentiated carefully from each other for clarity, because confusion arises if distinctions are not made between the *local* GVHRs (which are highly artificial circumstances) and the GVHRs produced by marrow or lymphoid cell transplants which are somewhat less so. The former are often induced in privileged sites or unusual organisms.

### Chorioallantoic membrane

Perhaps the simplest *in vivo* model involves the situation in which allogeneic adult chicken lymphoid cells are inoculated onto the chorioallantoic membranes of chicken egg embryos. Each pock so formed was shown by Burnet[88] and by Coppelson and Michie[125] to represent the site at which a single lymphoid cell alighted and reacted against the host tissue. Here, only a fraction of the cells are of donor origin, suggesting immediately the importance of recruitment of host lymphoid cells to the GVHR. This model apparently retains importance as the only one allowing direct enumeration of donor cell participants in an *in vivo* model.

### Phagocytic carbon clearance

J. Howard measured the rate of phagocytic clearance of carbon from the bloodstream by the reticuloendotrelial system (RES) and used it as an *in vivo* assay of GVHR.[299] The magnitude of RES activity measured in this way is a relatively nonspecific test, however, since infection and other stimuli can increase it.

### Spleen weight: The Simonsen assay[587]

Simonsen devised the widely used technique of weighing the spleens of rodents and fowls undergoing GVHR. The spleen weights at the peak of the reaction divided by littermate control weights yield a splenic index which bears a linear relation to the log of the dose of donor cells. As in the chorioallantoic membrane and popliteal node assays, however, host cells comprise the bulk of the new cell mass. Therefore, the assay mirrors not only donor cell dose, but additional important host inflammatory phenomena with considerably less immunological specificity, a theme which recurs throughout the field.

### Hepatic portal infiltrates

Another lesion which would seem *a priori* to be nonspecific but which retains a clear donor-cell, dose–response relationship is the number of *periportal hepatic mononuclear cell infiltrates* in mice and rats infused with allogeneic lymphocytes. In studies by Bain, the logarithm of the cell dose bore a linear relationship to the logarithm of the number of periportal infiltrates.[30] These lesions were randomly distributed and had to reach a threshold size to be countable. Donor–host contributions were unclear. No bile duct lesions were reported in these experiments such as those reported in several other species.

### Popliteal node assay

This assay, analogous to the spleen weight method, weighs the popliteal lymph nodes draining rodent footpads injected with donor lymphoid cells. The majority of cells in the enlarged node, whose weight is directly compared to that of the ipsilateral node, are of host origin. This assay was nearly 10 times as sensitive in detecting GVHD as was the renal subcapsular assay in the comparison carried out by Elkins.[176] Both donor and host cell proliferation are seen in this reaction whose full pathogenesis, although studied widely, is not completely understood as yet. Animals undergoing this reaction recruit host lym-

phoid cells from their entire bodies and also exhibit splenomegaly so that the reaction is not strictly a local GVHR. It is not comparable to the systemic GVHR in marrow transplantation because the full systemic syndrome does not develop. The various uses of this assay are reviewed by Grebe and Streilein.[264] Recently, Belldegrun, Belatsky, and Cohen[226] have been able actively and specifically to deplete lymphocytes reactive to specific antigens in mice by deliberately causing the recruitment of alloreactive cells to a popliteal node. These cells were then removed by the simple expedient of excising the lymph node in which the antigen-reactive cells were trapped, thereby significantly prolonging the survival of skin grafts. Although it may be difficult now to envision clinical application of this to GVHD, the study may be important. It shows that study of lymphoid traffic patterns in the immune response can yield completely new ways to manipulate immunity. It also shows that the recruitment phase of the immune response can be directly manipulated.

### Donor cell proliferation measurements

As reviewed by Elkins,[178] several methods for assessing donor cell proliferation in GVHR have been developed. Nisbet and Simonsen[471] used mitotic rates in donor spleen cells in chicken embryos, using a formula incorporating spleen weight, mitotic rate, and percentage of donor cells. As a measure of alloantigenic responsiveness, Bennet[40] compared $^{125}$IUDR incorporation into the spleen and nodes of recipient mice with that of syngeneic controls. Such methods may be limited by the fact that donor cell proliferation alone does not adequately describe the GVHR, but they do provide quantitative measurements.

### Renal subcapsular GVHR model

Several important insights were derived from studies of the subcapsular renal GVHR carried out (primarily) by Elkins.[176,177] In this model, allogeneic lymphocytes are injected under the renal capsule of host rats. A pronounced lymphoproliferative reaction ensues which can destroy a quarter of the kidney. Donor cell proliferation closely parallels lesion size. The histopathology and course both strongly parallel those of renal allograft rejection. When the allogeneic differences are weak, presensitization of the donor to host antigens has a profoundly enhancing effect. This is identical to the findings in human and canine marrow allograft rejection,[629,630,633,734] although a curiously and paradoxically opposite effect occurs in renal transplantation.[482] Additional analysis of this model strongly suggested a necessary interaction between donor lymphoid cells and host mononuclear cells. Elkins and Guttman[177] showed in an $F_1$ hybrid system that allogeneic host mononuclear cells alone could provide the necessary antigenic stimulus for damage to renal parenchyma syngeneic to the donor lymphoid cells. This study provided additional important evidence supporting the passenger leukocyte or innocent bystander theory originally proposed by Steinmuller.[618] The suggestion that ridding a graft of certain leukocytes might improve graft survival led to experimental animal work in thyroid and thymus transplantation which tended to confirm a role for alloantigen-bearing leukocytes in graft rejection and/or GVHR in some systems.[367]

## Local cutaneous GVHR in hamsters

Streilein, Grebe, and Billingham conducted experiments on local cutaneous GVHR that can be induced in many species.[264] They focused on the hamster model in which bulla formation and a positive Nikolski sign with a toxic epidermal necrolysis (TEN) syndrome develop after local intracutaneous injection of allogeneic lymphocytes. The syndrome is not induced by marrow transplantation in this model. Later studies by Elson[181] and van Bekkum[710,711] in the gut GVHR tended to confirm this innocent bystander principle. Streilein's group[647,649] was able to show, by experimental designs similar to those of Elkins, that the local reactions depend very much on the presence in the skin of host leukocytes bearing alloantigens which provide adequate antigenic stimulus.

### MODELS OF GVHD IN WHOLE ANIMALS

Because these models constitute several variations on a theme, they are discussed briefly and individually.

## Runt disease

As reviewed by Seemayer, GVHR was probably first described by Murphy[456] and Dancha-

koff.[138] The first whole-animal runting syndrome models were described in the course of splenic transplant rescue experiments after lethal irradiation. Between 1955 and 1959 several important studies were published which established: 1) that a distinct delayed syndrome apart from radiation sickness occurred in animals rescued by splenic or hematopoietic transplants; 2) that this had a cellular immunological basis; and 3) that genetic disparity was important. Barnes, Loutit, Billingham, Brent, and Simonsen, among others, contributed important pieces of this puzzle.

The runting syndrome is clinically defined by failure to thrive, alopecia, emaciation, lymphoid atrophy, diarrhea, and death. It was clearly related to genetically disparate lymphoid cell grafts, although it is notable that even in these early studies some murine syngeneic graft recipients, under certain conditions, were reported to show wasting.[33–35] This has been attributed to a lack of functional lymphoid cells and has recently been rediscussed in light of the immunoregulatory circuit dysregulation hypothesis in GVHD.[491]

## Secondary disease

"Secondary disease" is loosely defined as the disease which occurs following irradiation and allogeneic lymphoid grafting. It includes both the GVHR and its sequela, GVHD, and ensuing infections. Some authors equate it with the term GVHD. Elkins has recently urged reintroduction of the term "secondary disease" as a way of avoiding confusion with syngeneic events and other phenomena which have never been formally proven to be of allogeneic origin.[180] We prefer a three-part definition in which the GVHR is confined to the lymphoreticular events, the GVHD to the epithelial target organ events which can be seen apart from demonstrable infection, and "secondary disease" as an inclusive definition encompassing also superinfection, wasting, and death.

## $F_1$ hybrid disease

This disease is an important and frequently used model of GVHR in which the first generation ($F_1$) hybrid animal serves as a marrow or lymphocyte donor and the parent serves as a recipient. The $F_1$ hybrid of an AXB cross will fail to recognize the parental (i.e., AA) lymphocytes as foreign and will accept their graft. These cells in turn, however, will recognize the AB hybrid as foreign and a vigorous GVHR will ensue if the genetic differences are great enough. This classical model continues to be of importance to immunobiology.[240,241]

## Parabiosis intoxication

Parabiosis intoxication[126] is the special case in which the graft is induced, usually in an $F_1$ hybrid situation, by connecting the circulation of donor and host. This has not only demonstrated aggressive alloreactions by circulating lymphocytes, but has also been used to show that lymphoid stem cells sufficient to engraft the host marrow space circulate in the peripheral blood of several species including, for example, baboons.[638]

## Fetal liver transplantation

That the fetal liver is a rich source of hemopoietic stem cells, any pediatric pathologist is aware, and exploitation of this fact has engendered a large body of transplantation literature in mice, horses, and even humans. Lowenberg's monograph[393] details extensive murine studies. Human fetal liver transplants for aplastic anemia and other conditions are reviewed in the 1980 *Transplantation Proceedings*. Exemplifying the data obtained are studies of Arabian foals by Perryman and colleagues which have established that liver cells from sufficiently immature fetuses can be infused without inducing GVHD, but if the cells come from too young a fetus, immunologic reconstitution is not achieved.[496,497]

### SPECIFIC ANIMAL MODELS

## The chicken

Ivanyi and colleagues[303,665] have done considerable studies of GVHD models in whole chicken embryos as well as in $F_1$ hybrid 12-day-old chicken radiation chimeras. They developed an assay for GVHD based on the degree of follicular depletion in the folds of the bursa of Fabricius in the host bursa. Similar features could be induced by lipopolysaccharides from *Serratia*. In this model, as in others, endotoxin and allogeneic lymphoid grafts both seem able to deplete B-cells and act synergistically.

## The mouse

The mouse is distinguished by the most extensively studied mammalian immune system, and from it came the earliest runt models and splenic shielding experiments. The pathology is reviewed by Rappaport et al.[519] Minor histocompatibility differences can produce a GVHD in mice, termed chronic, as detailed by several authors, including Hamilton et al.[278] The spectrum of pathology in GVHD is similar to that seen in several other species. However, a "true" chronic GVHD syndrome, similar to that seen in rats by Stastney[615] and Beschorner,[54,55] and in humans by several authors, has not been readily induced or sustained in mice.

Van Bekkum[713] attributes to Barnes and Loutit in 1955 the first recognition in radiation chimeras that something other than radiation toxicity was occurring. Others confirmed that this was due to a cell graft and not to a humoral factor. A number of papers on this problem appeared in the late 1950s, including the study by De Vries and Vos[150] which reported dermatitis, pneumonia, hepatitis, and colitis in mice 3 or more weeks after hemopoietic cell transplantation. The importance of lymphoid atrophy as a lesion preceding the target organ lesions, and possibly being phenomenologically separable from them, was reported as early as 1962 by Loutit and Micklem.[390] Congdon emphasized the lymphoid atrophy as causative and possibly due to host GVHR. He opposed the graft-vs.-host hypothesis for several years based on these lines of thought.[713]

The mouse has emerged, particularly in the $F_1$ hybrid system, as a very important model for GVHD. Extensive studies in the $F_1$ model by Gleichmann et al., for example, have given rise to interesting hypotheses about the nature of drug-induced autoimmune and viral disease, suggesting an analogous reaction to that of GVHR.[239] The same hypothetical mechanism has been applied to the development of malignant lymphoma, a rich area of continuing research to be discussed in Chapter 10.

A detailed sequential study of the pathology of mouse irradiation chimeras transplanted with both $H_2$-compatible and -incompatible hemopoietic cells was reported by Rappaport et al.[519] These authors define acute GVHD as that occurring in histoincompatible combinations. They describe four phases of the acute syndrome; namely, 1) transient aplasia, 2) repopulation, 3) proliferation of lymphoid cells, and 4) acute organ damage which is a terminal disease. Chronic GVHD, defined as that in histocompatible pairs, has the same first 3 phases as acute, plus phases 4) chronic immunologic organ damage, and 5) repair and development of scleroderma-like lesions in some of the organs. Models of mouse GVHR in minor histoincompatible combinations have also been studied by Hamilton et al.[278]

The studies of Lapp and Seemayer on mouse GVHD have focused particularly on the interesting hypothesis that damage to thymic epithelium may be a generic pathological event leading to subsequent severe immunodeficiency. The thymus is an unusually labile and sensitive organ, and much care was needed in designing the studies in order to rule out several nonspecific or nonimmune mechanisms which could be responsible for thymic changes. They controlled their studies for the acute stress involution secondary to increased cortisol levels by adrenalectomy.[573,574] Injury to thymic epithelial cells by GVHR as the proximal cause of a number of possible events is postulated by these authors. First, the severe immunodeficiency occurring in GVHD may be due to this injury, besides injury of other functional units of the immune system. This, in turn, could result in imbalance among immunoregulatory cells which might increase the host's susceptibility, not only to infection but also to the oncogenesis produced by viruses. Similarly, neonatal or *in utero* GVHRs are invoked as possibly etiologic for severe combined immunodeficiency (SCID), di George syndrome, congenital biliary atresia, and even primary biliary cirrhosis. The potentially fundamental impact of this hypothesis justifies considerable additional testing.

Another valuable contribution from the mouse has been the demonstration in leukemic mice of the clear antitumor effect of a deliberately induced but partially controlled GVHR. The hypothesis reported by Boranic[70,71] was that tumor cells should bear host tumor antigens which could serve as targets for the GVHR in an immunotherapeutic model. A number of adoptive immunotherapy models have attempted to use the GVHR as a mechanism for enhancing antitumor effects. One of many examples is the study of

Einstein et al.[170] which was able to show increased GVHR induction by mouse spleen cells sensitized *in vitro* to allogeneic tumor.

### The rat

Stastny, Stembridge, and Ziff[615,616] published the classical description of cutaneous and systemic GVHD in the rat. They describe inflammatory acute and chronic cutaneous lesions highly suggestive of lupus erythematosus and scleroderma. Systemic changes included a migratory polyarthritis characterized histologically by a mononuclear cell infiltration of the synovia. A myocarditis of similar composition and cardiac valvular degeneration were described. Lymphoid depletion, followed by plasmacytosis and fibrosis, was described, as were slight mononuclear infiltrates in the kidneys. This was perhaps the first major suggestion that a useful analog to naturally occurring autoimmune diseases might be made available by animal GVHR.[239,240] The rat model continues to be useful, as emphasized by recent studies of Tutschka and Beschorner.[697] They studied a spontaneously arising syndrome in ACI/Lew radiation chimeras which could be induced by a tolerance-breaking regimen consisting of reirradiating the chimeras and giving a booster dose of ACI bone marrow. In this model, the animals showed dermatitis, alopecia, and dermal scarring. Corneal ulceration is frequent as in humans, although this may be a secondary or superinfection process. Salivary and lacrimal periductal infiltrates were described similar to those in humans, and chronic active hepatitis occurred in about one-third of those with skin involvement. These authors also found antisalivary gland antibodies in the serum of the animals with cutaneous and salivary gland infiltrative lesions.

### The rabbit

Porter induced GVHD in rabbit radiation chimeras, a model of particular interest to the question of liver disease because he discovered a lesion closely resembling primary biliary cirrhosis in only those animals with secondary disease.[507,508] The presence of a biliary parasite, coccidiosis (*Emeria stiedae*) appeared to be a pathogenetic factor in the cirrhosis, but was also found infecting the uninvolved animals. Only the animals with secondary disease developed the severe jaundice and biliary cirrhosis. This, plus the fact that the more severe cholestatic lesion with bile ductular cirrhosis has been reported primarily in radiated or chemotherapeutically preconditioned subjects, suggests that an additional, possibly specific, liver injury may be needed to induce full-blown biliary damage in GVHD.

### The dog

Canine cardiac, renal, and hepatic transplantation have also contributed much to transplant biology. Autologous and allogeneic marrow transplantation technology in the dog was developed rapidly in the late 1950s by Thomas and colleagues.[208,209] This model has become the most useful large animal model for marrow transplantation, partly because dogs are much more easily cared for than are primates. Radiation, intravenous therapy, anesthesia, and surgical techniques also are readily carried out. The advent of histocompatibility DLA-matching techniques further increased the value of this model in the canine, which is an outbred species like humans. Although immunogenetic studies are more logistically difficult than those in smaller animals, the other advantages have assured the continued importance of this model. Many of the significant advances allowing clinical application of marrow grafts to humans were courtesy of the dog: two

examples will suffice to make this point. One advance was that which showed the striking importance of tissue typing for marrow donor selection. Furthermore, the first clear experimental demonstration of the importance of blood transfusion presensitization to the rejection of marrow grafts was accomplished in dogs. The acute graft-vs.-host syndrome occurring in dogs bears many resemblances to that in humans and other species; the ablation of the normal morphology of the lymph nodes, spleen, and thymus is an example. Skin, liver, and gut disease can be described using the same general terminology and grading system as those applied to humans (Figs. 1–4). For example, a controlled study of canine liver lesions suggested a strong association of small bile duct lesions with a mismatched allograft of bone marrow. Subsequent studies suggested amelioration of this lesion by methotrexate (MTX) or by the use of histocompatible bone marrow.[352,546]

States of prolonged tolerance in stable canine radiation chimeras are established with relative ease, using matched littermates. Such tolerance can be dramatically broken by infusion of sensitized donor lymphocytes.[735] Recent studies also show that tolerance can be induced with cyclosporin, a new immunosuppressant derived from fungi. This tolerance is exquisitely sensitive

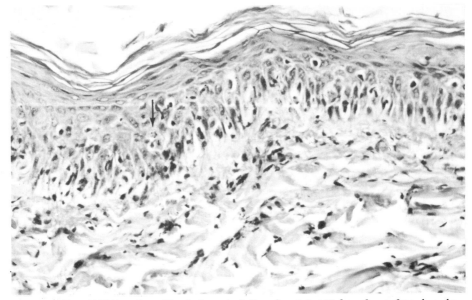

**Figure 1.** (Dog A243) Dorsal ear skin of mismatched allograft recipient 16 days after grafting shows lymphocytic infiltrates of epidermis, spongiosis, necrosis of epidermal cells (*arrow*). Lesions this severe (Grade II–III) can progress to total denudation (Grade IV), as was the case with the inner surface of the same dog's ear. (Reproduced with permission from Kolb et al.[352])

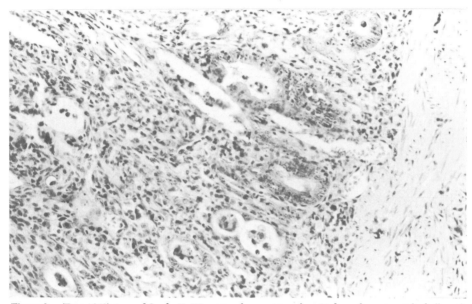

**Figure 2.** (Dog A249) Area of Grade II–III gut involvement in colon, 21 days after mismatched allograft. Multiple crypt abscesses occur followed by loss of crypts. (Reproduced with permission from Kolb et al.[352])

to continued serum levels of the drug. Some dogs develop a chronic syndrome which resembles the chronic syndrome in humans[23] (Fig. 5). The hepatic and cutaneous involvement are prominent features, just as in humans. Studies of the canine lip biopsy suggest a particular sensitivity for the subclinical disease in long-term survivors of allografting.[146]

We have found some supporting evidence in dogs for the thymic damage hypothesis in mice of Lapp and Seemayer.[573,575] Acute damage to the thymus occurs in all irradiated dogs, and the lesions do not distinguish allografted from autografted animals in the first 3 weeks after grafting. Thymuses of allografted long-term survivors have been uniformly atrophic whether the animals had

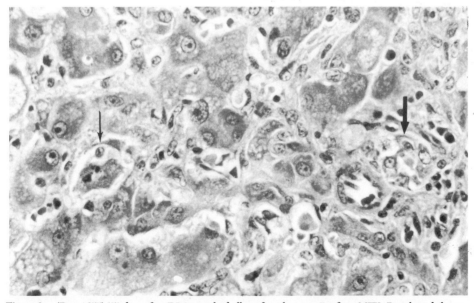

**Figure 3.** (Dog A255) 151 days after DLA-matched allograft without postgrafting MTX. Portal triad shows abnormal bile ductule with atypia and individual cells degeneration (*large arrow*). Individual hepatocyte necrosis (*small arrow*) tends to be scattered throughout the lobule. Often lymphocytic infiltrates mark areas of such dropout. (Reproduced with permission from Kolb et al.[352])

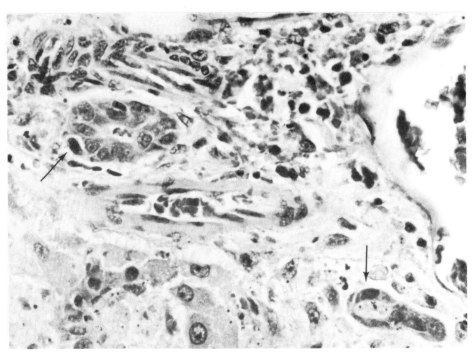

**Figure 4.** (Dog A156) Liver, 18 days after mismatched allograft. Abnormal bile ducts in portal triad (*arrows*) with adjacent lymphocytes and plasma cells. Atypia (anisonucleosis and altered nuclear–cytoplasmic ratios) is characteristic of GVHD. Often inflammatory cells invade ductal epithelium. Necrosis of individual small bile-duct cells with shrinkage and karyolysis, and karyorrhexis producing conspicuous nuclear dust, are often observed. (Reproduced with permission from Kolb et al.[352])

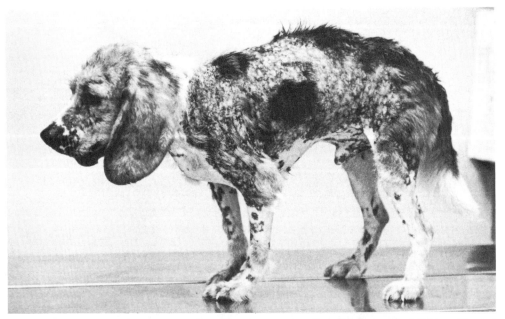

**Figure 5.** Chronic GVHD in a beagle, 610 days after bone marrow allograft from unrelated DLA-nonidentical donor. The host received a short course of intermittent MTX therapy, followed by daily oral CYA until day 100. Chronic cutaneous GVHD then developed, with alopecia, scaling dermatitis, reticulate hyperpigmentation, and failure to thrive.

clinical GVHD or not. By the end of 6–8 weeks, however, autografted dogs had a thymic morphology which is entirely normal (see Chapter 10). Thymic damage, therefore, does seem to occur as a uniform phenomenon in allografted dogs but does not correlate with clinical events. Perhaps adjunctive factors are necessary to induce clinical disease in the allografted dogs. This subject cannot be well studied *in vivo* without controlling for adrenal and other factors, as in the studies of Seemayer et al.[574]

Many canine irradiation recipients develop chronic pancreatic fibrosis and wasting disease. This occurs with equal frequency in both allografted and autografted dogs, however, and is unlikely to be due to GVHR. We have observed infiltration and necrosis of pancreatic ducts and of the larger biliary radicles of liver in both dogs[23] and humans, but only in unusually severe GVHD, and never with adequate severity to produce obstruction of these larger-order ducts.

Chronic interstitial lymphocytic and plasmacytic infiltration is a relatively frequent, naturally occurring canine renal lesion. We have not established any data showing this to be more frequent in recipients of allogeneic bone marrow.

A bronchial lesion in humans, associated with GVHD, was termed "lymphocytic bronchitis," and described by Beschorner et al.[50] A similar lesion was described in dogs by the group in Leiden.[770] We have been unable to confirm this association in large or small airways in either humans or dogs[272,476] (See Chapter 9).

## The horse

In 1973, McGuire and Poppie described a primary SCID syndrome in Arabian foals.[422] Subsequent studies by Perryman, McGuire, and associates established that this disorder involves severe dysfunction of T- and B-cells and results in early death from infection (usually within months of birth), and this high-prevalence syndrome (2.3% among Arabian foals) probably is inherited in an autosomally recessive pattern. This is the only naturally occurring animal counterpart of SCID (which occurs in human children) and has much economic importance to the Arabian horse industry. After they had established the type and degree of immunodeficiency, these investigators set about devising replacement immunotherapy based on some of the available

transplantation models in other animals and humans.

An initial study of six affected foals reported successful immune reconstitution after transplantation of fetal liver and thymic tissues. The gestational age of the donor fetus was found to be an important determinant of the resulting immunological function of the graft. For example, three of four foals grafted with fetus cells of 90 days' or more gestation developed severe GVHD. Another foal, given fetus cells of 80 days' gestation, developed lymphocytes which responded to mitogen and exhibited synthesis of the four major classes of equine immunoglobulins. A sixth foal, which received fetus cells of 68 days' gestation, showed no demonstrable effect whatever of transplantation. A subsequent paper added three foals to the first series and confirmed most of the impressions regarding the effect of gestational age. These data imply that considerable functional maturation of the equine fetal immune system occurs between the 68th and 94th days of gestation. They are consistent with similar data in the mouse and other species which imply that mature effector cells are needed to implement GVHD.

We were privileged to collaborate with this group by examining the autopsies of the horses in the initial study.[496] The full range of lesions observed has been subsequently published.[497] The skin lesions are less severe than those in humans but almost identical histologically. Mononuclear cells focally and diffusely involve the dermal–epidermal junction, associated with spongiosis, necrosis, and satellitosis of basal and suprabasal epidermal cells. Involvement of hair follicles is evident, with dilation of follicles and atrophy of lining epithelium (Fig. 6). Although the colon shows evidence of minimal involvement, the esophagus has the most striking predilection for this process, based on the series studied. Particularly noticeable is the invasion by mononuclear cells, with squamous metaplasia, of the ducts of the esophageal glands, with lesser involvement of the overlying surface squamous mucosal epithelium (Fig. 7). Numerous examples of the necrosis of epithelial cells and satellitosis by mononuclear cells around them are noted.

The most profound changes are seen in the liver. Figure 8 illustrates the intense portal infiltrates, expansion of tracts, fibrosis, bile ductule

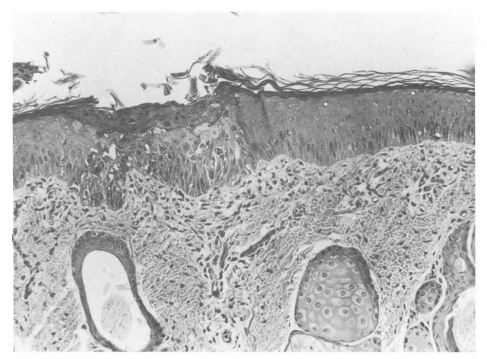

**Figure 6.**  Skin of Arabian foal who died 55 days after transplantation of fetal liver and thymic cells. The epidermis is involved, with infiltrating mononuclear cells. The hair follicle is dilated. (Reproduced with permission from Perryman and Liu.[497])

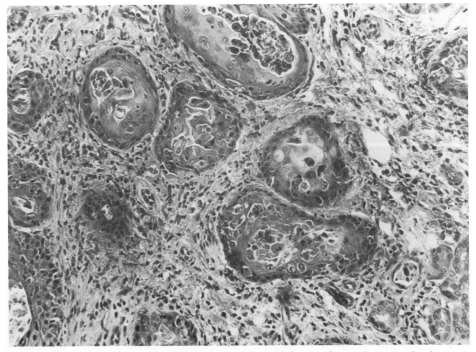

**Figure 7.**  Esophageal GVHD in foal 55 days after fetal liver and thymic cell transplant. Note florid necrosis of cells in those ducts draining the esophageal mucosal glands. In our experience this picture is more pronounced than that seen in humans or dogs. (Reproduced with permission from Perryman and Liu.[497])

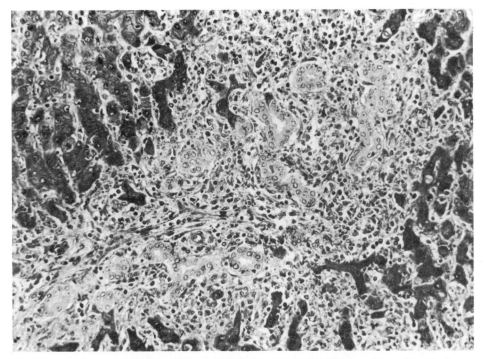

**Figure 8.**   Startling portal infiltrates, fibrosis, and bile duct lesions in foal 55 days after grafting. Such cases provide some of the strongest evidence for the analogy to primary biliary cirrhosis. (Masson-trichrome.) (Reproduced with permission from Perryman and Liu.[497])

destruction, and bile ductular proliferation which were seen in the foal. The changes bear a startling similarity to those seen in the early phase of primary biliary cirrhosis in humans and provide some of the strongest evidence supporting such an analogy.

The lymphoid tissues of untreated SCID horses show no plasma cells or germinal centers and are generally lymphocyte-depleted, particulary in paracortical (T-dependent) regions. Transplanted foals without GVHD show the development of normal lymph node and spleen morphology; i.e., lymph nodes at 12 months show well-developed primary and secondary follicles with germinal centers and well-populated paracortical zones. However, those foals which develop GVHD exhibit lymph node and spleen morphology very similar to that reported in dogs, humans, mice, and other species. Germinal centers return late (3–12 months after grafting), if at all. The nodes show no follicles or only rudimentary primary follicles. Paradoxically, however, plasma cells and immunoblasts (probably of B-cell type, primarily) are numerous in both the cortical lymph nodes and the periarteriolar splenic sheaths. In all these species, the impression is that of incomplete restoration of function as well as unregulated proliferation of some cells, particularly B-cells. In humans and dogs, this impression is buttressed by polyclonal hypergammaglobulinemia.[472,477]

### Nonhuman primates

De Vries et al.[151,152] reported pathological changes in irradiated monkeys treated with bone marrow. Twenty-six monkeys were treated with TBI; all 26 died within 100 days. Seven were ungrafted controls, two were autografted and 17 received homografts. Fourteen of the latter showed marrow engraftment. The allografted monkeys developed a GVHD syndrome much like that of mice and rabbits. Gross skin lesions were macular erythema of periorbital and peroral regions, in some cases extending to anterior chest and abdomen. Some showed extensive dry peeling and scaling of the ears and face. Histologically, acanthosis, hyperkeratosis, and plugging of hair follicles with patchy follicular atrophy were frequent. Eosinophilic necrosis of basilar and suprabasilar epidermal cells was common, with mononuclear cell infiltrates. Sweat duct involvement was indicated by squamous metaplasia.

Liver lesions in this study were individual and grouped parenchymal cell necrosis, with triaditis. Small bile duct abnormalities were very clearly described: "The epithelium of the smaller bile duct showed swelling and increased eosinophilia of the cytoplasm, nuclear pyknosis, and occasional mitoses." As early as 1961, therefore, destructive lesions of small bile ducts had been clearly described in both rabbits and monkeys and had been alluded to briefly without detailed description in mice.[150]

Gross gut lesions attributed to GVHR singled out the distal ileum as the predominant site of damage along with large intestine and, occasionally, stomach. The histologic lesions were crypt-cell death and desquamation with cystic dilation. Areas of crypt necrosis were focal, alternating with areas of active regeneration.

Occasional evidence of individual cell necrosis in allograft recipients was found in several organs, including liver, intrahepatic biliary ducts, adrenal cortex, pancreatic acini and islets, salivary glands, and renal pelvis. These were not discussed in detail. Van Bekkum, in reviewing the literature, included the hypothesis that the mechanism of damage of skin, liver, and gut cells might be by cytotoxic activity of donor lymphocytes against epithelial cells of host target organs.[708]

Woodruff et al.[760,761] published detailed light- and electron microscopic-observations of GVHD in rhesus monkeys which focused particularly on the nature of the necrosis of individual epithelial cells in the target tissues. The term "satellite cell dyskeratosis" has been used to describe the eosinophilic change of individual epidermal cells associated with closely apposed mononuclear cells. The hypothesis was again advanced that these lesions constitute the major target tissue phenomenon of GVHD. The mononuclear cells were given the name "aggressor lymphocytes." The authors proposed that these aggressor lymphocytes are either directly killing epithelial cells in these target organs or that they are dying and releasing a toxin, such as a lymphokine, by which killing might be mediated. The latter, more passive role for the lymphocytes is proposed for the lesions in the intestine, whereas their role in oral mucosa or epidermis is thought more likely to be a direct killing process.

Close contacts between lymphocytes and the putative target epithelial cells were demonstrated in the electron micrographs presented in the second of these papers.[760] Neither the genetic origin (*viz* donor versus host) nor the precise type (lymphocyte subset versus monocyte, etc.) of these putative aggressor cells has been fully elucidated. This study confined itself to monkeys sacrificed between days 4 and 10 post-transplantation, a period within which considerable residual irradiation damage complicates the problem of interpretation of some of the lesions, particularly those in marrow and gut. Nevertheless, there were distinct differences between the allografted and radiation-control populations.

Merritt et al.[431] studied eight irradiation control monkeys given autografts, nine given allografts alone, and 11 given allografts followed by horse or rabbit antilymphocyte serum. The antilymphocyte serum, particularly that raised in the rabbit, prolonged survival and lessened the severity of GVHD, results similar to those reported previously in other primates and other species. One untreated monkey showed particularly severe skin disease, with a syndrome resembling toxic epidermal necrolysis. This had been reported previously in mice and humans, although it is, in fact, unusual.

# Chapter 4

# Immunologic studies of human GVHD

**Mang-So Tsoi, Ph.D.**

## Introduction

Graft-vs.-host reactions (GVHR), according to the classical description by Billingham,[59] have the following basic requirements for initiation: 1) genetically determined histocompatibility differences between the graft donor and the recipient; 2) the presence of immune competent cells in the graft which can recognize the foreign histocompatibility antigens of the host and mount an immunologic reaction against such antigens; and 3) the incapability of the host to react against and reject the graft. These requirements clearly define the immunogenetic basis of GVHR which may bring about graft-vs.-host disease (GVHD), a major risk of allogeneic bone marrow transplantation (BMT) in man.[245,645,653,669] As described in detail elsewhere in this monograph, the clinical and pathological findings of GVHD are highly complex. Although alloaggression due to histocompatibility differences may be the underlying mechanism, the subsequent immunologic events that bring about the expression of the disease and associated phenomena such as autoimmunity, immunodeficiency, and immune dysfunction are not entirely clear.[180]

Numerous immunologic studies of GVHR and GVHD in animal models have dealt mainly with differences at the major histocompatibility complex (MHC) between donor and host. These studies were reviewed by Grebe and Streilein[264] several years ago. The present review is confined to immunologic studies of GVHD in humans. Unlike most studies in animal models, almost all immunologic studies in clinical GVHD are relatively recent, deal exclusively with donors and hosts who are MHC-identical or phenotypically similar for HLA loci, and use only *in vitro* techniques.

### HUMORAL IMMUNE MECHANISMS

As in animal systems, antibody response is believed to be less important than cellular immunity for the pathogenesis of clinical GVHD. Nevertheless, a few authors have considered the involvement of humoral antibodies and GVHD in humans.

### Antibodies against epithelial cells and skin

Mediation of skin GVHD by humoral immune mechanisms was first investigated by Merritt et al.[431] They described a complement (C')-dependent cytotoxic IgM antibody against epithelial cell lines (HeLa and Hep2) but not against lymphoid cells in the sera of three recipients of marrow transplants from HLA-identical siblings. The appearance of this antibody coincided with the onset of clinical acute GVHD. Saurat et al.[557] describing a lichen planus-like eruption in five cases of early chronic GVHD, reported the presence of serum IgG antibodies specific for the basal cells of the skin in 2/4 patients studied by the indirect immunofluorescence technique. They also reported Ig (class not described) deposits in the skin from 2/4 patients studied by the direct immunofluorescence technique. By direct immunofluorescence, Ullman et al.[705] found deposits of IgG, IgA, IgM, and C′3 at the dermal–epidermal junction and in blood vessel walls in two patients, one with acute GVHD and one with chronic GVHD.

By direct immunofluorescence, we studied the immune deposits in the skin of 88 patients with and without GVHD who received allogeneic marrow grafts.[688] Data from skin biopsies obtained before transplantation, from biopsies of patients with syngeneic grafts, and from healthy marrow donors served as controls. We found that IgM and C′3 deposits in the dermal–epidermal junction were significantly associated with GVHD. The frequency and intensity were related to the duration or type of GVHD: 86% of patients with chronic GVHD showed dense granular IgM deposits (Fig. 1) and 39% of patients with acute G8VHD showed faint deposits. No IgM deposits were seen in the skin of four recipients of syngeneic grafts, and faint deposits were present in only 11% of healthy marrow donors, in patients before grafting, and in allogeneic marrow recipients without GVHD postgrafting. Sequential studies in individual patients showed that there was an increment in IgM deposits during periods of active GVHD. Results similar to those with IgM, although less striking, were found for C′3 deposits: those patients with chronic and those with acute GVHD showed, respectively, the highest and next highest incidence and intensity.[688] In a blind study, Sullivan et al.[654] investigated the relationship of these immune deposits to the subsequent development of chronic GVHD. Fifty-one patients without symptoms of chronic GVHD at day 100, who then subsequently developed chronic GVHD, were compared in a proportional hazards' analysis with 84 patients who, at all times, were free of any symptoms of chronic GVHD. Those patients showing dermal basement membrane deposits of C′3 were found to have a 2.8-fold increased relative risk of developing subsequent chronic GVHD (*p* was less than 0.002). It suggested that

the deposits might be related to the pathogenesis and not be simply epiphenomena.[656]

The finding that syngeneic recipients and allogeneic recipients without GVHD showed few or no Ig deposits at the dermal–epidermal junction suggests that deposits found in allogeneic recipients with GVHD were antibodies produced in response to antigenic differences between donor and host. The nature of the antigen system(s) involved is unknown. Merritt et al.[431] suggested the involvement of: 1) minor histocompatibility antigens expressed only as epidermal cell-specific antigens, 2) cross-reactive viral antigens or epidermal cell surface antigens altered by a latent viral presence, or 3) hidden epidermal antigens, exposed by the GVHR, provoking the formation of "autoantibodies" against epithelial cells. The absence of IgM deposits in the skin of the syngeneic recipients and in most of the allogeneic recipients without GVHD argues against the involvement of cross-reactive viral antigens or altered epidermal cell surface antigens induced by viral infection, since these patients experienced a spectrum of viral infection similar to that of allogeneic recipients with GVHD. Moreover, the ultrastructural study of Gallucci et al.[229,230] showed no virus in the tissue of patients with GVHD.

By indirect immunofluorescence, Saurat et al.[559] demonstrated antibodies in sera of patients with chronic GVHD that reacted to antigens in the cytoplasm of keratinocytes. These antigens seemed to reside in the basal (proliferative) layers and might represent differentiation antigens no longer expressed or available on the stratum spinosum (maturing layers). Despite these findings, there is no conclusive evidence yet that skin antigens are targets of the humoral immune response in GVHD.

**Lymphocytotoxic antibodies**

Jeannet et al.[315] first described the presence of a cold IgG lymphocytotoxic antibody during acute GVHD in a patient grafted for SCID. This antibody lysed 25–70% of unrelated but not donor or recipient lymphocytes. Gluckman et al.[242,244] reported two studies of cold auto- and allolymphocytotoxic antibodies directed to the non-HLA antigens of the B- and/or T-lymphocytes in the serum of 50% of marrow recipients. In their first study, they found a correlation between the pres-

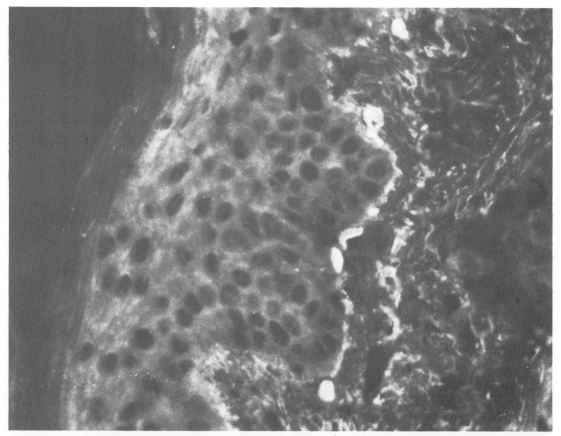

**Figure 1.** (UPN 789) A 33-year-old white male allograft recipient for ANL, transplanted 2½ years previously. Skin biopsy frozen section shows membranous and cytoid body staining with IgM at basal layer of epidermis. This patient had acute GVHD by skin and rectal biopsies and abnormal liver function tests by day 49. (Furnished by Dr. Keith Sullivan.)

ence of lymphocytotoxic antibodies and GVHD, but not in the second study. They attributed the conflicting results to differences of sample size and of conditioning regimen for transplantation. They suggested that the production of antibodies in graft recipients was the result of profound disturbances of immune regulation similar to those seen in patients with autoimmune disorders or cellular imbalance due to chemo- or radio-therapy-induced thymic dysfunction. Opelz et al.[481] also detected lymphocytotoxic antibodies in approximately 50% of 41 marrow-grafted patients. These IgM antibodies, reactive at 4°, 20°, and 37°C, were developed postgrafting against non-HLA antigens on lymphocytes of donor and chimera (i.e., the patient after transplantation) and, possibly, of host. There was no statistically significant correlation of the antibodies with GVHD, although a relationship between patient survival and development of antibodies against

chimera lymphocytes might exist. In contrast to the findings of Gluckman et al. and Opelz et al., Warren et al.[732] found no lymphocytotoxic antibodies against donor lymphocytes (chimera and host lymphocytes not studied) in patients with sustained engraftment, except in two cases with mixed donor–host chimerism.

In summary, results of studies of lymphocytotoxics after allogeneic marrow transplantation are conflicting. Moreover, none has shown a relationship of these antibodies to clincial GVHD.

### CELLULAR-IMMUNE MECHANISMS

Based on studies in laboratory animals, GVHD in humans has been assumed to be initiated by a cellular mechanism; i.e., the generation of alloreactive T-lymphocytes in recognition of antigenic differences, followed by lymphocyte-mediated damage to host target cells or organs. The interaction of effector lymphocytes and target cells has been inferred by the finding of close contact of lymphocytes with target cells by light microscopy and in ultrastructural studies in the skin and gut.[229,591,761] At present, there are only limited *in vitro* data concerning cell-mediated immunity in human GVHD due to the inherent difficulties of working in the human system and the unavailability of sensitive or appropriate *in vitro* assays to test immune responses to non-HLA antigens. Despite these restrictions, advances have been made in the *in vitro* study of cellular immune mechanisms of clinical GVHD.

## T-cell profiles
Peripheral E-rosetting T-cell profiles in marrow recipients were examined by investigators from several BMT centers. Elfenbein et al.[171] found that the percentage of T- and B-lymphocytes fell at 1–1½ months after grafting, then rose to pregrafting levels at 2–3½ months. Storb et al.[636] and Noel et al.[472] reported that patients after transplantation had T-cell numbers in the low normal range for 3 months and were normal thereafter. B-cell numbers were normal following the postgrafting nadir. No difference was found between patients with or without GVHD. Gale et al.[225] also found normal percentages of circulating T- and B-lymphocytes by day 50 and no correlation between the levels of T- or B-cells and GVHD. Later, using a xenogeneic antiserum detecting suppressor T-cells expressing $TH_2$ markers, Reinherz et al.[524] found that three patients with acute GHVD lacked $TH_2^+$ cells, and that of six patients with chronic GVHD, two lacked, and four had, increased $TH_2^+$ cells. Recently, Elfenbein et al.[172] detected peripheral blood cells (depleted of monocytes) that bound peanut agglutinin in allogeneic marrow recipients early after grafting. Since peanut agglutinin binds only thymocytes but not mature peripheral lymphocytes, the authors speculated that these cells were immature T-cells.

The recent production of hybridoma monoclonal antibodies to human T-cell surface antigens has made it possible to identify T-cell subsets. Using these antibodies, investigators from three independent laboratories have recently analyzed the peripheral T-cell profiles in marrow recipients.[22,142,221] Their data, in general, were in agreement with each other, but disagreed with those of Reinherz et al.[524] Like the E-rosette studies, they found that the total number of T-cells had approached normal post grafting. De Bruin et al.[142] reported an abnormally high number of immature T-cells early after transplantation, while the others did not test for such T-cells. The cytotoxic-suppressor to helper-cell ratio that is normally 1:2 (as defined by OKT8 or Leu-2 and OKT4 or Leu-3 antibodies, respectively), was found by all to be reversed in patients' peripheral blood. This reversed ratio was seen in all patients after transplantation whether or not acute or chronic GVHD developed. Their reports differed in the descriptions of the normalization of the T-cell phenotypes. Friedrich et al.[221] reported that the cytotoxic-suppressor to helper-cell ratio returned to normal in patients with an uncomplicated course or with resolved acute GVHD, but the reversed ratio persisted in patients with active GVHD. Atkinson et al.[22] reported that T4 (helper) cells were low and stayed so for over 2 years, and that T8 (cytotoxic-suppressor) cells began to recover within 3 months postgrafting and subsequently remained at normal or high levels for years. De Bruin et al.[142] observed that normalization followed a variable course. The results of these studies depict the imbalance of T-cell subset development postgrafting. However, they bear no relevance to the development of GVHD.

## Lymphocyte-proliferative responses
By conventional criteria, lymphocyte-proliferative reactivity in the mixed leukocyte culture (MLC) assay is governed by determinants of a chromosomal locus or loci within the MHC. Siblings who inherit the same two parental major histocompatibility haplotypes will not show cellular stimulation with one another in MLC except in the rare instance of a crossover. Thus far, only a few reports have described the detection of low-grade, unidirectional proliferation of lymphocytes from individuals sensitized *in vivo* against non-HLA antigens by blood transfusions and/or marrow rejection.[316,441,442,676]

In studies done early in the postgrafting period using HLA-identical donors, both Oplez et al.[480] and Tsoi et al.[690] were unable to detect proliferative responses of chimeric lymphocytes of donor-marrow origin from patients with or without acute GHVD to cryopreserved pretransplant host cells. However, in patients with chronic GVHD studied between days 211 and 1089,[690] chimera lymphocyte proliferation in response to host non-HLA antigens was detected. Lymphocytes from 14/22 recipients of HLA-matched marrow with chronic GVHD showed unidirectional lymphocyte proliferative reactivity to host cells cryopreserved before transplantation, manifested as high stimulation indices (SI) and relative responses (RR). Lymphocytes from only 1/12 long-term chimeras without GVHD showed a low-grade reactivity to host cells. Statistical analysis showed that lymphocytes from patients with chronic GVHD displayed antihost proliferative responses significantly more often than did those from marrow donors ($p < 0.001$) or from patients without GVHD ($p = 0.03$).

We have since extended our study to 100 patients with chronic GVHD tested between days 83–2932, including 20 who were diagnosed early (days 83–200) and 18 who had only subclinical chronic GVHD (unpublished data).[690] We found that cells from 30 of the 100 patients had positive MLC responses to host cells (SI was $\geq 2.2$, RR was $\geq 2.6$), whereas cells from only 2/22 patients without GVHD tested between days 309–1460 had proliferative activity ($p < 0.05$). If we excluded all patients who had acute leukemia in relapse or chronic myelogenous leukemia in blast crisis or in accelerated phase (in order to rule out that the lymphocyte reactivity seen was a response to leukemia-associated antigens), the number of patients with chronic GVHD who had antihost MLC response was 21/77 (27%), compared to 1/19 without chronic GVHD ($p < 0.05$). Sex differences between the marrow donors and recipients had no correlation with the MLC responses. Our conclusion is that after marrow transplantation, cells from some patients with chronic GVHD develop cellular immunity against host non-HLA antigens.

## Cytotoxic responses

*Autocytotoxic Null Cells.* Parkman et al.[491] investigated the *in vitro* capacity of chimera lymphocytes during acute GVHD to lyse donor, host, and control fibroblasts labeled with $^{14}C$ amino acids in a 24-hour assay. They found that unfractionated donor lymphocytes did not lyse the target cells, whereas unfractionated cells

from the chimera with acute but not chronic GVHD lysed all the targets, suggesting that target antigens were expressed on all the target cells tested. The cells responsible for fibroblast lysis were not T-cells, but null cells bearing C′3 receptors. They were present in the blood of normal individuals and were reactive when separated from "regulator" or suppressor cells on discontinuous gradients of bovine serum albumin. Based on these findings and those of Reinherz et al.[524] that peripheral lymphocytes from patients with acute GVHD lacked suppressor cells, and that cessation of acute GVHD coincided with the appearance of suppressor cells, Parkman et al.[491] postulated that acute GVHD was produced by donor autocytotoxic null lymphocytes when the level of suppressor cells was low. They further argued that acute GVHD could also be developed in other clinical settings; for example, the administration of chemotherapy or infusion of autologous or syngeneic bone marrow into irradiated recipients, in whom the manipulation of the immune system produced a deficiency in suppressor cells which could no longer regulate the autocytotoxic effector cells. These conclusions need to be reassessed in view of recent observations that ample numbers of cells with the suppressor phenotype are present early postgrafting.[22,142,221]

*Natural Killer (NK) Cells.* The relationship of NK-cell activity and acute GVHD has been investigated. First, Lopez et al.[389] described NK activity against fibroblasts infected with herpes simplex virus type 1, NK (HSV-1), in 13 patients before transplantation. Seven patients with normal NK activity developed GVHD post grafting and six with low NK activity had no incidence of GVHD. The authors suggested that the NK response pregrafting might be predictive of a patient's risk of developing GVHD post grafting, and that the assay reflected host-dependent GVHD stimulator cell function. Since the degree of positivity of NK did not correlate with the grade of GVHD, this function might reflect the capacity to trigger GVHD and not the effector function mediating GVHD. Livnat et al.[388] measured NK activity against a K562 myeloblastoid cell line, NK (K562), in a large number of patients at various intervals from day 30. They found that about a third to half of the patients were deficient in NK activity before grafting, and that NK activity was normal in all patients between days 30 and 100 after grafting, and was deficient in about 20% of the patients beyond 1 year. There was no association between NK activity and acute or chronic GVHD. Later, Lopez and Livnat pooled their data for an analysis of the relation between NK (K562) activity before transplantation and GVHD following transplantation.[389a] No such correlation was found, but the significant correlation between NK (HSV1) and subsequent development of GVHD, as reported earlier, continued to hold. They believed that there were different effector cell populations mediating NK (HSV-1 and K562) and that there might be cells among the NK (HSV-1) effectors providing allogeneic stimulation to the transplanted marrow. The problem with the latter hypothesis is that at the time of transplantation, the patient's circulating mononuclear cells all have been depleted by the conditioning regimens and, thus, can no longer serve as stimulators.

More recently, NK (K562) activity was studied by Dokhelar et al.[157] in 24 human marrow recipients starting at day 9. Again, NK activity was consistently decreased before grafting and restored after grafting, thus arguing for a donor-marrow origin of NK progenitors and not of the host. In patients with acute GVHD, peripheral NK activity remained low during the first month after transplantation, then rapidly increased and reached normal values, usually between days 30 and 50. In patients with acute GVHD, strikingly high NK values were observed early after transplantation. There was a strong correlation between high NK values and acute GVHD occurrence during the first month postgrafting. The authors suggested that cells involved in GVHD were able to exert NK activity at some stage of their mutation, or that NK cells played a role in the pathogenesis of acute GVHD.

Since infections, especially cytomegalovirus (CMV), frequently occur following grafting, the level of NK activity may be an indicator of infection status but not of GVHD. Indeed, Quinnan et al.[515] demonstrated a marked difference between NK and CMV-specific cytotoxicity of patients who died from CMV infection and that of patients who recovered from the infection. Both NK and CMV-specific cytotoxicity were absent or in very low levels in blood from fatal cases. In

contrast, NK activity near onset of infection in patients who eventually recovered was readily detected, and their lymphocytes later became cytotoxic for CMV-infected target cells. These results suggested that these effector cells were involved in the immune response to CMV infection. In contrast to these findings, Livnat et al.[388] did not find a significant association between NK activity and infection in patients, while Dokhelar et al.[157] found a drastic fall in NK values associated with all seven cases of severe viral infections (fatal in four). The difference in results from these laboratories may have been due to their emphasis on different analysis parameters.

*Antihost Cytotoxic Cells.*   In our laboratory, we have searched for specific antihost cytotoxic cells associated with GVHD. Several years ago, using DLA-identical canine donor–recipient pairs, we established that the microcytotoxicity assay was useful in detecting *in vivo* sensitization to non-MHC skin or leukocyte antigens.[686] We postulated, therefore, that this *in vitro* test might detect cytotoxicity during acute GVHD. Our first study in 28 human chimeras post grafting from HLA-identical siblings involved the testing of cytotoxicity (cellular inhibition) of skin fibroblasts from the host and donor by mononuclear leukocytes from chimeras, donors, and/or unrelated individuals.[687] We found that cytotoxicity to host fibroblasts and serum blocking of cytotoxicity rarely were seen in long-term stable chimeras, suggesting that maintenance of stable graft-host tolerance in chimeras did not depend on the presence of serum-blocking factors. In about 50% of the short-term chimeras tested, cytotoxicity of chimera lymphocytes to host fibroblasts and serum-blocking effect were observed, but no correlation was found between cytotoxicity and the occurrence of acute GVHD.

Subsequently, we studied 51 patients sequentially after transplantation to clarify the trend of cytotoxicity of chimera cells against host fibroblasts and the role of serum-blocking factors early after grafting (Table 1).[694] During the first 2 months post grafting, mononuclear leukocytes from about half the patients were cytotoxic to host fibroblasts with or without serum-blocking activity. As more time after transplantation elapsed, the percentage of patients without cytotoxic lymphocytes significantly increased. At the end of 1 year, 89% of the patients tested had neither cytotoxicity nor serum blocking, while the remaining 11% showed both activities. Early in post grafting, there was a suggestive correlation between the presence of *in vitro* cytotoxicity by chimera cells to host fibroblasts and the occurrence of acute GVHD. Cells from 14/20 patients with acute GVHD were cytotoxic to host fibroblasts, compared to those from 7/18 patients with no GVHD (*p* was less than 0.08). However, there was no correlation between the presence or absence early in the postgrafting period of serum-blocking factors and acute GVHD. We then attempted to improve the sensitivity of the test system with a $^{51}$Cr terminal-labeling assay described by Tamerius et al.[661] Results of our recent studies showed a significant association of chimera cytotoxic cells to host fibroblasts with acute GVHD.[695a] This assay appears to be useful in detecting *in vitro* specific antihost cytotoxicity that might be involved in GVHD *in vivo*.

### Suppressor cells

*Nonspecific Suppressor Cells.* Immunodeficiency is common in patients during the first 4 months or longer after receiving allogeneic marrow.[171,197,225,277,462,472,636,757] Later, patients without GVHD generally recover their immune function, while those with chronic GVHD remain immunologically impaired[472,530,757] and have increased infections.[19] Disorder in immunoregulatory cells may be the basis for the profound immunodeficiency associated with chronic GVHD.

We investigated nonspecific suppressor cell functions in long-term survivors after transplantation. Mononuclear cells from 120 long-term patients were tested for their ability to inhibit MLC

reactivity of their donor-marrow cells to unrelated alloantigens (unpublished data).[689,693] Results (Fig. 2) indicated that cells from only 1/40 long-term patients with no chronic GVHD showed suppression as compared to cells from 35/80 patients with chronic GVHD (*p* = 0.0001). Cells from short-term patients with and without acute GVHD, tested between days 28–142, however, rarely showed nonspecific suppressor activity.[691] This latter result agreed with the negative findings of Gale et al.[225] and Elfenbein et al.[173] who also used the lymphocyte proliferation assay. However, results of studies using the pokeweed-stimulated Ig synthesis assay demonstrated suppressor cell activity in short-term marrow recipients.[359,485,757]

The suppressor cell activity in MLC was shown to be significantly correlated with clinical events in that the nonspecific suppressor function was associated with active chronic GVHD. Cells from patients with resolved chronic GVHD and those with limited symptoms usually did not have suppressor activity (unpublished data).[691] Furthermore, it was noted that the acquisition of late varicellazoster infection was more likely to occur in patients with chronic GVHD whose

**TABLE 1**
Summary of Sequential Cytotoxicity Tests

| Median Day of Test after Marrow Transplantation | Number of Patients Tested | Number (and Percent) of Patients Showing | | |
|---|---|---|---|---|
| | | −CT[a] (−BL)[b] | +CT +BL | +CT −BL |
| 45 | 38 | 17 (45) | 19 (50) | 2 (5) |
| 90 | 32 | 19 (59) | 10 (31) | 3 (9) |
| 145 | 23 | 19 (83) | 3 (13) | 1 (4) |
| 389 | 18 | 16 (89) | 2 (11) | 0 (0) |

[a]CT = cytotoxicity; BL = serum blocking.
[b]In the absence of CT, BL could not be measured and was presumed to be negative.

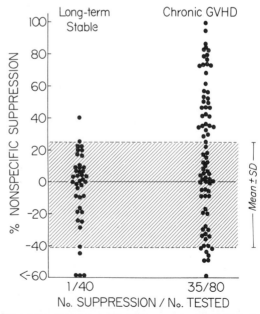

**Figure 2.** Percent nonspecific suppression of mixed leukocyte response of the marrow donors to unrelated alloantigens by cells from patients with chronic GVHD. The shaded area represents the mean value of suppression ± the standard deviation observed in long-term patients without GVHD.

lymphocytes displayed nonspecific suppression.[21]

Characterization of the suppressor cells in patients with chronic GVHD showed that in most cases they were nylon-wool-nonadherent T-cells with the T8 phenotype (unpublished data). Suppression could be abolished by 1600 rad *in vitro* irradiation.[689] The addition of helper or amplifying factors to suppressor cell cultures abolished suppression (unpublished data).[691] The helper factor was obtained from supernatants of 1-day MLCs[479] involving marrow donor or third-party lymphocytes responding to irradiated unrelated lymphocytes. In contrast, the supernatants obtained from MLCs involving chimera lymphocytes as responders failed to abrogate nonspecific suppression. The results suggest that: 1) the mechanism of suppression may be through competitive absorption of helper factors by the suppressor cells, such that T-cell proliferation is inhibited due to insufficient mediators. The presence of excess helper factors may thus overcome the effect of suppression. A second interpretation of these same data would be that targets of suppression are T-helper cells that produce helper factors (and, thus, the addition of helper factors bypasses the action of these suppressor cells); and 2) chimera cells are deficient in helper factor production.

Recently, we investigated the cell-mediated lympholysis responses in 40 marrow recipients.[449] The results showed that peripheral blood mononuclear leukocytes from patients with either acute or chronic GVHD had impaired cell-mediated lympholysis responses but not those from patients without GVHD. The cellular impairment seen in patients with acute GVHD would be corrected by adding helper factors (in the form of interleukin 2) to the cultures, indicating that defective helper factor production might be the basis of the impairment. On the other hand, the impairment seen in chronic GVHD could not be corrected by the mere replacement of helper factors, implying the involvement of other cellular defects, possibly in addition to helper factor deficiency. These additional defects might reside on the level of the effector cells, or might be due to the presence of nonspecific suppressor cells which inhibited cytolytic effector cells, probably through competition for helper factors.

Other investigators have also observed regulatory cell abnormalities in patients with chronic GVHD. Reinherz et al.[524] found increased suppressor T-cells in two patients with chronic GVHD inhibiting *in vitro* proliferative responses of cells from the patients and their marrow donors to mitogens and soluble antigens. Lum et al.[396] studying pokeweed mitogen-stimulated polyclonal Ig secretion, found a variety of defects causing depressed Ig secretion in patients with chronic GVHD. These defects included suppressor T cells capable of suppressing normal Ig synthesis, failure of B-cells to secret Ig in the presence of normal helper T-cells, and deficiency of helper T-cell activity. Using the pokeweed system, Saxon et al.,[562] Korsmeyer et al.[359] and Pahwa et al.[485] also demonstrated suppressor T-, helper T- and B-cell abnormalities in patients with chronic GVHD. These findings provide further support the possibility that immunoregulatory disorders exist in chronic GVHD.

*Specific Suppressor Cells.* Long-term stable chimeras without GVHD, in general, lack cellular immune responses against the host; i.e., they show neither lymphocyte proliferative activity against host cells stored before transplantation,[690] nor cytotoxic activity against cultured host skin fibroblasts.[692] In addition, they do not have Ig or C' deposits in the dermal–epidermal junction,[688] nonspecific suppressor T-cell activity,[689,691,693] nor abnormal activities of B-cells[396,530] and helper T-cells.[397,398,562] In summary, donor cells in long-term stable chimeras are tolerant to host antigens and display normal or nearly normal immune functions.

We ruled out the role of serum-blocking factors in the maintenance of graft–host tolerance in stable human chimeras.[687] Recently, we found evidence of specific suppressor cells in stable chimeras with HLA-identical marrow grafts.[692,693] Mononuclear leukocytes from 37 long-term chimeras (23 with and 14 without chronic GVHD) were tested for their ability to inhibit the reaction in MLC of donor lymphocytes to: 1) trinitrophenyl (TNP)-modified host leukocytes stored before transplantation (specific suppression); 2) unmodified unrelated cells (nonspecific suppression); 3) TNP-modified donor cells (control); and 4) TNP-modified unrelated cells (control).[693] The results showed that cells from 13/14 healthy stable chimeras without chronic GVHD had specific suppressor activity compared with those of only 5/23 chimeras with chronic GVHD ($p < 0.0005$), and the suppressor effect could be abrogated by 1600 rad *in vitro* irradiation. However, cells from none of the healthy chimeras had nonspecific suppressor activity compared with those of nine of the 23 chimeras with chronic GVHD tested ($p < 0.01$). In the controls, no differences in suppressor activity were detected between patients with and without chronic GVHD. These results suggest that stable chimerism in humans after HLA-identical allogeneic marrow grafting is maintained by specific suppressor cells, and that lack of them in patients with chronic GVHD may account for the *in vitro* anti-host immune responses and *in vivo* manifestation of GVHD.

## CONCLUSION

The preceding discussion has summarized the results of *in vitro* immunologic studies of cells from patients with or without GVHD. Although advances have been made in this complex and difficult area, the immunologic mechanisms of GVHD in bone marrow recipients are not entirely clear. Nevertheless, some conclusions can be drawn from the existing data.

Studies of T-cell profile seem to indicate that abnormality of T-cell maturation and imbalance of T-cell subsets may not be aspects related to GVHD but rather to conditions prevalent after grafting. These conditions may result from adverse effects of primary disease and conditioning regimens, thymic deficiency, infection, multiple drug treatment post grafting, and/or malnutrition. On the other hand, results of suppressor cell studies indicate that at least some aberrations of helper and/or suppressor cells are associated with GVHD. Yet, amid the disorder of immune regulation, donor cells in patients with GVHD can mount an antihost immune reaction as evidenced by the lymphocyte proliferation and the antihost cytotoxicity studies and, perhaps, also by the antiskin and antiepithelial cell antibody studies. The key difference between patients with and those without GVHD, therefore, is in immune regulation and alloimmunity. Further studies in these two aspects are needed to clarify the immunology of human GVHD.

# Chapter 5

# Pathology of acute and chronic cutaneous GVHD

**Howard M. Shulman, M.D.**
**George E. Sale, M.D.**

### Introduction

Most animals and humans affected by GVHD have involvement of the skin, the organ most useful and accessible for its diagnosis. The punch biopsy is quite safe and can be done frequently, even in immunosuppressed and thrombocytopenic patients. The histologic repertoire of the skin is limited, whereas the range of injurious agents which can mimic GVHD in this setting is large. Therefore, uniform histologic criteria for GVHD must be applied and other potential etiologies of inflammatory skin lesions carefully considered. More objective diagnosis is achieved if specimens are examined first without clinical information. The clinical data, which should include time after grafting, conditioning regimen, drug history, and observation of the gross rash, are then correlated. This chapter addresses the gross and microscopic differential diagnosis and pathogenesis of skin GVHD.

### ACUTE GVHD

#### Gross features

Acute GVHD has a variable gross appearance. The most common initial expression is a pruritic, morbilliform to erythematous, maculopapular rash. At first, GVHD usually involves the trunk, face, and palms, followed by ears and extremities (Figs. 1 and 2). A minority of cases of GVHD present with a punctate rash, corresponding to initial involvement of hair follicles (Fig. 3). Within several days, the rash becomes more confluent and the skin becomes dry and scaly. Progressive GVHD may display two kinds of desquamation. Less rapidly progressive cases show scaling of upper epidermal layers extending approximately to the lower stratum spinosum. Underlying epidermis may appear clinically improved with less scaling and erythema than at onset. This may be due to spontaneous waning of the reaction or to treatment. Infrequently, severe cases may show bullous ulceration with denudation resembling second degree burns (Fig. 1). In some of these cases, bleeding fluid loss, and superinfection can cause a serious management problem. Although such cases are infrequent, they can cause difficulty in diagnosis since they resemble the toxic epidermal necrolysis syndrome which is associated with a specific drug reaction or a known staphylococcal infection. However, the two conditions can usually be distinguished by serial biopsies.

#### Histologic features

Acute GVHD of the skin is by histologic pattern an interface dermatitis with a lichenoid reaction,

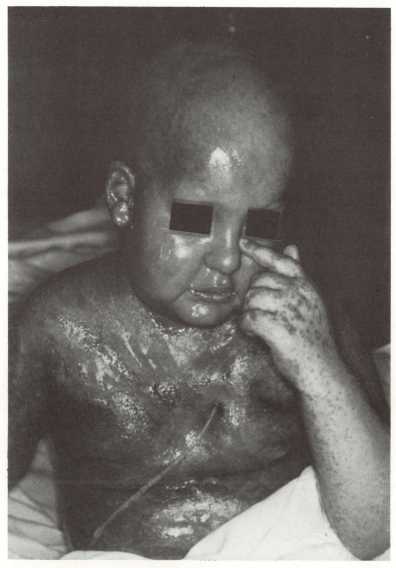

**Figures 1a and b.** (UPN 1132 Day 17) (*a*) Nine-year-old male allografted for ALL developed severe acute GVHD with grade IV changes. Photo exhibits transudation of plasma.

involving primarily the epidermis, pilar units, and superficial dermal venules.[2] Ordinarily, the epidermis and hair follicles will be involved simultaneously. Sweat duct involvement with individual cell necrosis and keratinization has been reported in acute GVHD in both humans and nonhuman primates, though it is more common in chronic GVHD. We have seen a few cases of acute GVHD present with isolated sweat duct involvement which then progress to definite and severe GVHD. The adnexal changes of GVHD are very similar to those of small bile ducts and salivary or lacrimal ducts (Fig. 4). The histologic grading scheme of acute GVHD proposed by Lerner et al.[379] was an attempt to grade the severity of the process, as follows:

*Grade I* is epidermal basal cell vacuolization accompanied by a slight mononuclear cell infiltrate around the superficial venules and/or in the epidermis (Fig. 5). Occasionally eosinophils are found in the perivascular space.

*Grade II* requires grade I changes (often more marked) plus findings of dead epidermal cells in the basal or suprabasal layers (Fig. 6). These

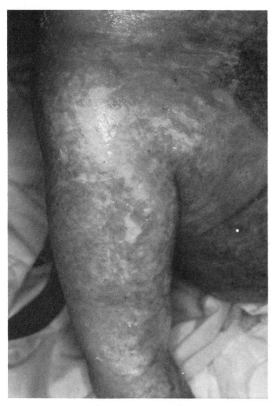

**Figure 1b.** Shoulder shows severe bullous changes.

dead cells have contracted, deeply eosinophilic cytoplasm with a pyknotic nucleus and have been referred to as "mummified cells,"[760] "dyskeratotic cells,"[545] and "apoptotic bodies."[733] They also may well be the same as sub-basilar colloid bodies. We now feel the term "dyskeratotic" is inappropriate since our ultrastructural studies have shown that these cells consist not only of keratinocytes, but also of Langerhans' cells and melanocytes which undergo active injury and contraction, rather than the normal process of keratinization. We, therefore, term them "eosinophilic bodies," and they may be surrounded by lymphocytes, forming the appearance of satellitosis around the dying cells. The term "aggressor lymphocyte lesions" was coined by Woodruff et al. to specify such findings.[759] Another term used is "mummified cell," the process of which is thought by Kerr and colleagues[345] to be identical to "apoptosis," a type of cell death associated with radiation, senescence, and alloreactions.

*Grade III* requires confluent regions of necrosis producing so much confluent damage at the

basal layers that bullae develop (Fig. 7).

*Grade IV* requires total denudation of the epidermis, producing a picture resembling toxic epidermal necrolysis (Fig. 8).

The lesions of GVHD can wax and wane. Acute GVHD may be evanescent with prophylaxis using low-dose, intermittent methotrexate (MTX), or may resolve under treatment with prednisone, antithymocyte sera, or cyclosporine (CYA). It is not uncommon to see histologic signs of active GVHD in random skin biopsies several weeks after resolution of the clinical rash. Under the influence of immunosuppressive therapy the lesions tend to be less inflammatory, often having only isolated "eosinophilic bodies." In cases of re-

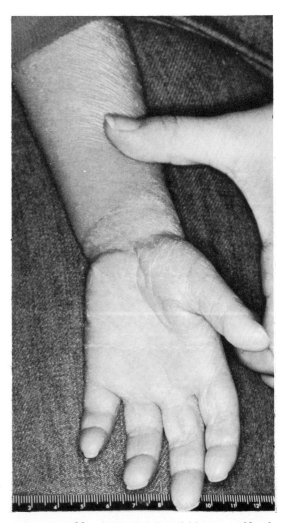

**Figures 2a and b.** (UPN 1007 Day 35) (*a*) Six-year-old male after graft for ANL. Acute GVHD shows scaling dermatitis of forearm.

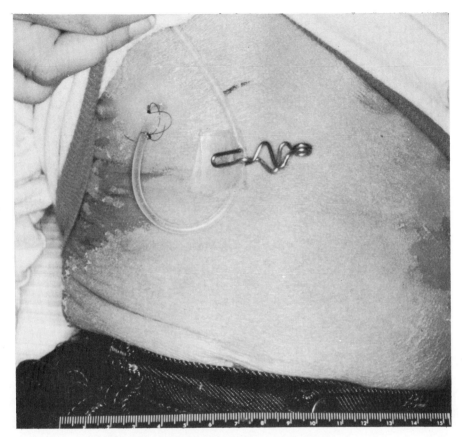

**Figure 2*b*.** Abdominal skin displays similar changes.

solved GVHD, residual changes include relative hyperkeratosis, hyperpigmentation, papillary damage, melanin incontinence, and epidermal atrophy without epidermal eosinophilic bodies, findings which characterize "quiescent" GVHD in the terminology of Slavin and Woodruff.[(592)]

Uncertainty in diagnosing GVHD is greatest in the first 3 weeks post grafting because of difficulty in separating the combined effects of chemoradiation therapy, infection, or GVHD in this early period. Since the reaction pattern of GVHD, particularly the earlier stages (grade I), is not pathognomonic, several other similar dermatitides must be considered.

### Chemoradiation pathology

The skin is relatively resistant to radiation and cytotoxic drugs when compared to organs with higher cell turnover rates, such as gut and bone marrow.[(95,194)] However, in the marrow transplant setting, the superlethal doses of cytotoxic drugs and irradiation used to ablate the host's marrow and immune system and/or tumor load are very large relative to previous experiences. Despite the fact that attendant cell and organ toxicity to the liver, gut, or lungs may be more limiting or life-threatening, skin toxicity can become serious when it produces desquamation. A variety of chemotherapeutic agents can produce skin toxicity. In general, the greater the number and dose of anticancer drugs used, the more likely that there will be a toxic reaction. Characteristic findings in some cases of toxicity are painful red digits, erythematous blistering, and Nikolsky's phenomenon of easy abrading of the epidermis.

Bleomycin provides an excellent example of early information about the problem of direct cytotoxicity to the skin. Initial trials showed skin toxicity to be the most frequently cited reason for discontinuation of the drug, although pulmonary toxicity has received much more attention. The skin lesions were characterized by pain, edema, and some bulla formation with epidermal loss, maximal in areas of pressure or friction, such as

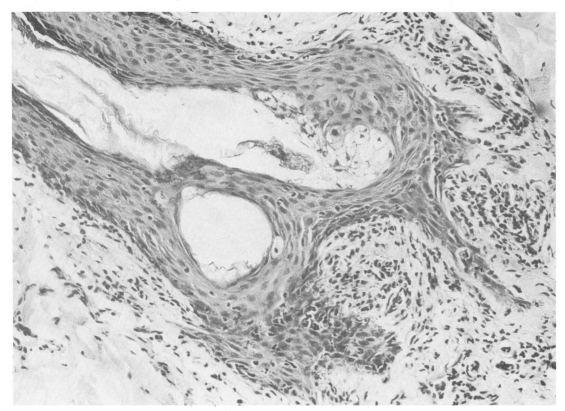

**Figure 3.** (UPN 569 Day 52) A 43-year-old man allografted for ANL who had no GVHD before day 52. Pilosebaceous unit involvement in rash appearing as a clinical folliculitis, which spread to a generalized maculopapular rash within a week. Patient later developed chronic GVHD.

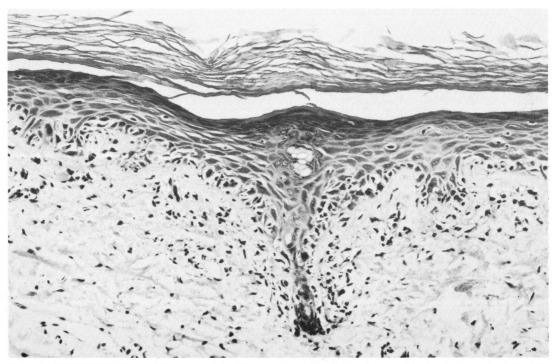

**Figure 4.** (UPN 1602) A 33-year-old man transplanted for acute lymphoblastic lymphoma with leukemia. Example of relatively early sweat duct involvement coincident with that of surface epidermal basal layer.

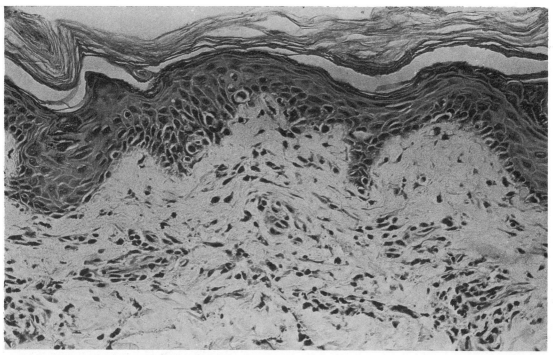

**Figure 5.** (UPN 567 Day 70) A 28-year-old woman allografted for ANL developed a rash that appeared nonspecific both clinically and histologically. A superficial perivascular dermatitis was present with eosinophils. The disturbances noted in the basal epidermis were not regarded as sufficient for a grade II diagnosis, hence no specific one was made at this time.

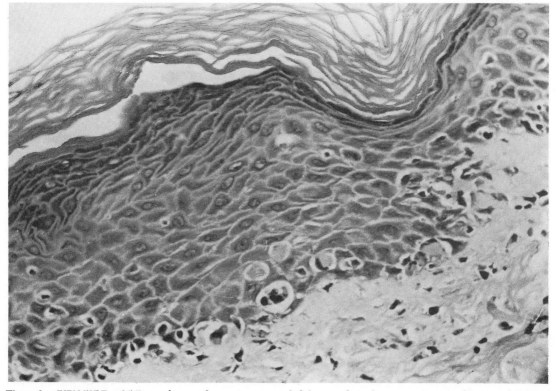

**Figure 6.** (UPN 567 Day 84) Repeat biopsy of same patient revealed these grade II changes, permitting a diagnosis of GVHD.

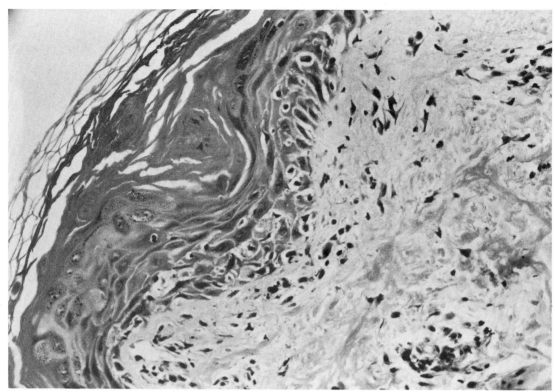

**Figure 7.**   (UPN 1418 Day 17) A 31-year-old male developed early severe GVHD after an allograft for ALL from a partially mismatched donor. The changes are grade II–III since multiple eosinophilic bodies are coalescing at the base of a rete ridge which is probably also perforated by a sweat duct. The imminent bulla would constitute the fully developed grade II lesion. The diagnosis of GVHD this soon after grafting is difficult even in mismatched marrow recipients.

the heels, palms, buttocks and knees. Previous reports[361] had emphasized that such agents have direct effects on epithelial cells of several sites, in addition to the gut. We have seen similar effects when cytosine arabinoside (Ara-C), or dimethyl-busulfan were given with cyclophosphamide (CY) and TBI (Fig. 9).

Koss et al.[360–362] discovered that busulfan affects the cytology of the cervix sufficiently in patients with chronic myelogenous leukemia or chronic lymphocytic leukemia to produce marked cytopathic damage which was difficult to distinguish from that of severe dysplasia or carcinoma. Furthermore, they examined the question in rats after the administration of CY and found similar cytologic atypia, not only in the bladder, gut, and marrow, but also in the skin. Similarly, in the hyperplastic epidermis of patients with psoriasis, low-dose MTX can produce individual cell necrosis of epidermal cells which is histologically similar to that seen in GVHD.[590,599,741]

Similar cytopathic effects on the normal epi-

dermis have been reported for bleomycin,[31,64,117] adriamycin,[542] for radiation coupled with actinomycin D or adriamycin,[140,265] and long-term hydroxyurea.[344] Our 1977 coded study of skin biopsies from autografted patients and patients receiving identical-twin grafts showed marked cytotoxic effects mimicking those attributed to GVHD (Fig. 10).[545] Some of these reactions can occur very early. For example, Figure 11 illustrates a skin reaction 6 days after autografting for Hodgkin's disease. Furthermore, we have occasionally seen tripolar mitoses in basal epidermal cells after intense preparative regimens, suggesting that direct damage to stem cells producing aneuploidy can occur even in the skin (Fig. 12).

The conclusion from our 1977 study was that the first 3 weeks after engraftment constitute a period of uncertainty. A skin biopsy taken between days 7–20 may show nonspecific interface dermatitis or even evidence of epidermal necrosis without requiring a diagnosis of GVHD. Our practice in these early (days 7–20) cases is to re-

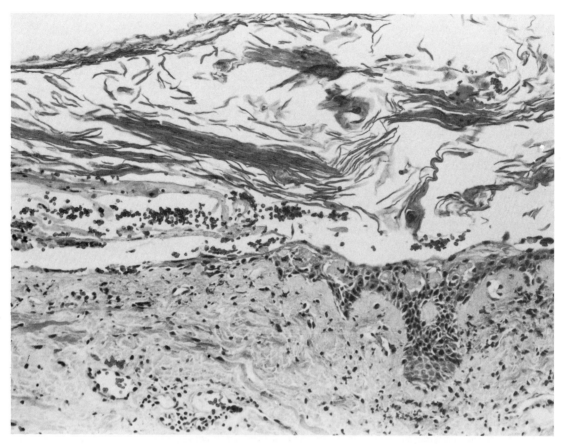

**Figure 8.** (UPN 1418 Day 36) Grade IV GVHD shows total denudation of epidermis at left, yet some parts of basal layer at right are spared.

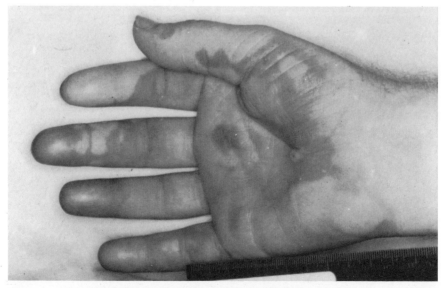

**Figure 9.** (UPN 957 Day 20) Hand of 36-year-old male with CML who received intensive chemoradiotherapy showing erythema, blanching, and early bulla formation of fingers and palms. Regimen was dimethylmyleran, CY, and TBI (200 rad ×6). Patient's erythema appeared on day 10 but was gone by day 31.

quest serial skin biopsies at intervals of 3–5 days. If the rash and the severity of the histologic changes are decreasing, no specific diagnosis is made. If the rash or skin biopsy changes persist or worsen and grade II changes are present, a diagnosis of GVHD is made. The clinical staff is made aware of the *relative* specificity of the findings and take this into account in diagnosis. We have concluded that a grade II lesion is necessary but not totally sufficient or specific for a diagnosis of GVHD and may be safely ignored, at least temporarily, if contradictory data are present. This approach acknowledges the uncertainties and concedes that mild and transient skin GVHD may be missed. Even if this entity were easily diagnosed, it would not always be treated, as the therapeutic agents are often toxic or experimental or both. Even as late as 30 days or more after grafting, residual chemoradiation damage may be detectable in the epidermis of some subgroups of patients. We reported such changes in the skin of 6/6 autografted CML patients, and attributed this to delayed recovery due to previous long-term chemotherapy with busulfan in such patients. Such therapy by itself often produces epidermal atrophy. This atrophy may be due to epidermal ridge and follicle stem-cell damage that decreases the reserve capacity for regeneration.

The precise pathogenesis of the damage associated with these cytotoxic agents is unclear. Assuming delivery of the drug or radiation to the epithelial cells, direct toxicity is the most likely hypothesis. Secondary effects of local vascular damage to endothelium are also possible. Another mechanism which has been discussed is the modification or unmasking of "hidden" antigens on plasma membranes by the agents, stimulating an autoimmune reaction. Parkman and Rappeport[491] have hypothesized that chemotherapy upsets the normal balance of immunoregulatory lymphoid cells, resulting in an excess of cytotoxic null or T-cells which produces an autoimmune reaction against epithelial cell targets. They and others[243,664] have reported "pseudo-GVHD" reactions in twin graft and autograft recipients. Their hypothesis, apparently is dependent on the modification or unmasking of "forbidden" antigens, as mentioned above. To test these balances in peripheral blood in the first 2-week period post grafting is impossible because insufficient lymphocytes are present for study. Its predictions for the imbalances later after grafting have not been confirmed. Atkinson and others showed that persistent long-term elevation of the suppressor–cytotoxic population occurs in all graft recipients regardless of the identity of the graft or the presence of GVHD.[19] The hypothesis also fails to deal adequately with the direct toxicity of drugs to epithelial cells and the fact that patients

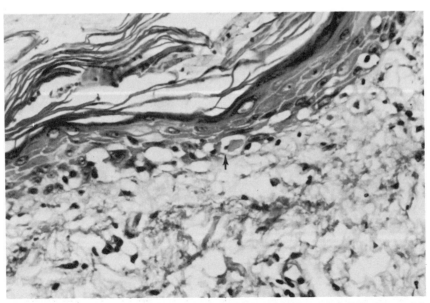

**Figure 10.** (UPN 364 Day 26) Skin histopathology of autograft recipient with CML. Eosinophilic body with lymphocyte nucleus (arrow). (From Sale et al.[545]; reprinted with permission.)

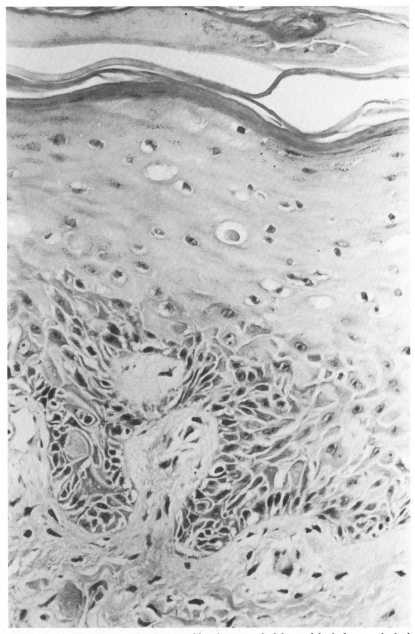

**Figure 11.** (UPN 1278 Day 6) A 37-year-old male autografted for Hodgkin's disease who had been treated previously with chemotherapy, then was given a pretransplant regimen including a total of 1800 rad TBI. The epidermis is hyperplastic and spongiotic. Necrotic epidermal cells are accompanied by sparse mononuclear infiltrate. Venules are dilated in papillary dermis.

infected with either viruses or bacteria can show clinical signs mimicking GVHD. Some authors also question the histological diagnosis in cases reported by Reinherz et al.[524] and by Rappeport et al.[520] because they did not report convincing grade II changes.[597]

It is important to evaluate critically reports of GVHR-like reactions occurring in syngeneic or autologous marrow recipients. The case reported by Gluckman and colleagues,[243] for example, clearly had CMV infection that could have explained the patient's entire course. Another case report involved an autograft recipient who not only had bacteremia but also had no evidence of

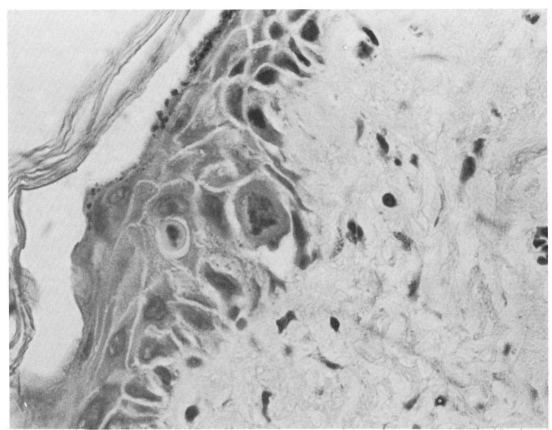

**Figure 12.** (UPN 767 Day 32) A 23-year-old male allografted for acute promyelocytic leukemia, preconditioned with dimethylbusulfan, CY, and 1000 rad TBI. Among the findings that suggest direct damage to epidermal stem cells by chemoradiotherapy are occasional bizarre mitotic figures. One such figure photographed here can be interpreted as tripolar, suggesting that aneuploidy has been induced by the preconditioning agents.

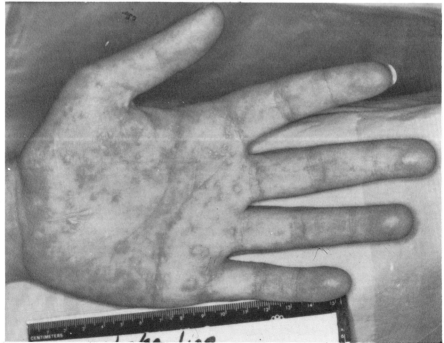

**Figure 13.** (UPN 1098 Day 100) Painful, raised, red to violaceous papulosquamous papules on the palms or soles represent early clinical signs of generalized chronic GVHD. Histologically, the papules represent lichenoid acanthosis.

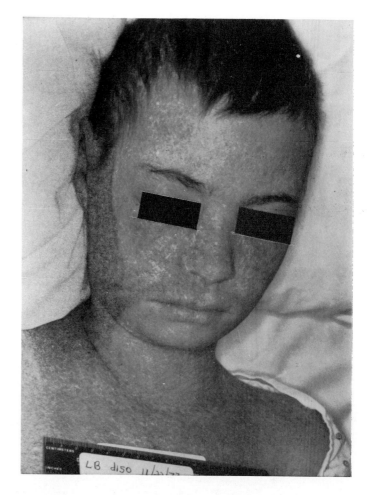

**Figure 14.** (UPN 705 Day 150) Forty days after *de novo* late onset of generalized chronic GVHD. There is diffuse erythematous desquamation.

graft at autopsy.[664] Neither of these cases seems fully convincing, even as an example of autoimmune reactions. We recently observed some skin lesions in a syngeneic recipient 1 year after grafting which had superficial and deep perivascular inflammation, dilatation, and edema of eccrine glands and patchy interface dermatitis. Further evaluation, however, revealed that the reaction, unlike generalized chronic cutaneous GVHD, was transient, and that the patient had probably been exposed to poison sumac.

So far, reports of "GVHD" in syngeneic recipients seem to have major disqualifying flaws. Even if syngeneic recipients occasionally exhibit

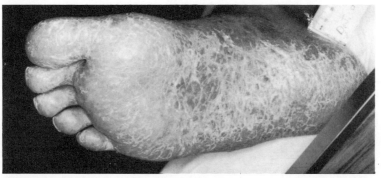

**Figure 15.** (UPN 814 Day 131) Painful, scaling, erythematous papules on soles, characteristic of early chronic GVHD.

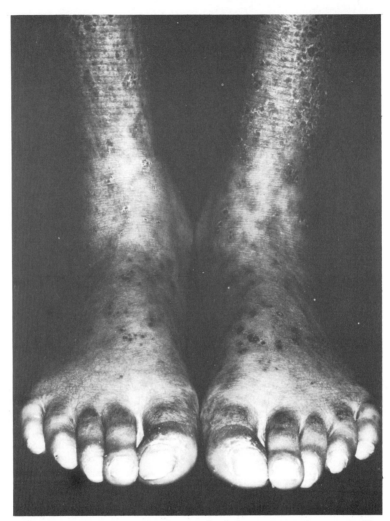

**Figure 16.** (UPN 520 Day 210) Early generalized chronic GVHD showing raised hyperpigmented papules, brawny edema, periungual swelling, and irregularity of nails. (From Shulman et al.[582]; reprinted with permission.)

true autoimmune reactions, two things seem certain at present. First, although theoretically interesting, the reactions are not of major clinical frequency;[200] and, second, they cannot, by definition, be called GVHR or GVHD.[179,180] Nevertheless, it is from the investigation of just such difficult paradoxes that new insights into autoimmunity may come (Chapter 2). Therefore, such cases should be thoroughly investigated and reported.

### "Drug" rashes, erythema multiforme, allergic rashes, etc.

Transplant recipients are exposed to many other drugs besides chemoradiotherapy. In addition to frequent use of multiple, broad-spectrum antibiotics, oral, nonabsorbable antibiotics are given to patients in laminar airflow (LAF) room isolation for the purpose of sterilizing the gut. The latter drugs are probably not associated with skin lesions except in the perianal region, secondary to mild diarrhea which these agents often may cause. Prophylactic sulfa drugs (trimethoprim sulfa: "Bactrim") are now routinely employed to prevent *Pneumocystis carinii* infection. The general guidelines for differential diagnosis of drug rashes must be used for these cases individually, with a logical analysis of both the clinical and histological data.

Most drug reactions are associated with a nonspecific interface dermatitis showing a perivascular edema with an infiltrate of mononuclear cells in the papillary and reticular dermis which mimics grade I GVHD. Occasionally, eosinophils will be seen in these infiltrates. These reactions are not difficult to differentiate from GVHD if the criteria for GVHD, grade II, are present. However, when drug reactions are severe, there is extensive necrosis of the basal layer, necrosis of eccrine ducts, and bulla formation, producing the histologic patterns of erythema multiforme.[2] Clinically, erythema multiforme will often present target-shaped lesions or will have other unusual clinical features helping to distinguish it from GVHR. Our experience with CYA has shown a peculiar early syndrome of facial and acral edema and erythema, apparently due to increased vascular permeability. The skin biopsy will reveal only vascular dilatation with pronounced perivascular edema.

## Infections

Infection is a fourth cause of skin rash in these patients, especially during the first 2–4 weeks after grafting. Bacterial and fungal infections can produce a variety of generalized cutaneous manifestations. Diffuse skin rashes occurring in such cases, possibly the effects of endotoxin, can mimic those of GVHD. Viral exanthemata, like those in children, are unusual. But infection with herpes viruses (especially CMV, herpes zoster, herpes simplex, and adenovirus) are common. Although skin infection by CMV has been reported in immunosuppressed patients,[385] we have not seen it in over 400 autopsies or in sev-

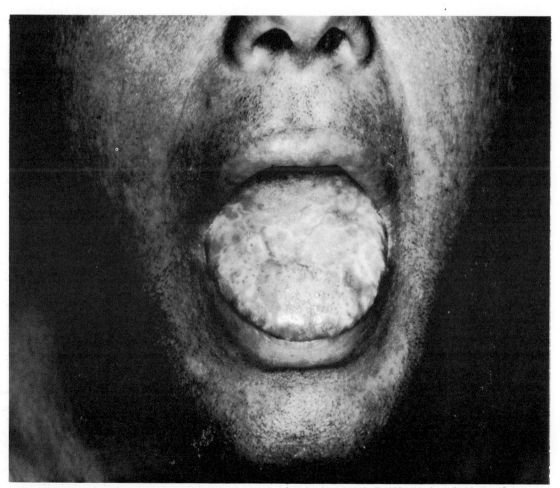

**Figure 17.** (UPN 756 Day 146) Oral changes of chronic GVHD with mosaic-like ulcerations and leukoplakia.

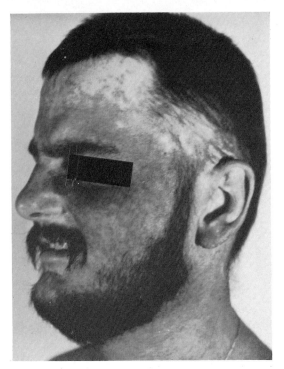

**Figure 18.** (UPN 677 Day 188) Irregular pigmentation with alternating areas of leukoderma and hyperpigmentation. The depigmentation usually corresponds to areas of inflammation.

eral thousand skin biopsies from immunosuppressed patients. Herpes zoster infections of the skin are a frequent problem in our patients but usually present in a classical fashion with crops of vesicles confined to a dermatomic distribution. Oral herpes simplex affects 40% of transplant recipients[440] and the herpetic lesions typically form in clusters or form ulcerations contiguous with mucous membranes.

The need for caution in histologic interpretation, even of skin lesions showing grade II changes, is illustrated by a recent case. A skin biopsy, submitted without clinical history, revealed mononuclear infiltrates, eosinophilic bodies, apparent satellitosis, and early splitting at the basilar to suprabasilar layers of the epidermis. Subsequently, it was learned that the lesion had come from the edge of a vesicle. A Tzanck preparation was positive for multinucleate giant cells with inclusions and viral culture revealed herpes zoster.

### CHRONIC GVHD

Chronic cutaneous GVHD has a "dynamic" histology evolving from an inflammatory into a

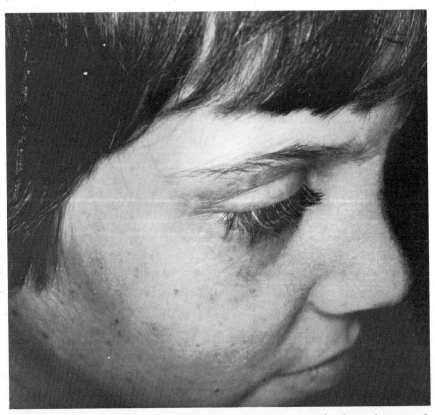

**Figure 19.** (UPN 644 Day 958) Symmetrical periorbital pigmentation and vitiligo with graying of eyelashes.

fibrosing dermatitis. A single biopsy taken at one point cannot convey the complex chronology of the disorder. A full appreciation of the dermatopathology of chronic GVHD required studying many patients over several years with serial photographs and biopsies. The natural history of chronic GVHD was compiled before the more recent advent of early diagnostic staging and therapeutic intervention which has lessened, modified, or prevented the typical features. Several points should be remembered when studying chronic cutaneous GVHD. First, the choice of biopsy site is important since histologic findings are often not uniform. Second, biopsies are often taken to assess response to immunosuppressive therapy and activity rather than to classify lesions histologically as early or late chronic GVHD. Since there is a preexisting background of older injury, it is important to biopsy recent or changing lesions, since these are more likely to show whether the process is still active. Third, the biopsy should include a full thickness of dermis and some subcutaneous fat, since much of the characteristic pathology involves eccrine units and the dermal subcutaneous interface. Elliptical biopsies and larger samples taken at autopsy have helped to present a much more graphic understanding of the pathology. Even within these larger samples, there may be some variability with some alterations being found only within focal areas.

In our initial report of 19 patients with chronic

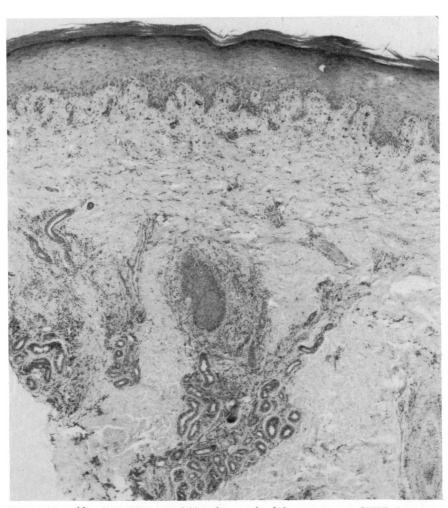

**Figures 20a and b.** (UPN 736 Day 225) (*a*) Early generalized chronic cutaneous GVHD. Low power shows lichen-planus-like epidermal changes as well as inflammation about dermal pilar units, sweat glands, and neurovascular bundles.

cutaneous GVHD,[582] we characterized two separate types: generalized and localized, each with different clinical and pathological features (Table 1). Our experience with over 200 patients with chronic GVHD still indicates that this dichotomy predicts the biological behavior and guides the need for immunosuppressive therapy. Also, we have learned that the distinction between these two types may be very difficult to discern in long-standing cases or in patients who experience re-exacerbation after cessation of immunosuppressive therapy. For didactic purposes we divide this continuum into early and late stages. We have not found the histologic grading of either type of chronic cutaneous GVHD, according to the degree, amount, and location of inflammation, to have prognostic significance.

### Generalized chronic GVHD

Most patients with cutaneous chronic GVHD (75–80%) have the generalized or inflammatory (lichen planus-like GVHR)[561] type, involving large, continuous areas of the skin and all aspects of the integument (including the nails and mucous membranes) with considerably more inflammation and epidermotropism than that with the localized variant. In Sullivan's study[653] 9/47 patients (19%) had the initial involvement or activation of generalized chronic GVHD in areas of sun exposure (reminiscent of lupus erythematosus) or

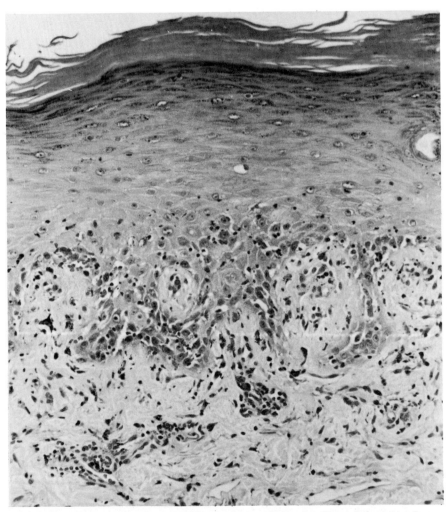

**Figure 20*b*.**  Higher-power view of epidermis shows compact lamellar orthokeratosis, hypergranulosis, and hyperplasia, a lichenoid reaction with sawtoothing and irregularity of rete ridges, and individual cell necrosis of epidermal cells. The infiltrate, primarily lymphocytic with a few eosinophils, is less than that of classical lichen planus. The papillary dermis is edematous and contains incontinent melanin pigment.

**TABLE 1**[a]

Guidelines for Diagnosis of Cutaneous Chronic GVHD

Clinical criteria
  Generalized type, early phase
    Continuing erythema, desquamation, increasing hyperpigmentation, vesiculobullous change, or papulosquamous plaques, plus at least one additional manifestation in the eye (conjunctivitis or sicca), the mouth (focal leukoplakia, cheilitis), or the nails (periungual edema or onychosis)
  Generalized type, late phase
    Poikiloderma with hidebound skin and/or contractures
  Localized type
    Hyperpigmentation and hypopigmentation and scaliness with nodular subepidermal induration involving a limited area of skin
Histopathologic criteria
  Generalized type, early phase
    Lichenoid acanthosis with syringitis and panniculitis or neuritis
  Localized type
    Focal reticular dermal fibrosis; epidermis with only mild inflammation or basal vacuolization
  Late phase (both types included)
    Epidermal atrophy with replacement fibrosis of papillary and reticular dermis and subcutaneous fat with or without continuing inflammation involving deep adnexal structures and subcutaneous fat

[a] Reprinted with permission[584]

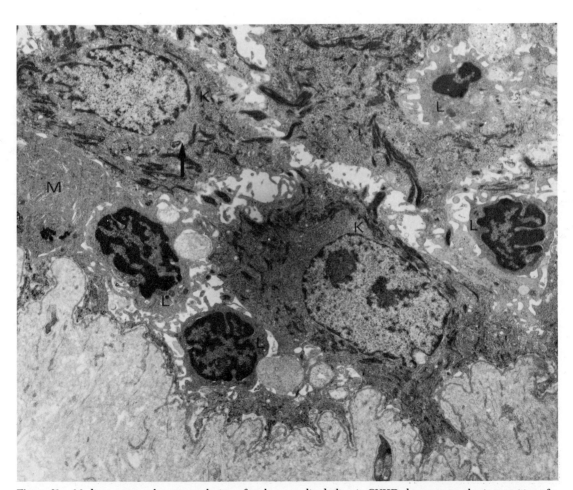

**Figure 21.** Medium-power, ultrastructural view of early generalized chronic GVHD demonstrates the juxtaposition of a prominent lymphocytic infiltrate (L) and occasional macrophages (M) in basal portion of epidermis. Keratinocytes (K) have disrupted and shortened tonofibrillar system, electron-lucent cytoplasm, markedly widened intercellular space, and autophagosomes (arrow). The convoluted basal lamina is replicated (×5600.) (From Gallucci et al.[229]; reproduced with permission.)

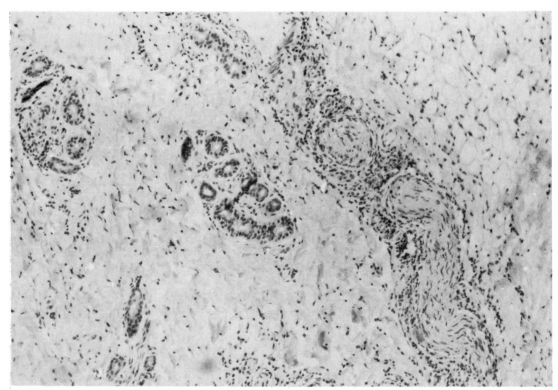

**Figures 22a and b.**   (UPN 512 Day 226) Early generalized chronic cutaneous GVHD. (a) Medium-power view of lower dermis shows lymphoplasmacytic inflammation about eccrine coils and large nerve trunks.

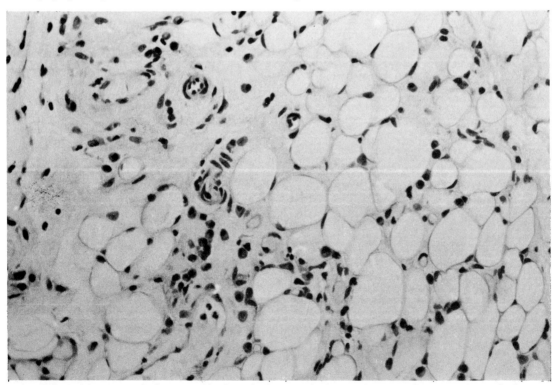

**Figure 22b.**   Higher-power of subcutaneous fat shows focal perivenular lymphoplasmacytic deposition of ground substance, and degeneration of adipocytes.

in areas of trauma or venous stasis. Other studies have reported distribution of generalized chronic GVHD in an area of measles exanthem[203] or limited to an area of previous irradiation.[771] These phenomena may cause a nonspecific activation of the immune system, or alternatively, some modification of epidermal antigens leading to initiation of GVHD. For example, studies have shown that exposure of living cells to ultraviolet light can produce epidermal breakdown with the formation of thymine dimers and polymers from altered nuclear macromolecules.[600] As Gilliam has pointed out: "when these altered nuclear macromolecules are released into the circulation, antibodies of different specificities are induced by the antigenic stimulation."[662]

## Clinical features of early generalized GVHD

Generalized chronic GVHD can be either gradu-ally or rapidly progressive. Typical features are painful, violaceous, flat-topped hyperkeratotic papules, particularly on the palmar and plantar surfaces (Fig. 13); mild, erythematous to violaceous scaling, particularly over the malar prominences of the face, and palms and soles (Figs. 14 and 15); periungual erythema with pitting of the nails; and brawny edema (Fig. 16). The erythema and papules usually spread to involve other parts of the integument within 4 weeks. This involvement may be confined to either the upper or lower half of the body and be predominantly pa-pulosquamous in one area and diffusely erythematous in another. Patients with an explosive onset usually have widespread involvement of the integument and mucous membranes (Fig. 17). After a month or more, diffuse pigmentary abnormalities develop as a consequence of disruption or destruction of the epidermal melanin

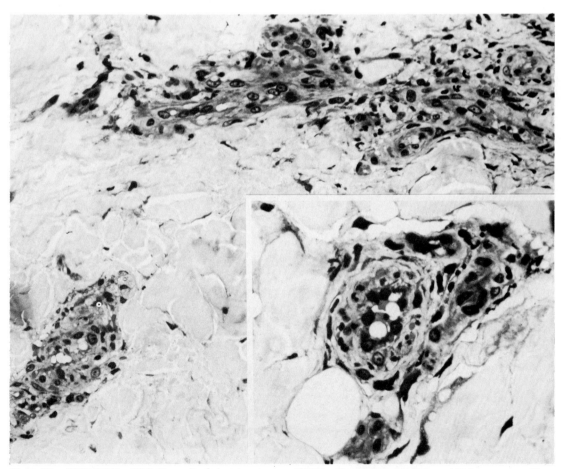

**Figure 23.** (UPN 734 Day 1054) Generalized chronic cutaneous GVHD with vasculitis. Medium- and high-power magnification (inset) of arterioles in reticular dermis with swollen endothelial lining and neutrophils within medial layer.

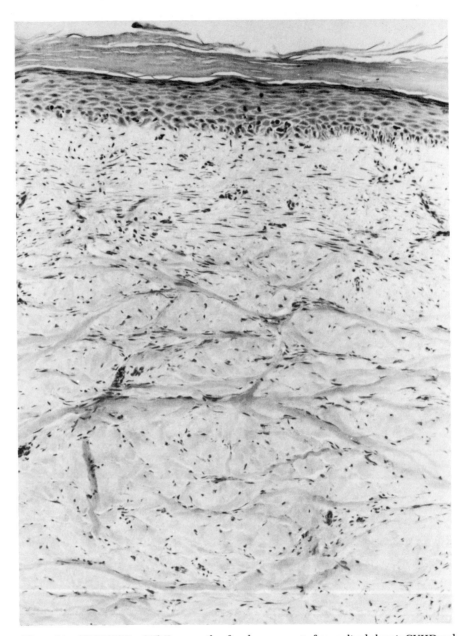

**Figure 24.** (UPN 705 Day 247) Four months after *de novo* onset of generalized chronic GVHD and 40 days after institution of immunosuppressive therapy. The signs of active GVHD are still evident with infiltration by lymphoid cells and injured basal cells. The rete ridges have been destroyed. The papillary dermis is widened by a fibroblastic proliferation, a finding quite dissimilar to scleroderma. Reticular dermal alterations include elongated, straightened, hypertrophic collagen bundles (interstitial collagenosis). The intervening bundles of collagen are broad, smudgy, and contain increased numbers of nuclei.

unit. Alternating areas of leukoderma from 0.5 centimeters up to several centimeters in diameter are juxtaposed with areas of diffuse hyperpigmentation, imparting a reticulate to cobblestone pattern (Fig. 18). A few patients have signs of true vitiligo, with the preservation of depig-mented patches of hair over the scalp, eyebrows, or eyelashes (Fig. 19). Hair on the scalp, axillae, and pubic regions becomes thin or fails to re-grow. On the scalp, a few patients develop focal or diffuse scaling alopecia and marked crusting. Other changes frequently associated with generalized chronic cutaneous GVHD are dryness of mucous membranes, conjunctiva, mouth, trachea, and vagina.

## Histopathology of early generalized chronic GVHD

Typical histologic features are usually first seen in biopsies between days 120–180, soon after the cessation of immunosuppressive therapy or after a triggering event. These features, however, may develop as early as day 50, as late as 1½ years post-transplant, and may vary with immunosuppressive treatment. Characteristic histology is seen best in the biopsy of a lichen planus-like, hyperpigmented papule (Fig. 20). The corneal layer has a true, lamellar hyperkeratosis overlying hypergranulosis. The acanthotic epidermis is composed of enlarged keratinocytes with glassy cytoplasm. The basal layer is partially obscured by a patchy to diffuse lichenoid reaction. The infiltrate in the basal layer is composed primarily of lymphoid cells and some monocytes. This infiltrate is usually greater than that in acute GVHD but less than in classical lichen planus. Rete ridges may have a sawtooth appearance, be completely destroyed, or be replaced by the ghostlike remnants of dead keratinocytes (eosinophilic or apoptotic bodies), with shrunken pink to orange cytoplasm with absent or centrally located pyknotic nuclei (Fig. 20b). Severe spongiosis and confluent liquefactive degeneration of the basal layers may produce separation from the dermal papillae with bulla formation and splitting of the basal lamina (Fig. 21). The lichenoid reaction produces lysis and thickening of the basement membrane zone, edema in the papillary dermis, and pigmentary disturbance of the epidermal melanin unit, resulting in melanin blockage. Coarse clumps of melanin lie between keratinocytes in the stratum spinosum while incontinent melanin pigment lies scattered in the papillary dermis or within macrophages.

Early chronic GVHD is distinguished from both acute GVHD and lichen planus by the inflammatory changes around the deep adnexal

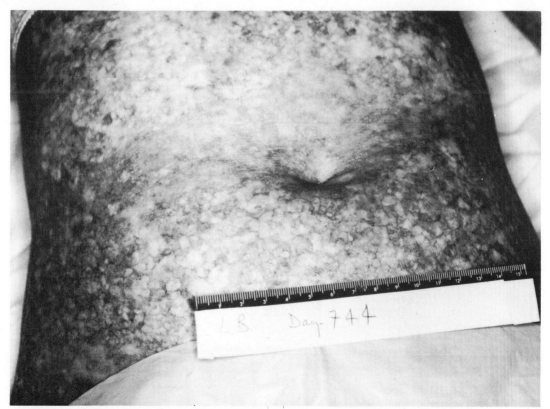

**Figure 25.** (UPN 705 Day 744) Characteristic reticulate changes of late chronic GVHD are telangiectasia and hypo- and hyperpigmentation. Dermal induration, tightness, and dyspigmentation have lessened or resolved over time.

flammatory changes around the deep adnexal structures in the reticular dermis (Fig. 22*a* and *b*). Besides inflammation about pilar units, there is a lymphoplasmacytic infiltrate scattered around eccrine coils and ducts and neurovascular bundles. Damaged eccrine ducts show squamous metaplasia and individual cell necrosis. Both superficial and deep dermal venules are often dilated and surrounded by a loose scattering of mononuclear cells, including eosinophils. Rarely, patients manifest signs of vasculitis showing leukocytoclastic debris and lymphocytes and neutrophils within vessel walls (Fig. 23).

After generalized chronic GVHD has been present for several weeks or months, there is some obvious widening of the papillary dermis by collagen, and sometimes a striking increase of fibroblastic nuclei (Fig. 24). Janin-Mercier et al.[313] have emphasized that this fibroblastic change in the papillary dermis of chronic GVHD is unlike scleroderma in which fibrosis begins in the deep dermis. The inflammatory changes also extend down to involve the interface of the dermis and subcutaneous fat (Fig. 22*b*). The adipose cells surrounding the eccrine coils and at the dermal–subcutaneous interface are replaced by an

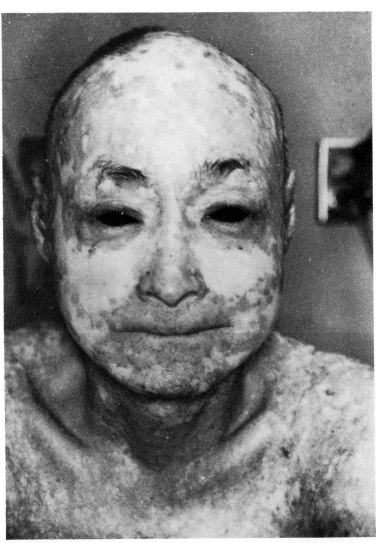

**Figures 26*a* and *b*.**   (UPN 294 Day 956) Late generalized chronic GVHD. (*a*) Irregular leukoderma hyperpigmentation tightness and scarring alopecia.

interstitial deposition of hyaline material. The latter stains only lightly with trichrome and not with PAS, acid mucopolysaccharide, or for amyloid.

### Clinical features of late phase

The cardinal features of the late phase are poikiloderma with reticulated telangiectasia (Fig. 25) with uneven, bronzed hyperpigmentation, and white, focally depressed scars. The dermis becomes inelastic and hidebound to the underlying fascial structures (Fig. 26). The loss of subcutaneous fat produces taut, parchment-like skin and facies with a beaked nose and protrusion of other bony prominences (Fig. 27). Some patients develop ulcerations in or loss of soft tissues of ears and digits. Frequently contractures form about knees and elbows, mouth and soft tissue, resulting in a loss of mobility. With the advent of immunosuppressive therapy, diffuse sclerodermatous-like changes and extreme contractures are uncommon. Instead, there is variable dermal atrophy and/or scarring with telangiectasis, pigmentary change, or prolonged erythema (Figs. 28 and 29).

### Histopathology of late sclerotic phase

Histologic changes which indicate progression from the early to the late phase are reversion of the epidermis from an acanthotic to an atrophic state, and progressive sclerosis of the deep dermis (Fig. 30a). The atrophic epidermis has relative hyperkeratosis and flattened keratinocytes. Rete ridges are blunted to absent. The dermal–epidermal junction is straightened, the basement zone is thickened (Fig. 30b), and the basal layer may have vacuolar degeneration. Inflammation or eosinophilic body formation is minimal to absent.

The initial fibrotic changes in the reticular dermis are a coarsening and crowding of the bundles which are straightened, elongated, and eosinophilic—changes referred to as "interstitial hyperplasia."[522] Fibrosis extends along the adnexal structures and then involves the entire reticular dermis (Fig. 30c). Most of the fibrosis occurs by diffuse replacement with dense, birefringement, nonwoven bands of collagen (substitutive hyperplasia) (Fig. 31a). Elastin stains reveal some coalescence of large fibers deep in the dermis and the destruction of smaller fibers in the papillary

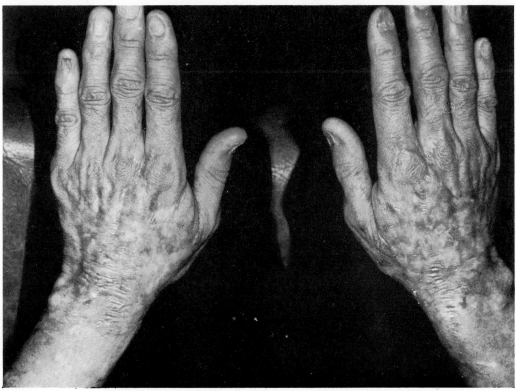

**Figure 26b.** Dorsum of hands with scarring, loss of mobility, and loss of nails.

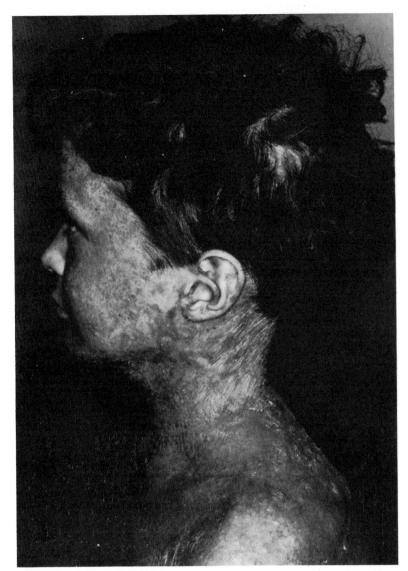

**Figure 27.**   (UPN 717 Day 381) Late generalized chronic GVHD with hyperpigmented, taut, atrophic skin.

zone. Eventually, both the reticular and papillary dermis are homogenized, and the subcutis may become organized and fibrotic. Within the expanded reticular dermis are entrapped nerves and arteries previously located within the subcutaneous fat. Fibrosis and thickened fibrous septa develop in the subcutaneous fat (Fig. 31*b*). Fibroses and thickened fibrous septa may also develop in the subcutaneous fat (Fig. 32). In long-standing chronic GVHD, histologic evaluation of activity is difficult because inflammation is only sparse or absent around the epidermis and

blood vessels. Basilar vacuolar degeneration or rare eosinophilic bodies, even in the absence of inflammation, are considered signs of active chronic GVHD.

### Localized chronic cutaneous GVHD

In 15–20% of patients with chronic cutaneous GVHD, lesions have a striking resemblance to localized scleroderma. Localized lesions of chronic GVHD have several appearances. At first, individual guttate lesions (clusters of small 0.5-to 2.0-cm deep pigmented patches) may ap-

The gross and histologic appearance usually distinguish localized from generalized chronic cutaneous GVHD. The localized type lacks erythema or papulosquamous plaques, and usually spares the nails and mouth. Widespread contractures are unusual and intervening areas of skin are grossly and histologically normal. Unfortunately, there are patients with chronic cutaneous GVHD in whom the clinical separation between the two types is more difficult. Such patients often have more widespread guttate lesions. Others have discoid or linear lesions as well as involvement of the nails and mucous membranes. The course of such patients is usually the more benign one of limited chronic GVHD. Some patients with generalized type

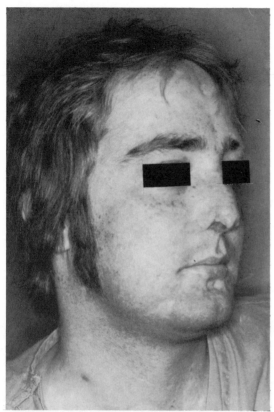

**Figure 28.** (UPN 863) After 2 years of immunosuppressive treatment for chronic GVHD, the cutaneous disease is static. Despite scarring and dyspigmentation, there is no induration or fixation. The esophageal and liver GVHD remain active, however.

pear as depressed hypopigmented areas up to a few centimeters in size and resemble lichen sclerosis et atrophicus or morphea. These clusters can spread out or coalesce to involve a large region, such as the back or abdomen (Fig. 33). The large depressions are surfaced by a thin and scaly epidermis, are first usually pigmented, and later depigmented. Geographic lesions may form firm, immobile bands whose distribution corresponds to tight undergarments (Fig. 34), while sun exposure seems to have little influence. The natural history of localized chronic cutaneous GVHD is usually that of an indolent or self-limiting process. Over a period of many months, the lesions soften and dyspigmentation lessens. At the same time, new crops of lesions may arise elsewhere. Localized chronic GVHD occurring by itself or in combination with only liver GVHD is considered to be limited chronic GVHD, usually not requiring immunosuppressive therapy.

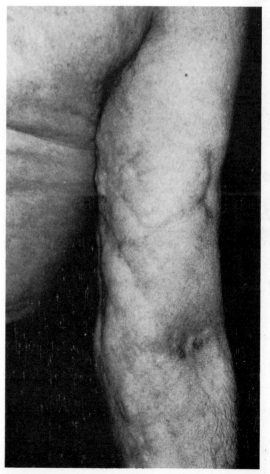

**Figure 29.** (UPN 734) A flare after 3 years of immunosuppressive therapy for chronic GVHD resulted in irregular dimpling, nodular scarring, and hyperpigmentation resembling eosinophilic fasciitis.

chronic cutaneous GVHD, who flare after withdrawal of immunosuppressive therapy, may also develop regional recurrences which resemble localized chronic GVHD.

## Pathology of localized chronic GVHD

The hallmark of this type is remodeling of dermal collagen. This begins within the reticular dermis with foci of broad, smudgy collagen replacing the normal pattern of curlicue woven bundles (Figs. 35*a* and *b*). Lymphoplasmacytic inflammation about eccrine coils, vessels, and pilar units is mild or absent. The epidermis has only an occasional eosinophilic body or vacuolar degeneration but lacks a lichenoid reaction. Because of the deep-seated and focal nature of early localized chronic GVHD, there is often a discrepancy between obvious gross lesions and the histopathology. This is particularly true when small, shallow

punch biopsies are obtained. Older lesions, greater than 1 year in duration, have diffuse dermal fibrosis (Fig. 36) which may involve the septa between lobules of the subcutaneous fat and the interstitium of cutaneous nerves. We have not seen fibrous extension into the underlying muscles, although this has not been thoroughly studied. Nor have we ever seen tissue eosinophilia, even though the gross and histologic appearance of some lesions might suggest the diagnosis of eosinophilic fasciitis, a condition which is probably part of the spectrum of morphea profundis.[651]

## Differential diagnosis

From the foregoing description, it is evident that comparison of chronic GVHD to other dermatological entities is dependent on the size, site, age of lesion, and type of chronic cutaneous GVHD.

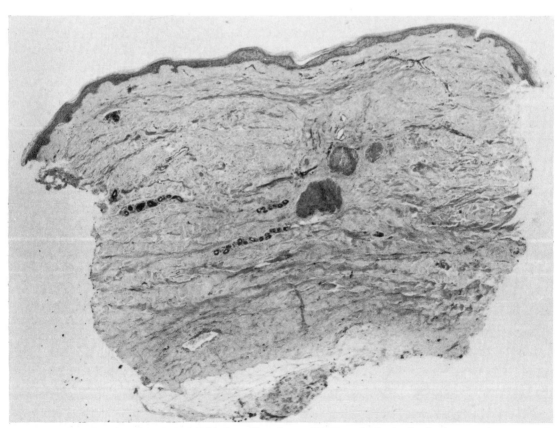

**Figures 30a, b, and c.** (UPN 734 Day 1503) (*a*) Flare of late chronic GVHD resulted in localized tightness on lower extremities. The histology has been modified by prolonged immunosuppressive therapy. The reticular dermis is widened beneath the entrapped eccrine coils. There is some hypertrophy and straightening of collagen bundles and the dermal subcutaneous interface is straightened.

Saurat[557,561] and Touraine[680] first called attention to the gross and histologic similarities of early generalized chronic GVHD to lichen planus. Though we find little difference between the epidermal changes of generalized early chronic GVHD and those epidermal changes showing the evolution of lichen planus lesions as described by Ragaz and Ackerman,[516] the term "lichen planus-like GVHD" is not always histologically appropriate. The histologic term "lichenoid" can be applied to most types and stages of cutaneous GVHD. Furthermore, some biopsies have epidermal changes of atrophy, vacuolar degeneration, spotty inflammation, and thickening of the basement membrane zone with positive direct immunofluorescence for IgM and C'3. In addition, the full-thickness skin biopsy of the lichen planus-like lesion usually discloses syringitis and sometimes panniculitis. Such features are more similar to hypertrophic lupus erythematosus or generalized morphea. The histologic differences between GVHD and these other entities are of degree rather than kind. For example, the panniculitis of GVHD is less than that of

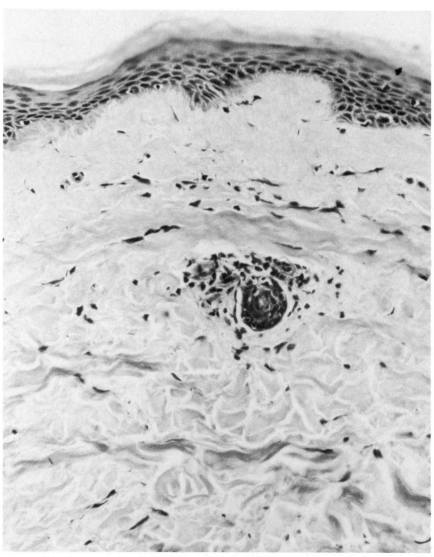

**Figure 30***b.* The atrophic epidermis rests on a thickened basement zone and sclerotic papillary dermis. A damaged sweat duct in the upper dermis is infiltrated by lymphocytes. (PAS).

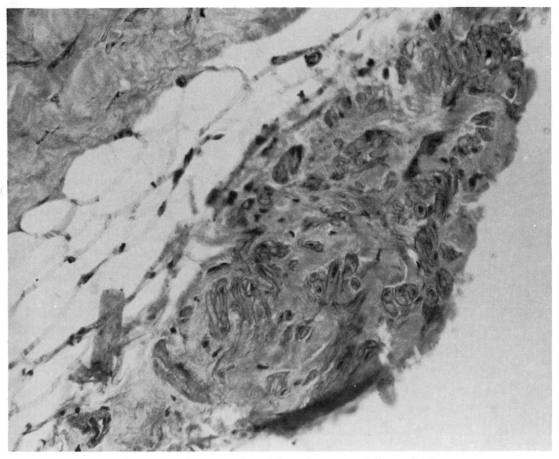

**Figure 30c.**  The nerve at base of dermis has interstitial fibrosis. (PAS).

lupus, while the lichenoid reaction and acanthosis are greater in chronic GVHD. If only the upper half of the dermis were examined, the widened and fibrotic papillary dermis beneath the atrophic epidermis of late-stage generalized chronic GVHD would resemble lichen sclerosis et atrophicus. Both the early and late stages of localized chronic GVHD have few differences from scleroderma.

**Pathogenesis of chronic GVHD**

As discussed in Chapter 4 by Tsoi, there is evidence that the humoral immune system may be involved with the pathogenesis of chronic GVHD. In particular, patients with generalized chronic GVHD showed deposits of IgM and C'3 along the dermal–epidermal junction. Since these deposits may actually precede the development of active skin GVHD, they may be involved in the pathogenesis.[654] The electron

microscopic studies of Gallucci, Grogan, Janin-Mercier, and Woodruff[229,269,313,760] noted that the lymphoid cells infiltrating the epidermis were in close contact with the membranes of keratinocytes and occasionally melanocytes and Langerhans' cells (Fig. 21). The lymphoid cells had zones of broad contact as well as elongated lymphoid cytoplasmic projections which involved small areas of membrane apposition (point contact) (Fig. 37). Although no breaks in the glycocalyx of the epidermal cells were observed on serial sections, we presume that this point contact represents a lymphocytotoxic effector mechanism. The damaged epidermal cells at first undergo cytoplasmic and nuclear swelling before undergoing condensation when they are seen as eosinophilic bodies. Desmosomal attachments are stretched and appear to be lying free in the intercellular space surrounded by lymphoid processes (Fig. 38). This is unlike pemphigus vul-

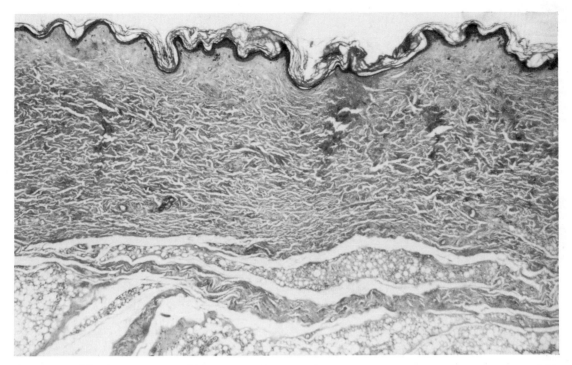

**Figures 31a and b.** (UPN 394 Day 350) (a) Late stage of generalized chronic cutaneous GVHD. Epidermis is now atrophic; both papillary and reticular dermal collagen are becoming sclerotic. The subjacent subcutaneous fat is undergoing fibrous replacement with incorporation into the dermis.

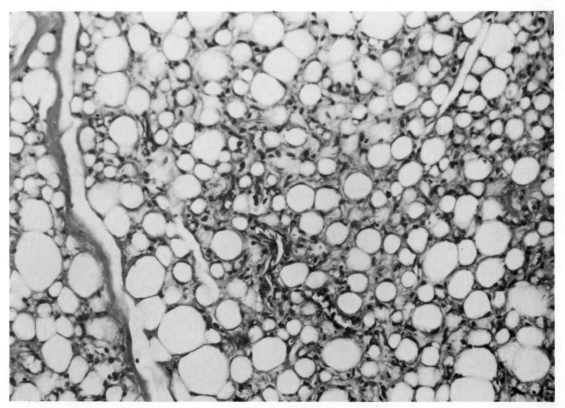

**Figure 31b.** High-power view of subcutaneous fat with involution of adipocytes, increased interstitial ground substance, and mild perivascular inflammation. The inflammation in the fat is much less prominent than in the panniculitis of lupus profundus.

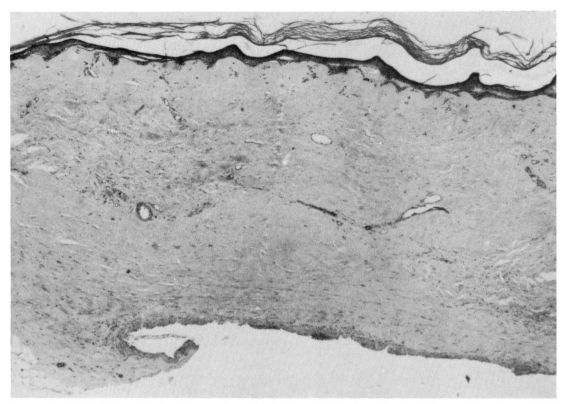

**Figure 32.** (UPN 274 Day 946) Late changes of generalized chronic GVHD. Beneath the atrophic epidermis is a markedly homogenized dermis devoid of appendages. Note that the lower third is actually incorporated fibrotic subcutaneous fat containing a large artery. The dermis was hidebound to the fascia with little or no intervening subcutaneous fat (PAS).

garis, another blistering disease in which there may be antibody-mediated acantholysis of desmosomes.

The similarity of chronic GVHD to scleroderma and other autoimmune disorders was first noted by Stastny et al.[615] in their murine model of chronic GVHD. More recently, Rappaport,[519] Beschorner,[54,55] and Atkinson,[23] have found several additional ways to produce radiation chimeric models of chronic GVHD rodents and dogs (Chapter 3). In these animals, as in humans, the skin changes of epidermal and periappendageal inflammation and panniculitis later evolve to dense dermal sclerosis resembling scleroderma. Fleishmajer[214] emphasized that initiating events of scleroderma occur in the early stages when mononuclear inflammatory cells surround vessels and eccrine coils in the reticular dermis and subcutaneous fat. These early lesions show injured endothelial cells and embryonic collagen fibrils in the areas of increased interstitial matrix lying in the reticular dermis and subcutaneous fat.[212,213]

At least two theories have been proposed as explanations for the fibrosis of scleroderma. One theory suggests that the primary event is related to vascular injury. This results in intimal hyperplasia and adventitial fibrosis, producing the characteristic concentric fibrointimal proliferation, narrowing or arterial lumina, and tissue ischemia with ensuing fibrosis.[92,533] Kahaleh et al.[331] have found a serum factor cytotoxic for endothelial cells in patients with scleroderma. It is of interest that Moraes and Stastny[446] and Paul et al.[493] have also found an alloantigen that resides on endothelium and monocytes but not on lymphocytes. This alloantigen may be involved in some instances of renal allograft rejection. Such alloantigens on endothelial cells could also serve as a minor antigenic target of chronic GVHD. In our electron-micrographic studies of the skin with chronic GVHD,[229] we found some

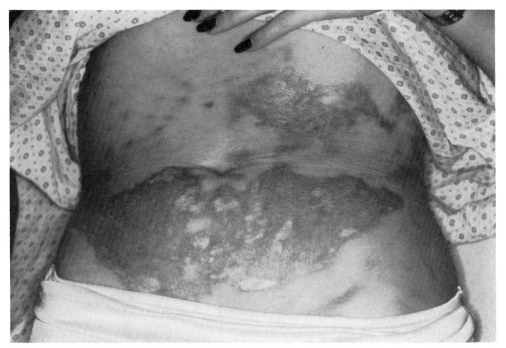

**Figure 33.** (UPN 684) Local chronic cutaneous GVHD with large geographic and smaller guttate lesions. The atrophic skin is indurated.

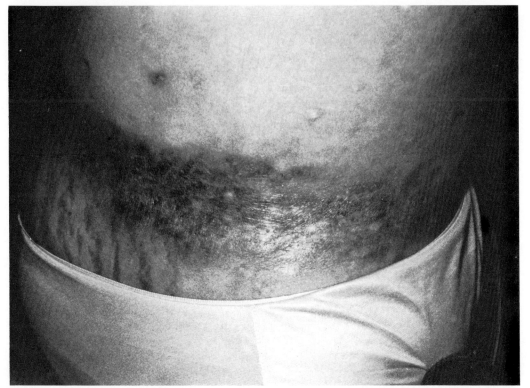

**Figure 34.** (UPN 963) Localized chronic cutaneous GVHD lesions 24 months following transplantation. Broad hyperpigmented contraction band has developed along the site of pressure from waistband of underpants. There are also smaller morpheic lesions and a similar contraction band beneath the brassiere line (not shown).

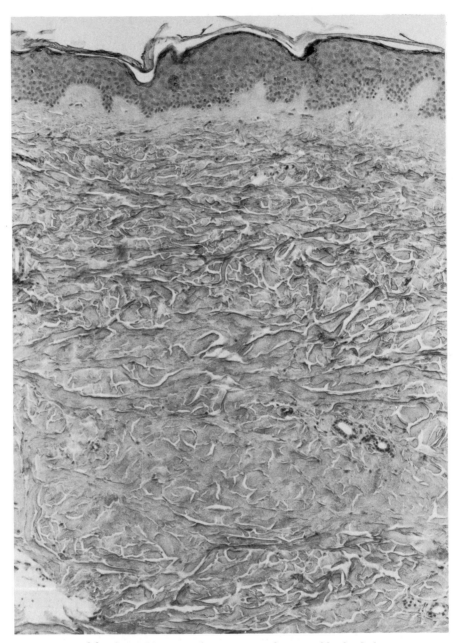

**Figures 35a and b.** (UPN 759 Day 435) Two separate biopsies of localized chronic cutaneous GVHD. (a) Within the reticular dermis is a nodular area composed of smudgy, crowded, and hyalinized collagen bundles. The upper dermis and epidermis are relatively unremarkable.

capillaries with replicated basal lamina. These findings, however, do not indicate the cause for this injury. For example, we have found concentric and eccentric arterial intimal sclerosis in many organs, not only from autopsies of patients dying with chronic GVHD, but also in those patients who have received intensive chemoradiation conditioning therapy and who have no chronic GVHD.

The second explanation for the fibrosis in scleroderma and, by analogy, in chronic GVHD, may be from a selection process favoring the growth of high-collagen-producing dermal fibroblasts.[76] The selection process may be initiated by potent biological effects of cytokines released by dermal inflammatory cells and their interaction with connective tissue cells in the dermis. Johnson and Ziff[322] found that the supernatant from PHA-stimulated lymphocytes killed some embryonic lung fibroblasts, while others were stimulated to produce increased amounts of collagen. From their studies, the authors generated the hypothesis that the dermal remodeling and fibrosis in progressive systemic sclerosis may be secondary to locally produced lymphokines from the lymphoplasmacytic infiltrates surrounding dermal eccrine units. In similar studies in the guinea pig, Wahl et al.[728] described activation of fibroblast proliferation and collagen production by lymphokines produced by T-dependent lymphocytes after a challenge with a specific antigen.

Kondo et al.[355] reported that lymphocytes in patients with progressive systemic sclerosis, but not in normal individuals, responded to extracts of normal and sclerodermatous skin in a macrophage migration inhibition test. They also found that most lymphocytes in the skin infiltrates of diffuse scleroderma were T-lymphocytes. Their findings suggested that lymphocytes sensitized to skin extracts were present in patients with diffuse scleroderma and that an immunologically mediated reaction to the skin may be a factor in the pathogenesis of diffuse scleroderma. Macrophages also produce factors which

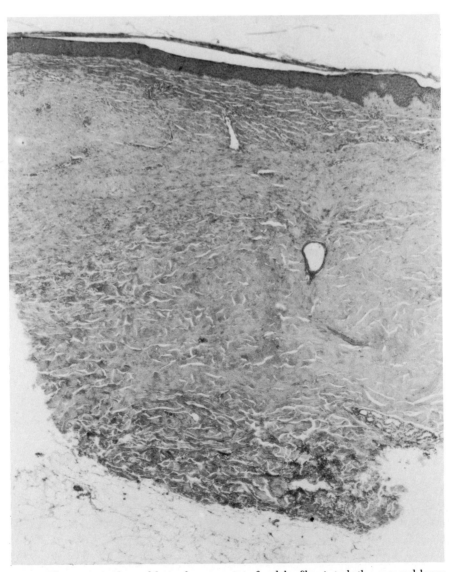

**Figure 35b.** A more advanced lesion has expansion of nodular fibrosis to both upper and lower reticular dermis as well as papillary dermis. The overlying epidermis now has loss of rete ridges.

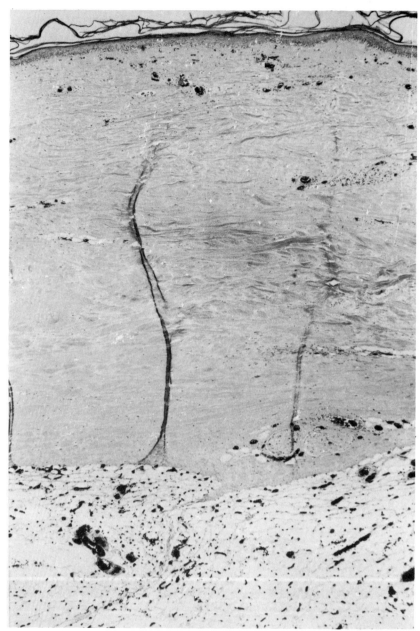

**Figure 36.** (UPN 366 Day 719) Late stage of localized chronic GVHD which resembles late generalized chronic GVHD. The expanded dermis shows homogenization and straightening of dermal collagen bundles and entrapped subcutaneous nerves near the straightened lower margin.

stimulate proliferation of fibroblasts *in vitro*.[355]

However, the effects of cytokines on fibroblasts are variable. Specifically, other studies have suggested that during the development of the inflammatory response, mononuclear cells and lymphocyte supernatant first stimulate fibroblast proliferation and collagen synthesis, and later cause inhibition.[318,358,463] Cytokines can also influence the local synthesis of prostaglandins by fibroblasts.[357] Prostaglandins can produce selective growth effects by either stimulatory or inhibitory action on protein synthesis. An additional factor which might modulate the production of cytokines and hence, fibroplasia, may be the patient's immunogenetic makeup. During the physiological degradation of collagen, indi-

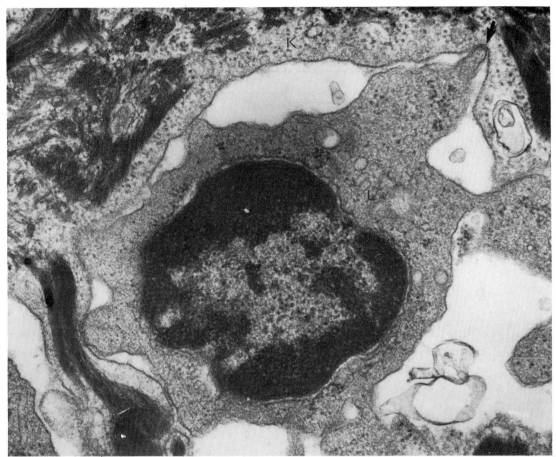

**Figure 37.** (UPN 512 Day 210) Early generalized chronic cutaneous GVHD. The glycocalyces of an intraepidermal lymphocyte (L) and keratinocyte (K) meet at the apex of an elongated lymphoid projection (arrow). (×42,000.) (From Gallucci et al.[229]; reproduced with permission.)

viduals are exposed to the (glycine–proline) determinants normally buried within the interstices of the triple helix of collagen. Those individuals with the HLA-DR4+ phenotype have T-cell-dependent reactivity to collagen. This expression of T-cell-dependent reactivity to collagen reflects the net balance of collagen reactivity versus collagen suppressor cells. As a result, in HLA-DR4+ individuals, collagen-specific suppressor cells are not generated, their activity is actively suppressed, or reactive cells are resistant to the effect of suppressor cells.[602,603]

Previous studies of qualitative and quantitative changes in the collagen produced by dermal fibroblasts in scleroderma have yielded discrepant results.[67,82,83,364,703] It should be remembered that these studies may be influenced by the culture conditions,[97] age of the lesions,[215,216] and the source of fibroblasts in the dermis: upper or lower dermis or whole dermis. Our own investigations of collagen production by dermal fibroblasts from several patients with chronic GVHD (Narayanan and Shulman, unpublished data) reflect this variability. Total synthesized collagen *in vitro* was measured by the incorporation of radiolabeled glycine and proline in fibroblasts obtained from full-thickness biopsies of dermis. Fibroblasts from one patient with untreated, late generalized chronic GVHD synthesized twice the amount of collagen as did his donor's fibroblasts. In addition, the ratio of the alpha-1 to alpha-2 chains in the patient was greater than 2:1, as is found in inflammatory states. Another patient with early generalized chronic GVHD had no abnormalities. Fibroblasts from a third patients with localized chronic GVHD would not

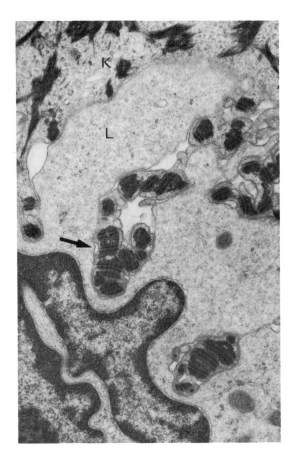

**Figure 38.** (UPN 262 Day 339) Early generalized chronic cutaneous GVHD. Keratinocyte (K) desmosomes (arrow) appear to be "pinched off" and surrounded by a lymphocyte (L). (×140,000.) (From Gallucci et al.[229]; reproduced with permission.)

grow on repeated passage. It is quite possible that the mechanisms of dermal fibrosis in generalized chronic GVHD, in which inflammation is more marked, may be quite different from those of localized GVHD, in which fibrosis occurs early, often in the absence of inflammation.

From the above discussion, it is evident that complex and sensitive mechanisms control the balance between stimulation and inhibition of fibroblast proliferation and collagen synthesis and degradation. Perhaps future studies may show whether in chronic GVHD these mechanisms are disturbed by altered lymphocyte function, or are merely appropriate responses to prolonged chronic inflammation.

# Chapter 6

# The human gastrointestinal tract after allogeneic marrow transplantation

George B. McDonald, M.D.
George E. Sale, M.D.

## Introduction

Few patients undergo allogeneic marrow transplantation without intestinal complications. The conditioning therapy used to prepare patients for transplantation causes mucosal damage; the intestine is a target organ in acute graft-vs.-host disease (GVHD); intestinal infections occur during prolonged immunosuppression; and the esophagus is a target organ in chronic GVHD. The clinical and histologic characteristics of these complications have been studied in the last few years but the major problems of differential diagnosis (usually GVHD vs. infection), pathogenesis, and therapy remain.

In this chapter, the intestinal disorders seen after marrow transplantation will be reviewed, using the term "GVHD" to describe a clinical syndrome found in humans. This field is confusing because of the inability to separate clearly the effects of lymphoid-mediated cell destruction, immunodeficiency, and infectious processes. Nonetheless, studies in human marrow graft recipients provide insight into the pathophysiology of intestinal disease after transplantation.

## EFFECTS OF RADIOCHEMOTHERAPY ON THE INTESTINE

Conditioning therapy preparatory to marrow grafting varies with the disease being treated. A cytotoxic drug such as cyclophosphamide (CY) is used alone prior to transplantation for aplasia to prevent rejection of the marrow graft by the host.[642,669] Chemotherapy with total body irradiation (TBI) is given to patients with leukemia since malignant cells must be eradicated.[669] Doses of TBI given as conditioning therapy are significantly lower than those given as primary radiation therapy for cancer, and alone would have only minor intestinal effects.[48] However, the threshold for intestinal damage by radiotherapy seems to be lowered by concomitant chemotherapy. Higher-dose conditioning therapy can produce fatal intestinal and liver necrosis,[583] but in most cases the intestinal damage is self-limited.[192]

The clinical symptoms resulting from conditioning therapy with CY and TBI (1000–1600 rad) are crampy abdominal pain and watery diarrhea. These symptoms generally subside within 10 days of conditioning therapy, but some patients persist in their symptoms for 3 weeks. The diarrhea is watery and may contain occult blood but is rarely grossly bloody. Protein loss is minimal.

We prospectively studied rectal histology in 13 patients undergoing marrow transplantation.[192] In contrast to normal rectal mucosal histology prior to conditioning, all 13 biopsies taken 7–10 days after CY and TBI conditioning were dif-

fusely abnormal. Crypt nuclear atypia was seen in all 13, flattened crypt epithelium in 10, abnormal surface epithelium in nine, and crypt cell degeneration in five. These changes persisted in some rectal biopsies taken 16–20 days after conditioning, but all biopsies taken after day 20 were normal unless GVHD had supervened (Fig. 1).[192] These microscopic changes in colonic mucosa are almost identical to those seen in the

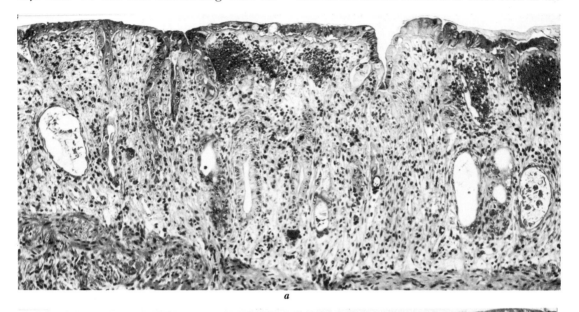

*a*

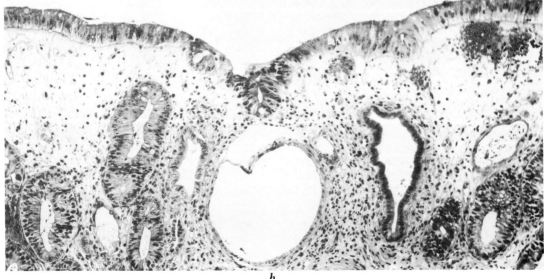

*b*

**Figures 1a, b and c.**   The effects of conditioning chemoradiation therapy on one patient's rectal mucosa are illustrated in these photomicrographs. Conditioning therapy consisted of CY, hydroxyurea, dimethylbusulfan, and TBI. Allogeneic marrow transplantation was done on day 0. (*a*) Day 7 biopsy showing diffuse destruction of crypts, resulting in crypt remnants with a cystic appearance, crypt dropout, and nuclear atypia throughout the mucosa. The surface epithelium has become cuboidal in appearance with loss of mucus. (*b*) Day 16 biopsy showing partial return of crypt epithelium. Distorted, cystic crypts remain in parts of this biopsy, but in others there has been regeneration. The surface epithelium is more normal, but devoid of mucus.

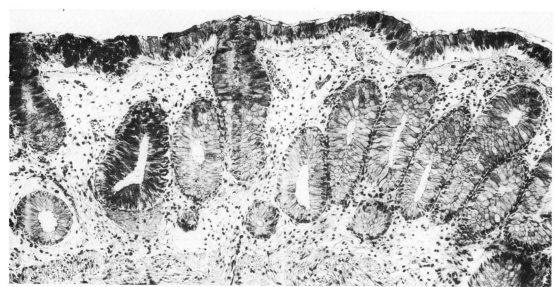

**Figure 1c.** Day 34 biopsy showing repopulation of epithelium with more normal-appearing crypts. Cystic crypts are absent and mucus has returned to both crypts and surface epithelium.

colon after higher-dose radiotherapy (Fig. 2).[48,744] We assume that the concomitant use of CY with TBI has increased the sensitivity of colonic mucosa to this dose of radiation.

The small intestinal mucosa is diffusely abnormal in marrow graft recipients who die before day 20 after transplantation. In an autopsy study, there were fewer crypt mitoses, nuclear atypia, and moderate abnormalities of villous architecture, all presumably due to the conditioning therapy.[53] This is not surprising since the mucosa of the small intestine is the most radio-sensitive part of the bowel due to its rapid mucosal replacement (normally 3–6 days).[48] After single doses of radiation, the mucosa returns to normal within 2–3 weeks, the same time required for resolution of conditioning effects on rectal mucosa and skin.[186,545] Prostaglandins may be involved in the genesis of intestinal injury from radiation as prostaglandin-synthesis inhibitors lessen intestinal damage.[429]

The stomach and esophagus are probably more resistant to conditioning therapy, but this has not been prospectively evaluated. The effects of radiation on the stomach have been well studied because this modality has been used widely to diminish acid secretion. With doses of 1500–2000 rad delivered to the stomach, there is necrosis of parietal and chief cells.[48] The esophagus responds to high-dose radiation by developing sub-mucosal edema and basal necrosis, an injury

pattern which also appears to be mediated by prostaglandins.[473] Chemotherapy reduces the tolerance to radiation in the esophagus,[265,469] but the effects of conditioning chemoradio-therapy and the time required for resolution are unknown.

Knowledge of the histology of the intestine after conditioning therapy is important in interpreting mucosal biopsies in the first 3 weeks after marrow transplantation. The effects of viral infection and GVHD may not be distinctive when they are superimposed on a conditioning effect. Furthermore, radiation and cytotoxic drugs used singly can produce vascular, neural, and smooth-muscle changes on a delayed basis, and it is possible that many of the changes we attribute to chronic GVHD could be a residual of conditioning therapy. This seems unlikely because of the absence of vascular changes in long-term marrow graft recipients who do not develop chronic GVHD, but the possibility deserves closer scrutiny.

### ACUTE GVHD OF THE INTESTINE

About 30–50% of allogeneic matched marrow recipients will develop intestinal GVHD.[738] Some will have only nausea, others will have water diarrhea, and others will have total intestinal denudation with cholera-like diarrhea and intestinal bleeding. The intestinal epithelium is a major target organ in GVHD, but the pathogenesis of enterocyte damage in this disease is not well understood. The comments which follow are based on published and personal experience with GVHD of the intestine in humans. A large literature about graft-vs.-host reaction (GVHR) in rodents, dogs, and nonhuman primates cannot be directly applied to humans because of species and transplantation-protocol differences, but does provide information about GVHR in those species. Similarly, experiments with intestinal allografts may not be analogous to GVHD in humans.

## Clinical features

The typical patient with intestinal GVHD has a red, macular rash involving the trunk, palms, and soles, and complains of watery diarrhea and lower abdominal cramping.[245,669,738] Some pa-

tients have intestinal GVHD without obvious skin or liver involvement.[192,577] Liver GVHD usually accompanies skin and gut GVHD and manifests itself by rising levels of serum alkaline phosphatase and bilirubin. Occasionally, anorexia, nausea, and vomiting are the presenting symptoms of GVHD, but unless an ileus is present, diarrhea will appear eventually. The abdominal pain is moderate in severity and worsens after meals and before diarrheal bowel movements. Intestinal ileus may occur, either spontaneously or coincident with opiate or anticholinergic drug use. Some patients have severe abdominal pain with peritoneal signs on abdominal examination, probably due to edema of the bowel wall (see below: *Radiologic and Endoscopic Appearance*). A patient with severe abdominal pain, ileus, and peritoneal signs on examination could have bacterial or fungal per-

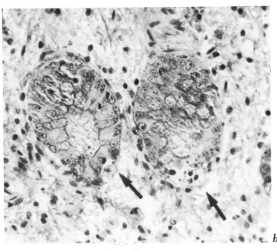
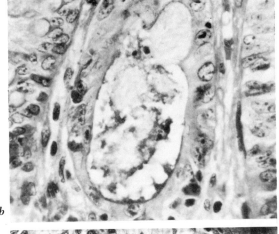

*a*

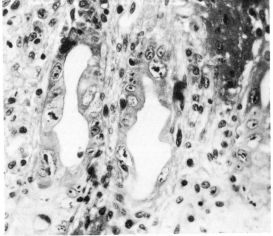

*b*

**Figures 2a, b, and c.** High-power photomicrographs illustrating chemoradiation therapy effects on rectal mucosa. (*a*) Day 6 biopsy after conditioning with CY and TBI, showing crypt cell degeneration and membrane-bound cell debris (apoptosis). (*b*) Day 14 biopsy after conditioning with CY and TBI, showing dilated crypt with flattened epithelium enveloping mucous and cellular debris. (*c*) Day 7 biopsy after conditioning with CY hydroxyurea, dimethylbusulfan, and TBI, showing nuclear atypia, enlarged nucleoli, flattened cells, and an increased mitotic rate. (Reprinted by permission of the publisher from the diagnostic accuracy of the rectal biopsy in acute graft-versus-host disease, by Epstein et al., *Gastroenterology, 78:764–771.* Copyright 1980 by The American Gastroenterological Association.)

*c*

itonitis due to bowel perforation, but this picture is also consistent with severe GVHD alone. The diarrhea is watery, usually contains occult blood, and varies in quantity from 200 ml to 15 l/day. Rarely, gross rectal bleeding occurs along with the watery diarrhea with a transfusion requirement of 1–5 units per day. Such bleeding may be from diffuse mucosal oozing in patients with low platelets, or from discrete ulcers in the intestine due to infection or stress.

Laboratory studies show leukocytes in the stool, but no fungal elements, parasites, or bacterial/viral pathogens are recovered unless there is an intestinal superinfection. Serum albumin levels can plummet from normal to 1–2 mg/dl due to intestinal protein loss which can be demonstrated by chromium[51] or alpha-1-antitrypsin studies.[127,245,745] Diarrheal stools are often a greenish color with large amounts of mucus, often passed along with cellular debris as long, ropy strands.

### Radiologic and endoscopic appearance

Radiologic studies of acute GVHD demonstrate mucosal and submucosal edema throughout the intestine.[211,537,564,580] When barium contrast x-rays are done in the acute phase of intestinal GVHD, the gastric folds are enlarged, small bowel folds are flattened, the bowel wall is thickened (often with a thumbprint pattern), and there is excessive luminal fluid (Fig. 3).[211] Transit of barium is rapid. Barium enema examination can demonstrate mucosal ulceration, loss of haustral folds, and mural thickening during the acute phase.[211,537,580] X-rays taken later (up to 12 weeks after the onset of intestinal GVHD) may show a ribbon-like appearance of the middle and distal small bowel with total effacement of folds (Fig. 4). However, when diarrhea and cramping resolve, the x-ray appearance returns to normal.

The acute phase changes are relatively nonspecific; similar changes are seen with cytomegalovirus (CMV) enteritis, Henoch-Schonlein purpura, acute radiation enteritis, and any condition which causes bowel-wall edema.[237,534,699] However, x-ray studies are quite useful in demonstrating that the intestine is the cause of abdominal symptoms and in suggesting a diagnosis of GVHD. A diffusely abnormal small intestine x-ray allows a confident diagnosis of GVHD when there is biopsy-proven GVHD of the skin and no

pathogens on stool examination. Small bowel and even rectal biopsies are dangerous in patients with low leukocyte and platelet counts, but a classic radiograph will often suffice. In contrast to the acute phase x-rays, however, the ribbon-like pattern of long-established intestinal GVHD is diagnostic in the marrow transplant setting (Figs. 4 and 5).[211]

Endoscopy of the upper intestine can be useful if there is widespread involvement with GVHD, but is more often done to rule out infections or peptic ulcer as a cause of pain, vomiting, or bleeding. With GVHD, the duodenal folds may be edematous and friable, and serpiginous areas of mucosal sloughing can be seen. Gastric mucosa is usually grossly normal at endoscopy, but isolated lesions of GVHD can be seen on biopsy. Sigmoidoscopy usually shows normal rectal mucosa even when biopsies are diagnostic of GVHD; occasionally, widespread GVHD produces an edematous, friable rectal mucosa. As in primate GVHD, widespread ileal and right-sided colonic changes are more severe in human GVHD but microscopic changes occur in both the proximal intestine and rectum.[547] For these reasons, biopsies of normal-appearing stomach, duodenum, and rectal mucosa may provide a diagnosis of GVHD when ileal tissue is inaccessible to biopsy.[186]

### Histology

Although the end stage of GVHD is total mucosal denudation (Fig. 5), an early stage of single mucosal cell destruction can be recognized by light microscopy. The sequence of events from individual cell necrosis to denudation is poorly understood.

*Colonic mucosa.* Rectal biopsies correlate well with mucosal damage in the cecum and ileum in GVHD and are useful in making a diagnosis in patients with unexplained diarrhea, abdominal pain, or nausea.[186,547] The earliest recognizable change of GVHD is that of individual crypt cell necrosis, which can be an extremely focal finding.[547] Membrane-bound debris from necrotic cells accumulates at the base or side of crypts, giving rise to such terms as "exploding crypt," "apoptotic body," and "karyolytic body" (Fig. 6).[230,379,547,593] This form of crypt cell necrosis is not specific for GVHD since it can be seen with chemoradiation therapy, inflammatory

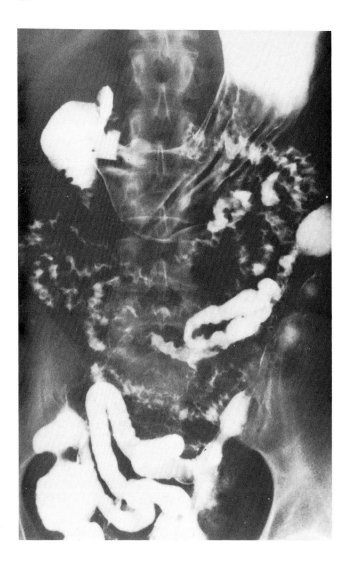

**Figures 3a and b.** Intestinal x-rays early in acute GVHD. (*a*) Barium outlines the stomach and most of the small bowel in this study done after 4 days of crampy abdominal pain, nausea, and diarrhea. There are thickened, nodular folds in the proximal small bowel and a rigid appearance to the ileal loops. (From Fisk et al.[211]; reproduced with permission.)

bowel disease, and infectious colitis.[155,254,484] Unlike the case in these other diseases, however, the crypt degeneration of early GVHD is not accompanied by widespread inflammation or other cell destruction. The location of crypt cell degeneration at the abluminal side of the mucosa, in the absence of bacterial or viral pathogens, suggests an immunologic mechanism for cell destruction.

A prospective study of this histologic feature showed it to be specific for GVHD if biopsies were done after day 20, the time required for resolution of the histologic features of chemoradiation conditioning damage. In the acute, early phase of GVHD, lymphoid cells were not increased in the lamina propria of rectal mucosa,

and the lymphocytes present appeared intact.

In contrast to these isolated lesions in otherwise intact mucosa, the histology of more extensive GVHD shows widespread cell destruction, particularly in the right colon and ileum.[352,547,591,593,708] These changes include cystic dilation of crypts, which often contain debris from lysed crypt cells, crypt abscesses, dropout of whole crypts, and, finally, absence of crypts (Fig. 6). At autopsy of patients with severe GVHD, sheets of bacteria, fungi, and exfoliated debris line the few epithelial cells which remain.[53]

A histologic grading system for intestinal GVHD published in 1979 did not include the finding of individual crypt cell degeneration, but

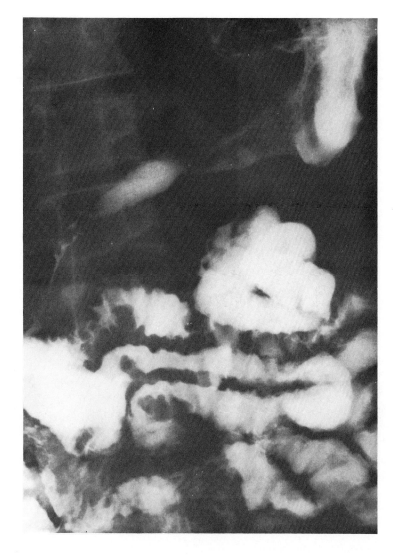

**Figure 3b.** This study was done in another patient after 6 days of vomiting, abdominal pain, and diarrhea. The gastric wall is thickened and nonpliable, and the folds and walls of the duodenum and jejunum are edematous. (From Fisk et al.[211]; reproduced with permission.)

rather, graded the more extensive mucosal damage.[547] A revised histologic grading system for intestinal GVHD is as follows:

Grade I.   Individual crypt cell necrosis
      II.   Crypt abscess, crypt cell flattening, with or without crypt cell degeneration
     III.   Dropout of one or more whole crypts in a biopsy
     IV.   Total denudation of epithelium

We have further simplified the intestinal histology into a "diagnostic" category (grade I change) and "consistent" categories (grades II–IV changes). The finding of extensive necrosis is less specific than the earlier "exploding crypt" lesion since many destructive processes could cause extensive necrosis.[738]

The histology of a rectal biopsy, the volume of diarrhea, the amount of protein lost in stool water, and intestinal x-rays all attest to the severity of a given patient's GVHD. Yet some patients with extensive mucosal destruction may have a primary viral or a toxic (e.g., *C. difficile*) enteritis. To make these diagnoses, we rely on stool microscopy and cultures, serology, toxin assays, and on careful examination of mucosal biopsies for inclusions typical of viral infection. The more common finding, however, is that of intestinal GVHD complicated by a superinfection, due to profound local immunodeficiency. (See below for

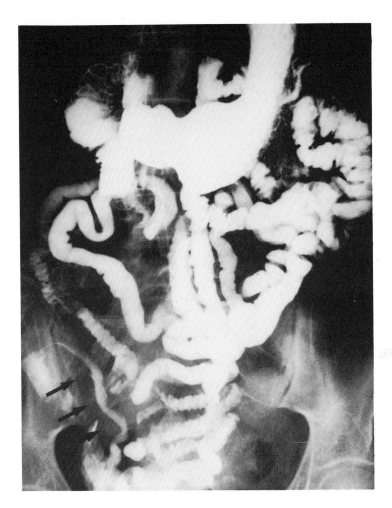

**Figures 4a and b.** Intestinal x-rays later in the course of acute GVHD. (*a*) This study of the stomach and small intestine was done after 15 days of profuse, watery diarrhea. The proximal small intestine is normal; the distal small intestine has thickened folds and walls, with a ribbon-like appearance to the terminal ileum (arrows).

a more complete discussion of infections and local immunodeficiency.)

*Small intestinal mucosa.* Prospective studies of morphologic changes in the small bowel are not available because the jejunum cannot be biopsied safely when platelets are low, and because the ileum cannot be biopsied safely at all. However, valid conclusions can be drawn from postmortem histology in humans and primates, from surgical specimens, and from endoscopic biopsies of the duodenum. On the other hand, models of GVHD in rodents are so dissimilar from the disease in primates that conclusions drawn from animal experiments must be interpreted with caution. Diarrhea is a variable phenomenon in rodent GVHD models and extensive morphologic changes in the small bowel are unusual despite "runting" in those animals.[401,453] In contrast, large-volume watery diarrhea is the *sine qua non* of intestinal GVHD in monkeys and humans.[245,547,708] In rodents, changes in intestinal flora alter the natural history of the GVHR,[122,287,324,707,710,711] whereas intestinal GVHD in humans is largely unaffected by prophylactic ingestion of nonabsorbable antibiotics.[85]

The most extensive small intestinal lesions in GVHD in humans and monkeys are in the ileum (Figs. 4 and 5), but the upper small intestine may show microscopic evidence of GVHD even when gross changes are absent there. Serial sections of properly oriented mucosa may be necessary to demonstrate these "exploding crypt" lesions which can be quite focal (Fig. 7).[192] In monkeys, the earliest lesion is widespread karyorrhexis and crypt cell disintegration, followed by cystic dilation of degenerating crypts.[593,709,760] Later severe changes are loss of surface epithelium and denudation of the entire mucosa. The lamina propria shows infiltration by lymphoid cells

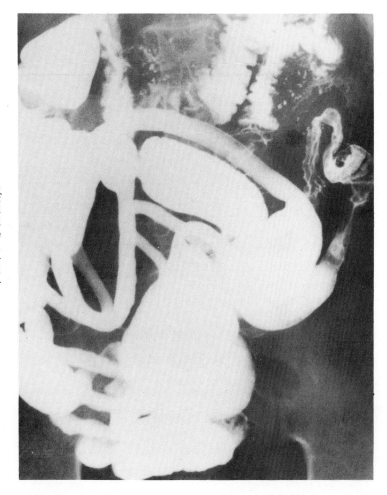

**Figure 4b.** This intestinal x-ray is from a different patient, after 13 days of crampy abdominal pain, nausea, and vomiting. The duodenum and proximal jejunum appear normal but the middle and distal small intestine show narrow, ribbon-like segments of bowel connecting larger, dilated segments. The distal small intestine was resected and is pictured in Figs. 5 and 9.

which migrate into the crypts. These monkey studies, however, include animals that died before day 20 along with those that died later, and thus may confuse chemoradiotherapy and GVHD effects on the mucosa.

Small intestinal morphology in patients with severe, protracted GVHD shows a markedly thickened bowel wall, loss of villus architecture and crypts, fibrotic submucosa, and edematous lamina propria, often with ulcerations deep into the submucosa (Fig. 8).[53,352,547,592,709] Both the lamina propria and smooth muscle can be heavily infiltrated with lymphocytes and plasma cells. With more extensive GVHD, the denuded epithelium may be replaced by a single, cuboidal-cell layer, or the submucosa may be covered by mucus, cell debris, and sheets of organisms (Fig. 9).[53,547] The "exploding crypt" lesions are disproportionately few in patients with such extensive mucosal destruction, leading to the hypothesis

that while crypt cell lysis may be the first lesion, the more extensive damage is related either to a lamina propria lymphoid reaction or to a local immunodeficiency, with bacterial invasion of the mucosa.[53]

*Stomach and esophagus.* Individual epithelial cell necrosis can be seen in stomach and esophagus during acute GVHD but has not been extensively studied (Fig. 10).[592] Esophageal infections due to viruses and fungi are common in the post-transplant period,[419] but the relationship of such infections to epithelial GVHD is unclear. On the other hand, the esophagus may be extensively involved in chronic GVHD.[416]

### Histology—Electron microscopy
The ultrastructure of intestinal GVHD has been described in chimeric monkeys and in humans.[230,592,760] Studies in monkeys demonstrated migration of lymphocytes into the crypts

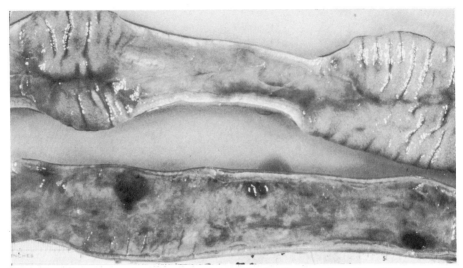

**Figure 5.**    Adjacent segments of ileum, resected shortly after the x-ray above (Fig. 4*b*) because of the development of intestinal bleeding and peritoneal signs. The ribbon-like segments seen on x-ray are devoid of mucosa and have a membrane of cellular debris and bacteria overlying hemorrhagic submucosa. The dilated segments have some preservation of circular folds but the mucosa is grossly abnormal (see Fig. 9).

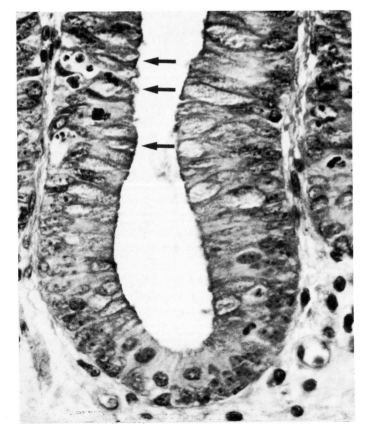

**Figures 6*a*, *b*, *c*, and *d*.**    High-power photomicrographs showing individual crypt cell necrosis (apoptosis) in rectal biopsies from patients with acute GVHD. There is a progression from single-cell necrosis to dropout of individual crypts. (*a*) The lateral wall of a crypt where membrane-bound cellular debris accumulates above the basal lamina at the site of the necrosis of 3 crypt cells (apoptosis). There is no lymphoid infiltration in the vicinity.

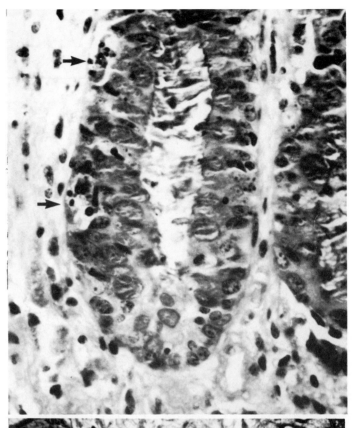

**Figure 6b.** Base of a crypt with several areas of cell necrosis (arrows), a loss of the normal crypt architecture, and extrusion of cell debris and mucus into the crypt lumen.

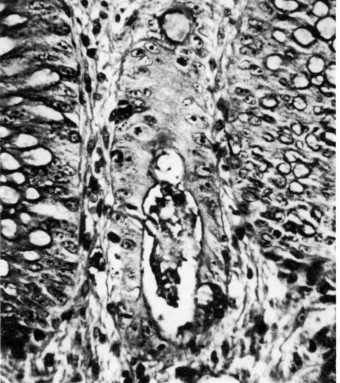

**Figure 6c.** Severely damaged crypt with a cuboidal appearance of remaining cells, nuclear atypia, and luminal debris. Note that adjacent crypts are relatively intact.

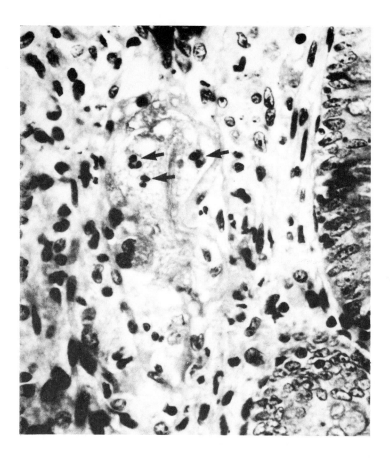

**Figure 6d.** Remnant of a crypt with several apoptotic bodies lying within confines of the former crypt's basal lamina. The adjacent crypt remains relatively preserved.

of both colon and small intestine, with necrosis of lymphocytes and crypt cells, and with sloughing of necrotic cells into the crypt lumen. However, these monkeys were studied during a time when the effects of conditioning therapy on the mucosa were probably still present, that is, within 3 weeks of conditioning. Our studies in humans were controlled since pretransplant and day 9-22 biopsies of rectal mucosa were compared to biopsies taken during acute GVHD. These studies implicate lymphocytes as effectors in the damage to crypt cells in GVHD. Lymphocytes indented the cytoplasmic membranes of crypt cells by point contact and extended broad pseudopods to their nuclear membranes (Fig. 11).[230] Damage to enterocytes resulted in both coagulative necrosis and the development of the characteristic membrane-bound cell fragments ("apoptosis"). These changes are similar to those described with GVHD of the skin and liver.[46,229] Most of the lymphocytes appeared viable, in contrast to the pancellular lymphocyte necrosis seen in monkey GVHD (Fig. 11).[592,760]

In an experimental $F_1$ hybrid murine model of GVHD, similar ultrastructural events were seen. Large lymphocytes passed through the epithelial basement membrane to contact crypt cells which became damaged and accumulated "autophagic vacuoles." Coagulative necrosis occurred when crypt cells were enveloped by pseudopods of "aggressor lymphocytes."[575]

## Intestinal immunodeficiency in GVHD

The intestinal lymphoid system is profoundly affected by allogeneic marrow transplantation, but little is known about the sequence of events leading to reconstitution, or even whether that reconstitution is complete. Older literature describes two processes in animals with GVHD, one involving an "aggressor lymphocyte" destruction of crypt cells, and the second a "lymphoid response."[761] The lymphoid response refers to a sequence of changes in lymph nodes, spleen, and Peyer's patches of the intestine. This sequence consists of early lymphoid proliferation, then lymphoid atrophy, then reconstitu-

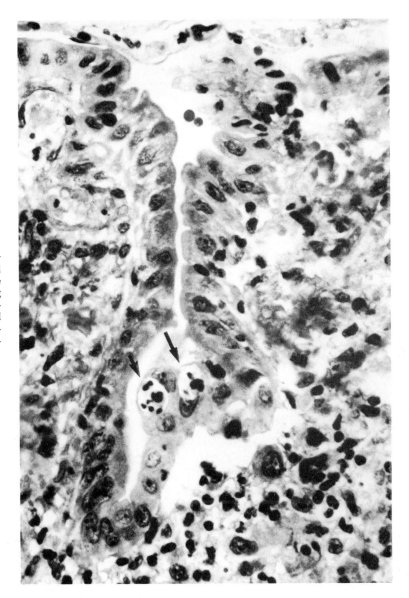

**Figures 7a and b.** High-power photomicrograph of small intestinal mucosa from patients with acute GVHD. (*a*) Jejunal biopsy showing two apoptotic bodies (arrows), abnormal crypt architecture, stunted villi, and abnormal surface epithelium. The lamina propria contains primarily lymphoid cells.

tion.[104,152,761] However, studies in dogs and man do not confirm lymphoid atrophy as a feature of GVHD in these species,[164,352,477] and suggest that conditioning therapy is responsible. A retrospective study of lymphoid populations in man showed that both allogeneic and syngeneic or autologous graft recipients had depletion of lymphocytes in Peyer's patches and mesenteric lymph nodes in the first 130 days after transplantation. In this study, severity of GVHD at autopsy was not related to intestinal lymphoid cellularity. In patients autopsied after day 130, cellularity in follicles and germinal centers of Peyer's patches and in the B- and T-cell regions

of mesenteric lymph nodes was normal.[53] Other studies have found that lymphoid morphology appears nearly normal about 7 months after marrow grafting.[164,352]

In contrast, there are differences in lamina propria plasma cell populations between patients with GVHD and those without GVHD. The former group had a marked depletion of IgA- and IgM-bearing plasma cells.[53] (A similar finding has also been reported in mice with acute GVHD.[249]) Control patients (recipients of syngeneic or autologous grafts) had numerous IgA- and IgM-bearing plasma cells in the intestinal lamina propria.[53] These studies suggest that the

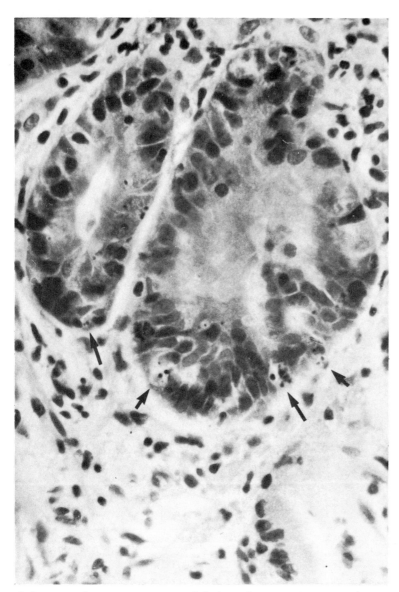

**Figure 7b.** Duodenal biopsy showing adjacent crypts with numerous cells undergoing necrosis (arrows). Brunner's glands deep to the crypts are uninvolved.

deficiency of secretory immunoglobulins plays a role in the mucosal destruction of GVHD by allowing the invasion of luminal organisms. The exact sequence of events cannot be reconstructed from autopsy material, and the relative importance of lymphocyte-mediated destruction versus damage from the lumen is unknown. One prospective study of marrow transplantation for leukemia in a protected environment that included ingestion of nonabsorbable antibiotics showed no differences in the incidence of GVHD between protected and control groups, but the onset of clinical GVHD was delayed in protected patients.[85] The severity of GVHD was the same in both groups. Animal experiments demonstrate

that germ-free marrow graft recipients and those "decontaminated" by ingestion of antibiotics have less severe GVHD.[122,287,325,707,710,711,726] A recent study of marrow transplantation for aplastic anemia showed that a protected environment was associated with a reduction in and a delayed onset of acute GVHD.[645] The interrelationship between the microflora of the intestine and GVHD is discussed in Intestinal Infections after Marrow Transplantation below.

### Abnormalities of intestinal function in acute GVHD

When the entire intestinal mucosa is denuded, it is not difficult to understand why gross malab-

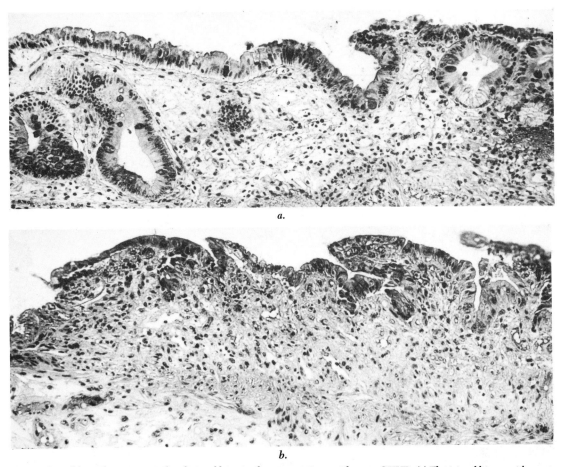

*a.*

*b.*

**Figures 8a and b.** Photomicrographs of jejunal biopsies from two patients with acute GHVD. (a) Flat jejunal biopsy with crypt dropout, distorted remaining crypts, and abnormal surface epithelium. Individual crypt cell necrosis (apoptosis) is not present in this biopsy. Lymphoid infiltration is sparse. (b) Abnormal jejunal biopsy showing blunted villous architecture, absence of crypts, and abnormal surface epithelium.

sorption of water, electrolytes, and nutrients occurs. However, disabling symptoms can occur with intestinal GVHD which is less extensive morphologically.[232]

*Water and electrolyte malabsorption.* Even in the normal fasting state, over 5 liters of fluid are presented to the intestine for reabsorption. This fluid comes from gastric, biliary, pancreatic, and intestinal sources. The normal intestine reabsorbs this endogenous fluid in an efficient manner such that only 1–2 liters of fluid are presented to the colon and less than 200 ml of stool water is excreted. "Absorption" in the intestine is really a net absorption, reflecting the sum of intestinal secretion and absorption. In acute GVHD, the profuse watery diarrhea could result from many lesions. Crypt cell damage alone could lead to massive secretion, and villous damage to dimin-

ished absorption and increased secretion; carbohydrate malabsorption would present an increased luminal osmotic load; ileal damage would lead to diminished retrieval of isotonic saline and bile salts; and colonic damage would lead to malabsorption of the fluid presented by the ileum. The cellular mechanisms of the often profuse watery diarrhea, which occurs without any oral intake in patients with intestinal GVHD, remain unexplored.

*Protein loss.* Hypoalbuminemia is a common occurrence when patients have intestinal GVHD.[245] This is clearly due to protein loss from the intestine, shown by radiolabeled albumin in animals and by stool antitrypsin measurements in humans.[127,745] The losses can be large, and despite parenteral nutrition with amino acids, negative nitrogen balance is the rule

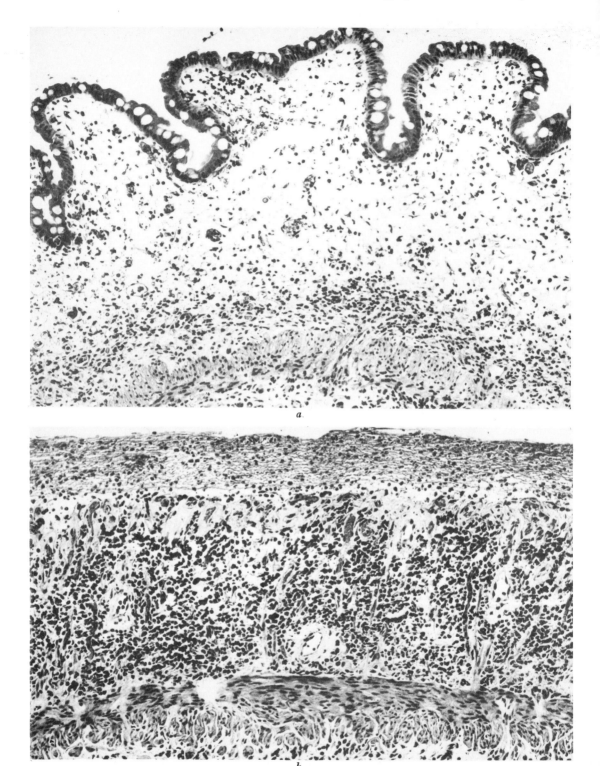

**Figures 9a and b.**   Photomicrographs of resected ileal mucosa from a patient with acute GVHD. The intestinal x-rays and a gross photograph of the resected ileum are illustrated in Figs. 4 and 5. (*a*) Ileal mucosa taken from the dilated but not denuded segment, showing absence of crypts, submucosal edema, and a lymphoid infiltrate. (*b*) Mucosa taken from a denuded area adjacent to *a*, above. There is a complete loss of epithelial cells, submucosal edema, and a membrane composed of proteinaceous material and cellular debris. There is a prominent lymphoid infiltrate throughout.

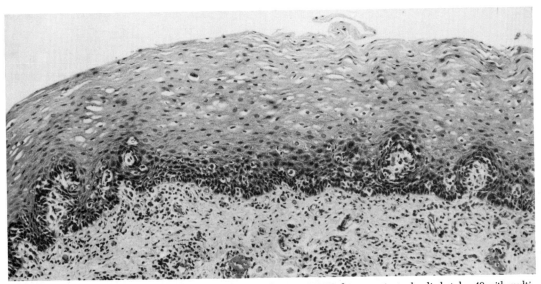

**Figure 10.** Photomicrograph of esophageal involvement with acute GVHD from a patient who died at day 40 with multisystem GVHD. There is lymphocytic infiltration into the basal layer of the epithelium with a lichenoid reaction and individual cell necrosis.

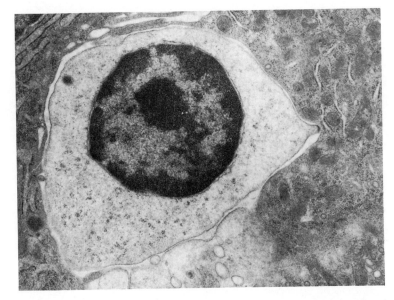

**Figure 11.** Electron microscopy of rectal mucosa from a patient with acute GVHD. The nucleated cell is a lymphocyte whose cytoplasmic projection invaginates the cytoplasmic membrane of an adjacent crypt cell. (Lymphocytes in biopsies from patients with acute GVHD appeared viable.)

in acute GVHD. The mechanisms for protein loss are unknown, but it seems likely that more than weeping of plasma from denuded surfaces is involved, since the losses occur early in acute GVHD in the absence of severe mucosal damage. The loss of immunoglobulins via this route may contribute to the immunodeficiency of acute GVHD.

*Carbohydrate, fat, and protein absorption.* When patients with acute intestinal GVHD eat any type of food, crampy abdominal pain and diarrhea usually result.[232] Sucrose- and lactose-containing foods are poorly tolerated, and in the face of severe intestinal GVHD, even glucose solutions are malabsorbed. This is a particularly frustrating problem during the recovery phase of intestinal GVHD when, despite return of appetite and cessation of diarrhea, eating is limited.[232] We assume that brush-border oligo- and disaccharidases are diminished in GVHD. This has been suggested in a mouse model of GVHD,[285] but studies in humans are lacking. Our patients with acute GVHD also malabsorb fat, as determined by qualitative analyses of stool;

this has also been demonstrated in a mouse model.[538] Ileal mucosal damage leads to bile salt malabsorption, perhaps worsening colonic retrieval of fluid. Bile salt depletion has been described in the runted mouse.[487] It is possible that absorption of intact antigens occurs when mucosal denudation is present; this has been described with inflammatory bowel disease, and the resulting circulating immune complexes may be relevant to the transplant setting.[527,749]

*Intestinal motility.* Two clinical observations deserve mention. First, rapid intestinal transit of barium and ingested liquid is common with acute GVHD and is often followed by crampy abdominal pain and diarrhea. Second, on the other hand, some patients develop anorexia, vomiting, and intestinal ileus when the only abnormality is GVHD. This may be related to transmural thickening of the bowel wall or perhaps to bacterial colonization and invasion.

### Natural history and treatment

In general, intestinal GVHD parallels skin and liver GVHD in its severity, but there are exceptions to this. The mortality from severe GVHD is significantly higher than from mild disease, and clinical grading systems have been devised to categorize patients.[669,738] If intestinal infections can be ruled out, diarrheal volume is a useful objective way of determining the severity of intestinal involvement with GVHD.[547] Treatment of established GVHD is a major problem especially for patients with severe disease. High doses of prednisone and antithymocyte globulin are useful in a small percentage of cases.[161,736] Cyclosporine and monoclonal antibodies (directed against T-cells) are currently being evaluated.[145,340,513] However, acute GVHD is often a finite illness, suggesting that the relationship between donor lymphoid cells and host epithelial cells changes with time. Most survivors of allogeneic marrow transplantation who develop intestinal GVHD resolve the symptoms of abdominal pain, cramping, and diarrhea within 3 months, but some have persistent symptoms for 6 or more months before slow resolution. Others die of progressive GVHD and infection.

### Pathogenesis

As mentioned in Chapter 2, three theories have been proposed to explain the pathogenesis of mucosal disintegration in acute GVHD in humans. These are the "immunodeficiency–superinfection" theory; the "innocent bystander" theory; and the "aggressor lymphocyte" theory. All three theories may have some validity in explaining mucosal denudation in human GVHD, but the primary event seems to be a direct, lymphocyte-mediated crypt cell lysis. Failure to replace surface cells (whose turnover is normally rapid) would quickly lead to an atrophic mucosa. Neighboring cells, such as enteroendocrine cells in the intestinal mucosa, may be damaged in the process. The immunodeficiency which results from depletion of lamina propria IgA- and IgM-bearing plasma cells may lead to bacterial colonization, further mucosal destruction, and sepsis. Further studies about the nature of the lamina propria lymphocyte population, the process of antigen recognition, and the local immune response seem crucial to an understanding of intestinal GVHD.

### INTESTINAL INFECTIONS AFTER MARROW TRANSPLANTATION

It is difficult to imagine a situation in which intestinal immune defenses are more deranged than after marrow transplantation, especially when GVHD is present. The intestinal mucosa is an extraordinarily complex barrier to microbial infection, but most of the known defenses are abnormal in intestinal GVHD.[415] Clinically, the diagnosis of GVHD is often difficult because many intestinal infections can mimic as well as coexist with GVHD. An accurate diagnosis of an infectious process, either primary or a superinfection of already damaged mucosa, becomes important because treatment of GVHD suppresses the immune response further.

### The intestinal microflora after marrow transplantation

The normal intestine contains a microflora of bacteria, fungi, and viruses, some of which are potential pathogens. The immune system is able to distinguish between "acceptable" and "nonacceptable" organisms, allowing a defensive response against pathogens while avoiding an inappropriate response against the microflora.[415] In addition, several nonimmunologic factors such as dietary carbohydrates, intestinal motility, mucus production, and cell-surface factors play a role in the symbiotic relationship between humans and their flora.[415] The upper small intestine contains small numbers of both anaerobes and aerobes which rise in number in the distal ileum, where anaerobic bacteroides and *E coli* are the most numerous organisms at $10^8$/ml. In the colon, bacterial counts reach $10^{11}$/ml, with anaerobes outnumbering aerobes by a large margin. There is a normal viral and fungal flora as well, but it is less well characterized.

Infections in patients with profound granulocytopenia are largely due to invasion of damaged mucosa by aerobic organisms and fungi, many of which are acquired from the hospital environment.[53,173,565,752] The concept of diminished "colonization resistance" has been invoked to explain bowel colonization by aerobic organisms.[714] In experimental animals, the anaerobic flora have the capacity to prevent colonization by new organisms. The use of antibiotics may suppress the anaerobic flora, removing the resistance factor and allowing colonization by aerobes and fungi.[565,566] This hypothesis appears to be valid in humans as well as in animals, since clinical trials of antibiotics, which selectively (rather than totally) suppress the normal microflora, demonstrate maintained colonization resistance and fewer mucosally derived aerobic infections.[723,746] Patients who receive marrow transplantation care in a protected environment, including nonabsorbable antibiotics by mouth, have less sepsis and fewer major local infections than control patients.[85]

## Bacterial infections

Enteric infections due to known bacterial pathogens (*Salmonella, Shigella, Yersinia, Campylobacter,* etc.) are unusual in the controlled marrow transplant environment, but bacteria-laden pseudomembranes are a common finding in patients dying of severe GVHD and/or sepsis.[53,547] Clusters and sheets of bacteria can be found in esophagus, small bowel, and colon, which, by their invasion of tissue, qualify as infections. Resistant aerobic, Gram-negative rods predominate (*Pseudomonas, Enterobacter, Serratia, Klebsiella, Citrobacter,* etc.).[85,173,752] Pseudomembranous colitis due to *Clostridium difficile* and its toxin(s) has been reported after marrow transplantation[764] but is uncommon in our experi-

ence. The clinical manifestations of *C. difficile* enteritis may be atypical in granulocytopenic patients. Recent reports of vancomycin-responsive enterocolitis *not* due to *C. difficile* have suggested that other toxin-producing organisms can proliferate in the intestine.[219,501]

## Viral infections

Cytomegalovirus (CMV) infections are the most common and difficult post-transplant infections to deal with, both diagnostically and therapeutically. The sources of CMV in transplant patients are more widespread than was realized at first. Activation of latent virus in the host, acquisition from donor cells, and infection from blood products, especially granulocytes, make CMV infections a widespread problem.[435,439,755] Older literature describes CMV as a secondary infectious agent occurring in abnormal mucosa,[255,563] but in an immunosuppressed host, CMV can be a primary pathogen causing intestinal ulceration, esophagitis, abdominal pain, watery diarrhea, protein-losing enteropathy, typhlitis, and diffuse colitis (Fig. 12).[93,218,658,699,706,748,748] In the esophagus, shallow erosions due to CMV can be seen at endoscopy, but diagnosis rests on finding cytopathic effects of CMV in brush or biopsy material or on viral cultures.[5,419] Gastric lesions due to CMV include both discrete ulcerations and diffuse gastritis with typical inclusions on biopsy.[26,93] Involvement of the small intestine with CMV is common in the post-transplant period. Symptoms range from epigastric pain to watery diarrhea (Fig. 12). Differentiating CMV enteritis from GVHD is difficult because CMV can cause a diffuse enteritis with massive protein loss and bowel-wall edema similar to GVHD of the intestine. Because acute intestinal GVHD and CMV enteritis are common, these two diseases often coexist (Fig. 13). Diffuse CMV colitis is seldom an isolated finding in our experience. However, in the renal transplant setting, typhlitis (ileocecal ulcerations) was due to CMV in a recent series.[499,658] Since GVHD also affects these areas, determining which came first may be impossible. Cecal ulcers due to CMV may bleed massively or perforate (Fig. 14).[103,658,748] Successful surgical resection of intestine ulcerated by CMV has been reported.[748] In many ways, however, the diagnosis of widespread intestinal CMV is moot, since effective treatment is

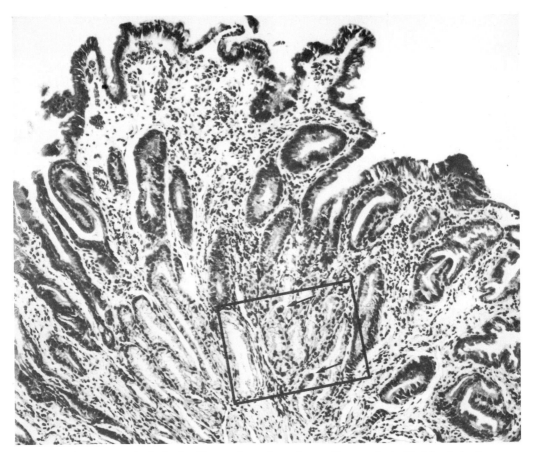

**Figure 12.**  Photomicrograph of a duodenal biopsy obtained at endoscopy from a patient with abdominal pain, nausea, and vomiting after marrow transplantation. (*a*) The crypts and villi are intact; there are no areas of apoptosis, but two cells in the Brunner's gland area demonstrate the typical cytopathic effects of CMV.

not yet available. The primary reason to find CMV is to avoid potentially fatal immunosuppressive therapy for GVHD.

Herpes simplex virus (HSV) also causes esophagitis which is similar to CMV in many respects (Fig. 15).[419,461] Early in the disease, vesicles are seen in the esophagus with shallow erosions evident in the later stages. It is not uncommon to find multiple pathogens (e.g., viruses and fungi) in infectious esophagitis in immunosuppressed patients,[419,461,535] but HSV may be treatable with antiviral agents.[646,724] Coxsackie virus, rotovirus, and adenovirus infections have also been described as causes of enteritis in immunodeficient patients, including those with marrow grafts.[556,681,764,765]

### Fungal infections

Intestinal fungal infections are common in immunosuppressed patients and are probably the most common source of deep fungal infection in marrow transplant patients.[174,193,439,753] Candida species are the most common by far, with most being *C. albicans* and *C. tropicalis*. Candida esophagitis usually presents as acute odynophagia, but persistent fever with only mild esophageal symptoms may occur.[325,351] Endoscopic brushings and biopsies will provide the diagnosis, but some patients will have mixed viral/ fungal and bacterial esophagitis. Mucosal lesions in the stomach and duodenum have been described: presenting symptoms are abdominal pain and vomiting.[336,498] Watery diarrhea can result from Candida involvement of the small bowel;[329,332,650] however, when GVHD is present, making this diagnosis is difficult. Small numbers of Candida can be cultured from the normal fecal flora, but when large numbers appear or when pseudohyphae are seen in stool specimens, Candida infection is probably pre-

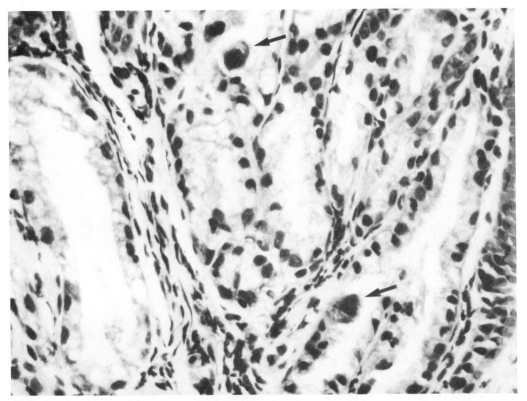

**Figure 12b.** High-power view of the Brunner's gland area enclosed above. Large intranuclear inclusions appear in glandular cells (arrows) but there is little cellular necrosis in the vicinity.

sent.[332,566] Such patients are usually febrile, leading to the use of systemic antifungal therapy in most cases. One reason for considering seemingly superficial Candida lesions seriously is the fact that yeast forms can pass through the human small intestine in a noninvasive manner by a process known as "persorption."[363,625] This may be the mechanism for cryptic deep fungal infections in immunosuppressed patients. Free bowel perforation and peritonitis due to Candida and other fungi have also been reported in immunosuppressed patients.[193,568]

### Parasitic infections

The intestinal parasites most commonly acquired by immunodeficient patients are *Giardia lamblia* and coccidia species.[80,98] Giardiasis is a common disease of the small intestine which causes abdominal discomfort and watery diarrhea, occasionally of very high volume. The small intestinal lesion may be patchy in distribution, with variability in the degree of villous appearance on biopsy. Diagnosis is most often made by finding trophozoites in stool and jejunal secretions. Three coccidia species are pathogens in humans: *Isospora belli*, *Isospora natalensis*, and *Cryptosporidium*. These organisms affect the small intestinal and colonic mucosa and produce watery diarrhea. Diagnosis depends on finding these tiny organisms in intestinal biopsies and fecal specimens.[98,427,470,700,743]

The activation of endogenous parasites is a major concern in patients who will be made immunodeficient by transplantation. Dissemination of intestinal protozoa and nematodes has been described, especially for strongyloides.[98,570] Patients arriving in Seattle from areas of the world where parasitic diseases are common are carefully screened prior to transplantation.

### CHRONIC GVHD OF THE INTESTINE

The syndrome of chronic GVHD differs from acute GVHD in many respects, among them the time of onset after transplantation, the target organs, and probably the pathogenesis.[583] Pa-

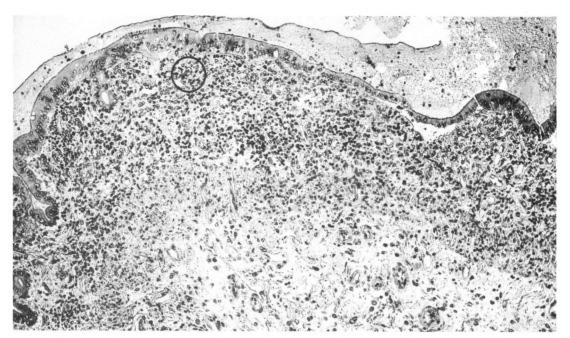

**Figures 13a and b.** Photomicrographs of jejunal mucosa taken at autopsy from a patient with acute GVHD and disseminated CMV infection. (*a*) Low-power view showing a flat mucosa with virtual absence of crypts, lymphoid and plasma cell infiltration, and scattered cells showing cytopathic effects of CMV. The area illustrated in *b* below is marked. (*b*) High-power view of one area showing typical CMV-infected cell (as marked) in the lamina propria just below the surface epithelial cells, which show atypia but no evidence of viral inclusions. The lymphoid and plasma cell infiltrate in the lamina propria is seen well here. (Fig. 14 is a more distal specimen from same patient.)

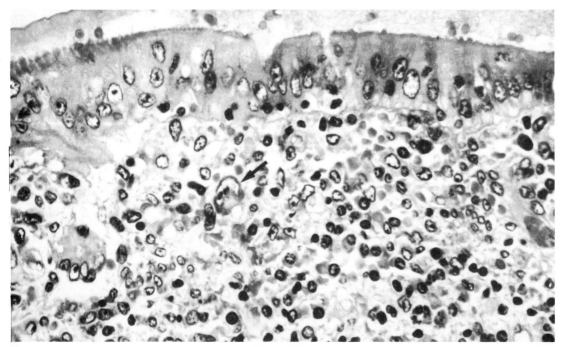

**Figure 13b.**

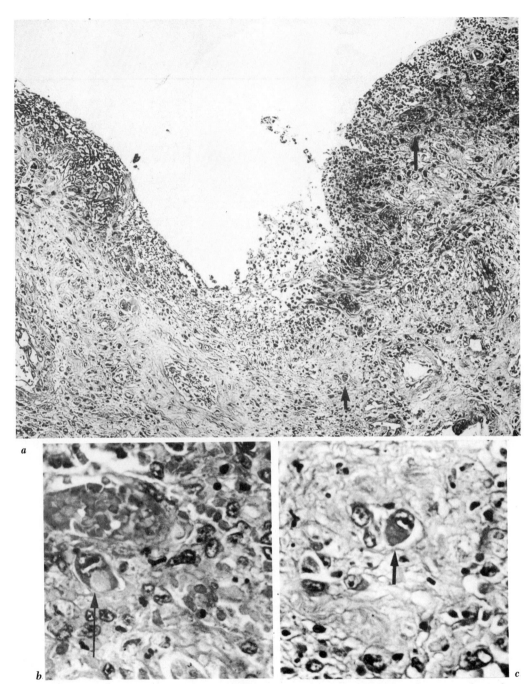

**Figures 14a, b, and c.** Intestinal ulceration due to CMV in patient with GVHD. The tissue is ileum obtained at autopsy. (*a*) Low-power view of an ulcer extending deeply into the submucosa of the ileum. The mucosa adjacent to the ulcer is devoid of epithelial cells. Numerous cells with CMV inclusions lie at sides and base of the deep ulceration. The areas illustrated in *b* and *c* are marked with arrows. (*b*) High-power view of the area to the upper right portion of the ulcer, showing both intranuclear and intracytoplasmic inclusions typical of CMV infection (arrow). (*c*) High-power view of the area beneath the ulcer, showing another CMV-infected cell (arrow).

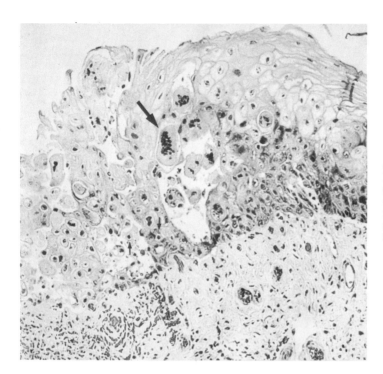

**Figure 15.** Photomicrograph of an esophageal biopsy, showing changes of herpes simplex virus esophagitis. The stratified squamous epithelium is disrupted by viral infection. Both large and multinucleate giant cells (large arrow) and smaller cells with Cowdry A intranuclear inclusions (small arrows) are seen.

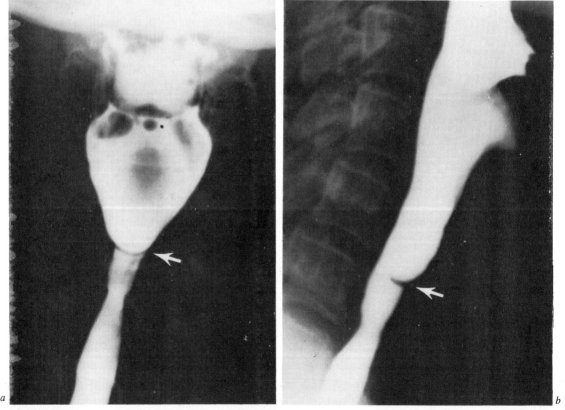

*a*                                                                                                          *b*

**Figures 16a and b.**   X-ray appearance of the upper esophagus in a patient with chronic GVHD. (*a*) Anterior view showing a thin upper esophageal web (arrow) below the level of the cricopharyngeal muscle. (*b*) Lateral view of the same web (arrow). In addition, there is a persistent narrowing of the lumen just below the web.

tients with untreatable acute intestinal GVHD develop a tubular, ribbon-like small bowel,[211] an irreversible process which usually leads to death. Most other patients who survive acute GVHD have resolution of intestinal symptoms even when developing chronic GVHD in other target organs. This resolution is usually complete in 3 months, but some have resolved only after 6 months. The more common symptoms of chronic GVHD are due to esophageal involvement, but, rarely, steatorrhea and panmalabsorption occur.[653]

### Esophageal involvement

We have seen 15 patients with esophageal pathology due to chronic GVHD.[416,417] The first patients with this complication had advanced chronic GVHD with extensive skin, eye, mucous membrane, and liver involvement.[584] We now recognize chronic GVHD at an earlier stage and lately have seen patients with more subtle GVHD involving the esophagus.

Symptoms in our patients developed 2–20 months after transplantation. Dysphagia and weight loss due to poor caloric intake were the most common symptoms, but other patients have presented with painful swallowing and excruciating chest pain. These symptoms were thoroughly investigated in our first eight patients.[416] All had a diffuse, desquamative esophagitis involving the upper esophagus, and in three patients there were distinctive upper esophageal webs (Fig. 16). Two additional patients had strictures, one in the midesophagus and one distally. Five of seven patients studied with manometry had abnormalities of peristalsis. Acid reflux was detected in all patients; two patients with severe pain associated with reflux could not clear the acid from their esophagus. Although x-ray was sensitive in detecting strictures, one web and all but one case of mucosal desquamation were missed by standard barium esophagrams.[416,417]

Biopsies of the desquamative esophagitis showed infiltration with lymphocytes and lesser numbers of plasma cells, neutrophils, and eosinophils. Individual necrotic squamous cells can be found in noninflamed esophageal mucus, analogous to findings in GVHD of the skin (Fig. 17). No infectious organisms were found in esophageal tissue in these patients. Esophageal

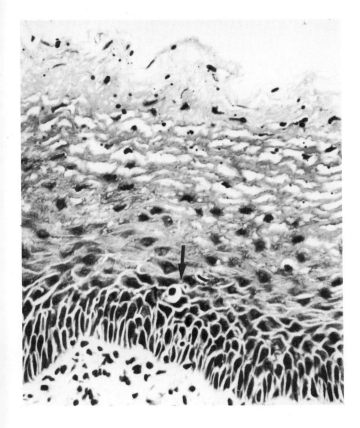

**Figure 17.** Photomicrograph of esophageal mucosa obtained by endoscopy from a patient with extensive chronic GVHD and upper esophageal desquamation. There is cytolysis near the basal layer (arrow) and exfoliation of surface debris.

histology from five autopsied patients showed no muscle or neuron abnormalities by silver stain or conventional light microscopy. There was, however, increased submucosal fibrosis associated with overlying mucosal inflammation and epithelial atypia.[416] Unlike the scleroderma esophagus, there was no muscle fibrosis in our GVHD cases.

The pathogenesis of this desquamative esophagitis is unknown, but there may be both cellular and humoral factors involved. Ultrastructural studies of chronic GVHD of the skin have shown a specific type of point contact between lymphocytes and damaged epidermal cells, suggesting a cytotoxic injury process.[229] Several humoral abnormalities have been described with chronic GVHD along with an imbalance of regulatory suppressor cells (see Chapter 4).

In summary, the esophageal epithelium is a target organ in acute GVHD, but esophageal symptoms are most prominent in patients with extensive chronic GVHD. Symptoms are due to webs, strictures, and an inability to clear acid from the esophagus. Treatment with both immunosuppressive and antireflux drugs is beneficial for established chronic GVHD and, when instituted early, probably prevents extensive organ damage.

### Intestinal changes

Although stomach, small bowel, and colon mucosa show striking changes in acute GVHD, these organs are generally spared in well-established chronic GVHD. Patients with severe acute intestinal GVHD that does not improve with treatment do not survive to develop chronic GVHD. However, we have seen two patients whose acute GVHD melded into a chronic GVHD picture and in whom widespread colonic submucosal fibrosis and mucosal calcification were present at autopsy.[583] Two additional patients had both small bowel and colon involvement, resulting in severe diarrhea, panmalabsorption, crampy abdominal pain, and pronounced malnutrition until death. In each, acute GVHD had resolved in the post-transplant period, and only later did signs of extensive chronic GVHD appear. Evaluation revealed gross steatorrhea (coefficients of absorption less than 50%) without obvious cause as small bowel x-rays and

peroral biopsies were normal, as were intraluminal digestion of a test meal, D-xylose absorption, and Schilling test with intrinsic factor. However, at autopsy there was focal fibrosis of the lamina propria and striking segmental fibrosis of the submucosa and serosa, extending from the stomach to the colon (Fig. 18). There was also hyalinization of serosal and submucosal blood vessels with subendothelial basal lamina replication. There was no degeneration or fibrosis of the smooth-muscle layers, in contrast to scleroderma of the small bowel. In view of these autopsy findings, we theorize that the severe malabsorption was due to lymphatic blockade of absorbed nutrients.

These two cases occurred early in our experience with chronic GVHD, however, we have not seen such malabsorption or submucosal fibrosis in recent years, despite screening all patients for malabsorption at regular intervals. The pathogenesis of the extensive submucosal fibrosis in these few patients is unknown. Whether it is a result of untreated chronic GVHD or the residual of severe mucosal acute GVHD, or perhaps due to conditioning therapy, is open to question. Fortunately, it is uncommon.

A fifth patient presented with milder chronic GVHD and malabsorption, and with coefficient

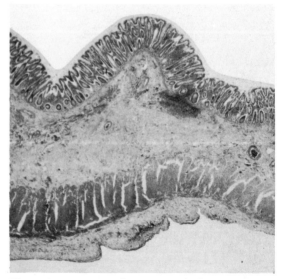

**Figure 18.** Low-power photomicrograph of intestine in a patient with extensive chronic GVHD of long standing. Section of colon showing extensive submucosal and serosal fibrosis. Similar changes were present in the small intestine. The overlying mucosa in both areas was normal. (From Shulman et al.[584]; reproduced with permission.)

of fat absorption of 62%. Intestinal x-rays and biopsies were normal, but cultures of jejunal fluid showed an overgrowth of *Pseudomonas* and *Candida* species. The steatorrhea responded dramatically to treatment with nonabsorbable antibiotics and nystatin, suggesting that bacterial overgrowth (stasis syndrome) was responsible for his malabsorption.

## Malnutrition in chronic GVHD

An analogy between runting syndrome in experimental animals and chronic GVHD in humans can be drawn, but in humans the cause of malnutrition is poor oral intake in most cases, rather than malabsorption. Oral mucositis, esophageal symptoms, and anorexia due to systemic illness seem to be the primary reasons for poor caloric intake. The exceptions are the two patients with gross steatorrhea mentioned above and one additional patient who had clear evidence for small intestinal stasis syndrome with bacterial overgrowth in the jejunum. Secretory immunoglobulin deficiency in patients with chronic GVHD has been described and may well occur in the intestine as well as in other areas.[304,306]

## SUMMARY

Intestinal complications of marrow transplantation are common. Symptoms of conditioning chemoradiation therapy resolve within 2 weeks, and the mucosa is morphologically normal at 3 weeks. Acute GVHD may present in several ways, the most common being crampy abdominal pain and profuse watery diarrhea. Intestinal x-rays and rectal biopsies are invariably abnormal when symptoms are severe. Isolated crypt cell degeneration is the earliest histologic finding and the most useful in terms of diagnosis. Intestinal infections (especially CMV and *Candida*) can mimic acute GVHD, but the major clinical problem is determining when infection and GVHD coexist in a given patient. Chronic GVHD involves the esophagus and liver more commonly than it does the intestine, but we have seen four cases with striking fibrotic change in the lamina propria of small bowel and colon. The interaction between lymphoid cells in the lamina propria, epithelial cells, and the intestinal flora in patients who have received marrow grafts deserves further study.

# Chapter 7

# Liver disease after marrow transplantation

Howard M. Shulman, M.D.
George B. McDonald, M.D.

## Introduction

Liver disease is a common and potentially lethal complication of bone marrow transplantation. The main causes of liver disease in this setting are chemoradiation injury and graft-vs.-host disease (GVHD), but drug-liver injury and infections (viral and fungal) remain important considerations. Several of these causes may coexist at any one time, blurring both clinical and histologic distinctions.

When faced with a seriously ill, jaundiced patient, the clinician must make a diagnosis in order to start the proper treatment. For example, should immunosuppressive therapy for GVHD be started in a jaundiced, febrile patient who might have fungal liver disease? Should drug doses be altered when venocclusive disease (VOD) is the cause of jaundice? The clinical and laboratory picture may suggest one specific cause for liver dysfunction, but when there are doubts, liver histology must be examined. Percutaneous liver biopsy can be done safely using the Menghini aspiration biopsy technique in patients with platelet counts over 60,000/mm³, a level which can be achieved with platelet transfusion if necessary.[578]

However, just as the clinical picture can be confusing, so can liver histology in the post-transplant patient. Much of the literature on human

hepatic GVHD is derived from autopsy tissue. This histology is often modified by specific immunosuppressive therapy, preterminal shock, or rapid autolysis in the presence of jaundice. Furthermore, at autopsy a high prevalence of systemic cytomegalovirus (CMV) infection occurs in patients with GVHD.[436] Larger-sized specimens obtained from antemortem open-wedge liver biopsies and autopsy tissue are advantageous for dealing with such spotty lesions as venocclusive disease (VOD), the bile duct injury of GVHD, and CMV inclusions. Yet, by careful analysis of needle biopsy material and by utilization of data from previous analyses of human and experimental studies of GVHD and VOD, we can usually provide accurate diagnoses of liver disease.

In this chapter, we present those liver diseases most commonly related to marrow transplantation, arranged in chronologic order of their appearance after transplantation. Discussion will center on the clinical, laboratory, and histologic features of these diseases.

### PRETRANSPLANT LIVER DYSFUNCTION

Abnormal liver tests are common in patients referred to our hospital for marrow transplantation for leukemia and other malignancies. For example, an abnormal pretransplant SGOT (aspartate aminotransferase) value was present in 89 of 255 patients transplanted for malignancy from 1978 to 1980.[418] Similar observations have been made in patients with acute myelogenous leukemia by several groups.[36,124,330] Histologic investigation usually reveals either nonspecific hepatitis[14] or chronic liver disease.[717] Although these patients are seldom symptomatic from their liver dysfunction, marrow transplantation results in a more serious liver disease, VOD, which affects about 20% of patients transplanted for leukemia and other malignancies after conditioning with cyclophosphamide (CY) and total body irradiation (TBI).[420] The single most predictive factor for development of VOD in such patients is an abnormal SGOT value before transplantation. That is, patients transplanted for malignancy who have active hepatitis incur a 3.4-fold risk of developing VOD after transplantation, as compared to patients with normal pretransplant SGOT values.[418,420] Pretransplant viral hepatitis preceded the onset of aplastic anemia in several patients; however, none of these developed VOD after marrow transplantation. The likely reason for this disparity is that their conditioning therapy involved only CY and not TBI.

The following case illustrates the problem of pretransplant hepatitis and the subsequent development of VOD.

> A 25-year-old male (UPN 1371) with acute myelomonocytic leukemia in first remission was admitted for marrow transplantation with an SGOT value of less than 3000 IU/dl. A liver biopsy showed a lobular hepatitis with moderate lymphocytic infiltration of the triads. Serologies for hepatitis viruses A, B, CMV, and EBV were negative, and a presumptive diagnosis of post-transfusion, non-A, non-B viral hepatitis was made. Marrow transplantation was delayed. Four weeks later when the SGOT was normal, he was preconditioned with a regimen of CY (120 mg/kg) and 1200 rad fractionated TBI. On day 11, he developed sudden weight gain, jaundice, and elevated SGOT (14 times normal). Over the next few days, deepening icterus (total bilirubin of 24 mg/dl), prerenal azotemia, and pulmonary edema preceded hepatic coma, and he died of liver failure 7 days after onset of his disease. His necropsy showed hepatomegaly with generalized centrilobular congestion, hepatocellular necrosis, and widespread lesions of VOD.

There are three main causes for liver dysfunction in patients referred for marrow transplantation. These are viral hepatitis, drug-liver injury,

and malignant infiltration. We feel that viral hepatitis is the most likely explanation because of frequent blood-product transfusions before marrow transplantation in these patients.[36,124] Non-A, non-B viral hepatitis can produce a smoldering liver disease with waxing and waning of transaminase and a progression to chronic hepatitis.[45,295] Recent studies suggest that hepatitis B (HB) and CMV infections are the cause of about 10% of the post-transfusion-related hepatitis. A recent study in patients with leukemia suggests that HB virus may be present in hepatocytes even in the absence of serologic markers for the virus.[717] It seems less likely that these pretransplant SGOT elevations are caused by drug injury, despite the fact that many chemotherapy drugs are hepatotoxic.[394] In our series of patients transplanted for malignancy from 1978 to 1980, there was no relationship between previous antineoplastic chemotherapy and SGOT elevations.[418] Others also have failed to note liver deterioration due to chemotherapy in patients with leukemia who had hepatitis.[124] Nonetheless, a few patients with leukemia have arrived for transplantation with liver-biopsy-proven VOD, a well-recognized complication of antineoplastic chemotherapy (see below). In our opinion, however, most have non-A, non-B viral hepatitis from prior blood transfusions.

## EFFECTS OF CHEMORADIOTHERAPY ON THE LIVER

Many different regimens are used to prepare patients for marrow transplantation, but most use chemotherapy (usually CY) or chemotherapy and TBI. Two liver lesions can result: VOD and pericentral hepatocyte necrosis. VOD is the most common liver disease in the first month posttransplant and a cause of liver failure and death.[51,260,309,420,423,583,720,762] Pericentral hepatocyte necrosis is a less distinct and a less severe illness.[583]

### Clinical features of VOD

In its most florid form, VOD presents with weight gain, right-upper-quadrant (RUQ) abdominal pain, hepatomegaly, ascites, jaundice, and oliguria. These findings usually develop early, within 1–3 weeks after transplantation and, infrequently, as late as 5–6 weeks.[420,583] Rarely, hepatic encephalopathy develops before the onset of clinical jaundice, which can be delayed in its appearance for several days. Transaminase and alkaline phosphatase levels may be normal initially, then may rise rapidly. Patients dying within days of the clinical onset of the illness succumb to fulminant hepatic failure. At the other end of the clinical spectrum is the patient who has none of the above signs or symptoms, but in whom the histologic picture of VOD is later found. In our recent report of 32 cases of VOD after transplantation, 13 cases had the florid, progressive presentation, 13 had an illness that was subclinical or obscured by other events, and six had a less severe illness characterized by jaundice and ascites but with a slow resolution of these signs over 1–4 weeks.[583] Our more recent series of 53 patients with VOD seen between 1978–1980 showed that 45% had a serious illness characterized by persistent jaundice and ascites, or death (usually before day 30). The remainder had a milder illness from which a clinical recovery was made. Those with the more serious VOD had higher average bilirubin levels (19.3 vs. 4.8 mg/dl), gained more weight, had higher SGOT levels, and were more likely to develop encephalopathy.[418,142] Death from VOD resulted from volume overload, intestinal bleeding, aspiration of gastric contents, coma, and azotemia.

We have found that a correct clinical diagnosis of VOD can be made in 90% of those patients who rapidly develop jaundice, hepatomegaly, and ascites in the first month after marrow transplantation. Often, the sudden onset of RUQ pain will herald the disease. Recognition of ascites lags behind a rapid weight gain, which is seldom initially recognized as caused by liver disease. A clinical diagnosis of VOD also rests on excluding unusual diseases which may present similarly, such as pericardial effusion producing passive liver congestion, pancreatitis with biliary obstruction and ascites, and bacterial peritonitis. Hepatic vein thrombosis (Budd-Chiari syndrome), although clinically indistinguishable from VOD without angiographic studies, has never been demonstrated at autopsy in our patients. The timing of the onset of illness and the profile of liver function tests usually differentiate VOD from GVHD of the liver. In our unit, VOD usually appears within 8–25 days after conditioning therapy, whereas liver GVHD usually devel-

ops after day 21 and follows the clinical recognition of liver dysfunction. Even when GVHD occurs earlier, ascites does not develop for many weeks.[583] Viral hepatitis seldom causes ascites and encephalopathy unless there is massive hepatocellular damage. On two occasions, however, we have mistaken severe intra-abdominal fungal infections for VOD. Peritoneal infections causing ascites, weight gain, and jaundice must be carefully ruled out by ultrasonic imaging of the abdomen, and paracenteses with cultures of ascitic fluid. Abnormal liver enzyme levels and jaundice due to total parenteral nutrition (TPN) may occur, but in adults this is not accompanied by ascites, encephalopathy, or liver failure.[727]

## Histology of VOD

Our analysis of 32 autopsy cases of VOD surviving from 2 to 86 days post-transplantation provided a chronologic sample of the liver histology. The histologic diagnosis of VOD is easily missed or sometimes difficult to prove unless special stains, which delineate the central veins, are utilized—in particular, the trichrome and reticulum stains. The changes are also greatly enhanced by embedding sections in plastic, or by using Carnoy's fixative (which lyses red cells) before embedding in paraffin. In our experience, the reticulum stain, although providing excellent contrast for black-and-white photomicroscopy, has less diagnostic usefulness than does the trichrome stain.

When patients died within 1 week of the onset of VOD, the H & E-stained sections of liver showed marked centrilobular hemorrhagic necrosis obscuring most terminal hepatic venules and sublobular veins (Fig. 1). The central veins are easily recognized on the trichrome-stained sections by their dense, wavy, continuous band of adventitial collagen, as compared to the haphazard bundles of collagen comprising the portal triads. The spotty pathognomonic venular changes in early VOD consist of concentric narrowing of the lumina of the affected small central veins by an edematous subendothelial zone containing wispy collagen fibers, fragmented red cell membranes, and hemosiderin-laden macrophages (Fig. 2). Hemorrhage into the space of Disse in pericentral areas was common. In some cases, clusters of hepatocytes lay within the lumen of portal veins and within the walls and

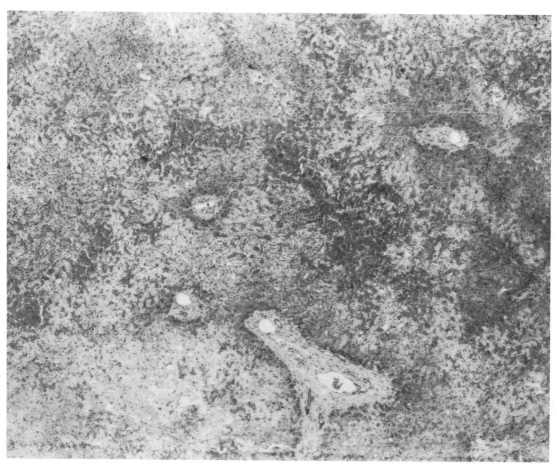

**Figure 1.** (UPN 1036) Fatal VOD 23 days after autograft. Low-power view of early changes. Punched-out zones of centrilobular hemorrhagic necrosis are easily overlooked unless VOD is considered and higher-power magnifications and/or connective tissue stains are examined.

lumina of central veins (Fig. 3). The hepatocyte embolization may arise from widespread injury to hepatocytes in zone 3 of the liver acinus, producing detachment with embolization dependent upon the direction of intrahepatic blood flow (portal or central). Much less frequently, hepatocyte embolization to central veins occurs with GVHD.

When patients with VOD survived more than 3 weeks from onset of the illness, the lumina of the affected central venules were often eccentric and partially or completely obliterated by concentrically arranged, subendothelial reticulum or collagen fibers (Figs. 4 and 5), admixed with foamy cells containing hemosiderin, bile, and lipofuscin pigments. The irregular and atrophic pericentral hepatocytes were surrounded by dilated sinusoids containing proliferated reticulum fi-

bers and collagen (Figs. 6 and 7). Some portal zones contained increased fibrous tissue and dilated lymphatics and portal venules.

There was a rough correlation between the number of central venules involved by VOD and the clinical course, particularly in patients dying with fulminant VOD.[583] In the livers of patients surviving longer than 3 months, there was often a patchy distribution of VOD lesions, with marked diminution in number and size of small central veins, widespread centrilobular hepatocellular cholestasis, and irregular spacing between portal and central zones. This may perhaps represent repair or functional heterogeneity of different liver lobules.

Our recent experience has shown that liver biopsy in patients with overt symptoms of VOD often show diagnostic histologic changes. Previ-

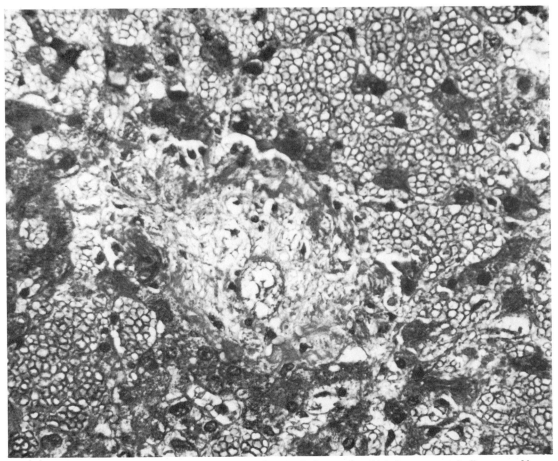

**Figure 2.** (UPN 1705) VOD diagnosed on liver biopsy on day 45. The lumen of a sublobular vein is markedly narrowed by an edematous subendothelial zone containing wispy collagen fibers and scattered cells. The surrounding lobule is disrupted by marked congestion.

ously, we reported that VOD was present in the liver biopsy from only two of eight patients shown to have VOD at autopsy.[583] However, most of these eight patients had subclinical or mild VOD. The accuracy of a clinical diagnosis of more severe VOD is high,[418] but when confirmation is needed, either ultrasound, CT x-ray,[27] or liver histology may provide a definitive diagnosis. When a patient with VOD later develops GVHD, liver biopsy can still be useful in confirming the latter diagnosis even before the centrilobular changes of VOD have resolved (Fig. 2).

## Pathophysiology of VOD

Three classes of agents produce hepatic VOD: pyrrolizidine alkaloids (*Senecio, Crotolaria, Heliotropium*),[424] ionizing radiation,[195] and many different antineoplastic drugs.[17,380,394] Many cen-

ters have described VOD as a complication of bone marrow transplantation in syngeneic, autologous, and allogeneic recipients.[41,51,260,309,423,583,720,762] To be more precise, the chemoradiotherapy used to prepare patients for marrow grafting is the proximate cause of VOD and could become a limiting factor in dose incrementation of cancer chemoradiotherapy. Our studies showed a clear and strong statistical association between the subsequent development of VOD and four factors: high-dose conditioning regimens, transplantation for leukemia, older age, and liver disease.[420,583] There was no association with sex, nutritional status, type of marrow transplant, or hepatic GVHD. The first reported cases of VOD after marrow transplant suggested a causal association of VOD with GVHD,[41] but this conclusion was probably due to an erroneous diagnosis of

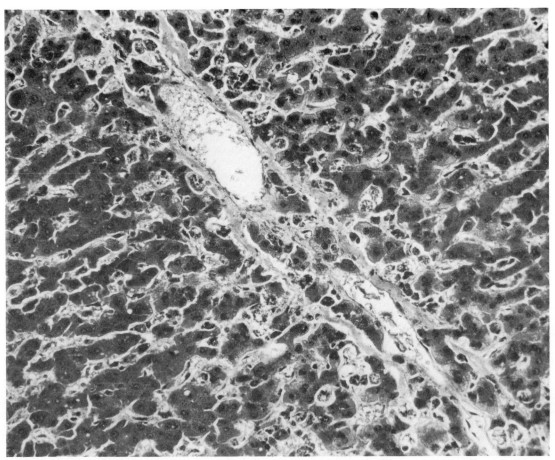

**Figure 3.** (UPN 1478) VOD day 57 after second bone marrow allograft. Embolized hepatocytes within the subendothelial zone of a sublobular vein.

GVHD. All subsequent studies have failed to find a relationship of VOD to GVHD, or an increase in prevalence of VOD among allogeneic vs. autologous or syngeneic transplant recipients. The doses of TBI (920–1525 rad) used in preconditioning are probably insufficient to cause VOD alone, as shown by animal studies[284] and reports in man of radiation hepatitis that required more than 3500 rad, fractionated, before producing VOD.[194] Of the drugs used in combination conditioning chemoradiotherapy, busulfan and dimethylsulfan seem to be the most toxic.[51,583] Others have reported VOD in autologous recipients after high-dose BCNU[423] and mitomycin C[260] plus TBI conditioning. Our recent series of 53 cases of VOD seen between 1978 and 1980 provides further insight into other risk factors for VOD;[418] i.e., an elevated pretransplant SGOT level increased the risk of subsequent VOD, and younger patients with ALL had a lower risk of VOD than did those with CML or AML.

Why should there be such striking centrilobular toxicity from chemoradiotherapy? When VOD occurs after irradiation, the primary site of injury is the venular endothelium, presumably because of the greater radiosensitivity of endothelium over hepatocytes. The $D_0$ (dose of irradiation that reduces the number of *in vitro* confluent cells in culture to 37%)[756] for rat hepatocyte is 249 rad.[319] Parallel studies of rat hepatic venular endothelium have not been reported. When VOD is produced experimentally by pyrrolizidine alkaloids, both the venular endothelium and centrilobular hepatocytes are injured.[6] Many antineoplastic drugs produce centrilobular hepatocyte damage as well as

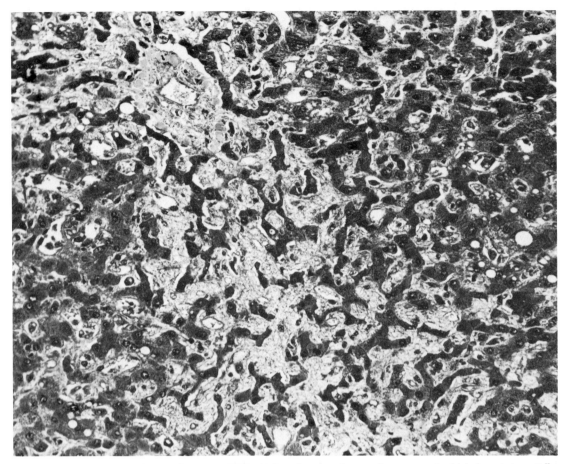

**Figure 4.**   (UPN 822) Later changes of persistent VOD, 49 days after clinical onset of symptoms. A sublobular vein is partially obliterated by subendothelial fibrosis. In the adjacent zone 3 of the liver acini, there has been extensive hepatocyte atrophy and dropout leading to compression of distances between adjacent central veins. (Masson trichrome.)

VOD,[394,428] but only when the synergistic or additive toxicity from conditioning regimens using chemotherapy and irradiation is present does the high incidence of VOD seen after marrow transplantation for malignancy occur. The centrilobular location of VOD may relate to the portal blood flow and functional heterogeneity of the liver lobule. Hepatocytes in the pericentral region have different metabolic capabilities from those in the periportal area.[271,488] We speculate that liver-activated metabolites of antineoplastic agents are concentrated in pericentral hepatocytes by the sinusoidal blood flow. Moreover, enzyme systems responsible for metabolizing these drugs may be concentrated in this zone. This latter mechanism has been suggested for the centrilobular necrosis seen with Senecio alkaloids and other hepatotoxins.[424,445,750] For example,

CY, the most commonly used preconditioning agent for marrow transplantation, is metabolized by microsomal mixed-function oxidases to aldophosphamide, which then yields highly cytotoxic metabolites.[428] The greatest concentration of these oxidases is in the centrilobular hepatocytes.[271] The absence of hepatotoxicity with CY alone may be due to the presence of enzymes in the liver which oxidize aldophosphamide to inactive metabolites. We speculate that pretransplant hepatitis may predispose patients to VOD by decreasing the activity of such aldehyde-oxidizing enzymes.

The end result of centrilobular and venular damage is obstruction of sinusoidal blood flow. Normally, liver sinusoids empty into the terminal hepatic venules through small pores that perforate the endothelial lining (Figs. 8 and 9).[452]

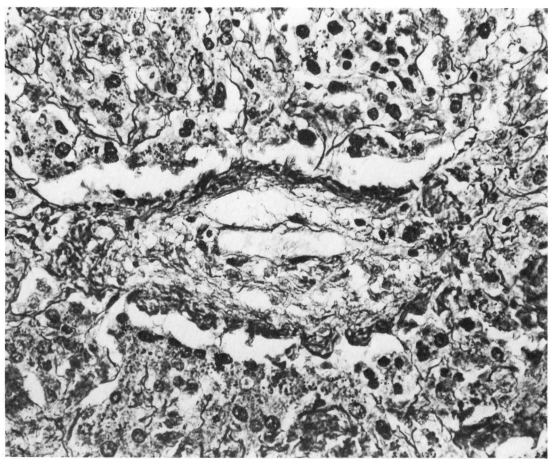

**Figure 5.** (UPN 560) Day 65 after syngeneic marrow graft with asymptomatic VOD. Central vein lumen is filled by loosely scattered reticulum pigment and pigment-laden cells. (Snook's reticulum.)

When these pores are obstructed by endothelial damage, there is intramural entrapment of fluid and cellular debris, including exfoliated hepatocytes, with eventual fibrosis of venous walls. The role of fibrin deposition in the genesis of the VOD lesion is unclear. In our studies, direct immunofluorescent stains failed to show fibrin or fibrinogen in the obliterated venules. Electron microscopy revealed small amounts of fibrin in two of six cases. This contrasts with other studies in which fibrin was regularly found enmeshed in the obstructed venules of later lesions.[195] One study of the use of prophylactic heparin in humans receiving liver radiation was inconclusive in demonstrating protection from VOD.[384] We feel that local thrombosis, unlike the situation with Budd-Chiari syndrome, is probably not the first event in VOD.

**Pericentral hepatocyte necrosis after marrow transplantation**

In the course of our retrospective analysis of liver histology from 204 marrow-transplanted patients, we described 12 patients with a liver disease resembling a mild form of VOD.[583] These patients developed jaundice without ascites in the first several weeks after transplantation, usually with modest elevation of bilirubin, SGOT, and alkaline phosphatase levels (to 3 and 5 times normal upper limit). Later autopsy liver histology demonstrated irregular centrilobular hepatocyte degeneration and dropout, sinusoidal fibrosis, and phlebosclerosis (a thickening of the adventitia without luminal narrowing or subendothelial fibrosis) (Figs. 10 and 11). We speculate that collapse of pericentral hepatocytes leads to eccentric fibrosis around central venules, although some

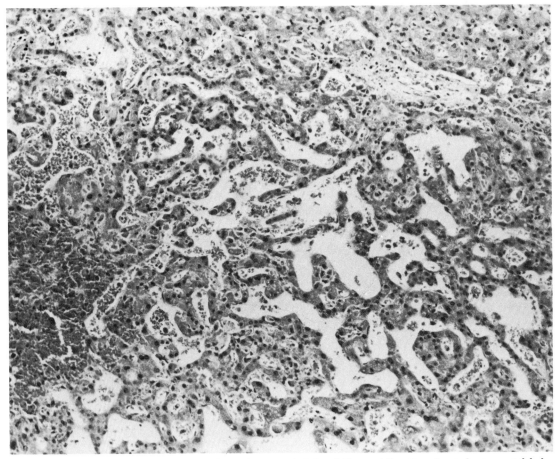

**Figure 6.** (UPN 1430 day 37) Later changes of VOD (at autopsy). Subtotal fibrous obliteration of central vein, centrilobular sinusoidal dilation, hepatocyte atrophy and dropout, and spotty central hemorrhage. (X20.)

cases of phlebosclerosis could represent older VOD lesions in which subintimal collagen had retracted or undergone recanalization. This process is probably a less severe form of chemoradiotherapy toxicity. Hepatocellular injury, reported after a number of antineoplastic agents,[12,394] may be centrilobular or panlobular in distribution.

### GRAFT-VS.-HOST DISEASE

#### Clinical features of acute and chronic GVHD
A typical patient with acute GVHD of the liver develops abnormal liver function tests coincident with or after GVHD arises in other target organs. The clinical picture is that of cholestasis with a hepatitis of varying severity. At the onset of liver GVHD, there may be occasional liver tenderness or darkening of urine, while a change in stool color, itching, or loss of appetite occurs infrequently. The bilirubin and alkaline phosphatase often rise roughly in parallel while elevations of SGOT are usually more modest (to 10 times normal). Alkaline phosphatase and bilirubin, both greater than 10 times normal, are found in more long-term cases, while SGOT may return to nearly normal levels. Severe hepatocellular dysfunction (prolonged prothrombin time, encephalopathy) is unusual, but bilirubin can reach levels of greater than 30 mg/dl without causing debility. Ascites occurs only after weeks of intractable liver GVHD. With severe multisystem GVHD, fever, anorexia, and malaise are prominent, but are less so with isolated liver GVHD.

#### Histology of GVHD
This account of liver GVHD is based on our clinical experience with over 150 human liver biop-

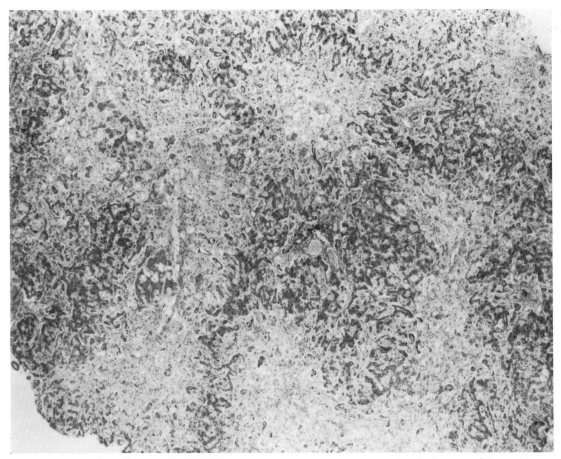

**Figure 7.**    (UPN 1458 day 83) Hepatic failure with submassive hepatic necrosis from both VOD and GVHD.

sies, several hundred autopsies, and published experimental studies of GVHD in dogs[23,352,546] and other mammals.[46,51,379,403,494,496,584,592,596,759] In most cases, we made a diagnosis of liver GVHD when liver dysfunction was accompanied by clinical and histologic signs of GVHD in other organs. Histologically, GVHD is characterized by a degeneration or paucity of small bile ducts and cholestatic hepatitis. We first describe the chronologic stages in well-established cases of GVHD, and then discuss the pathogenesis of liver GVHD in comparison to the findings in other immunologically mediated liver diseases.

*Acute GVHD.*    The earliest lesions (found in biopsies within 1–4 days of onset of liver dysfunction) demonstrate a mild nonspecific reactive or lobular hepatitis. The hepatocellular cords have only mild unrest, anisonucleosis and anisocytosis, and mild triaditis (Figs. 12, 14, and 15). Dropout

of individual hepatocytes and acidophilic body formation are present in only small numbers. Beschorner et al.[51] found a predominantly periportal location for the hepatocellular injury and acidophilic bodies in GVHD. In our experience and in others'[592] the acidophilic bodies found in GVHD have no particular zonal localization. Sinusoidal collections of proliferating Kupffer cells admixed with lymphoid cells are infrequent in the early lesions, and lesions of bile ducts are spotty.

Histology of liver biopsies obtained a week or more after the onset of liver GVHD show more prominent changes of hepatitis, cholestasis and degenerative changes of the small, centrally located interlobular or septal bile ducts (Figs. 12–17a). If the patient is not on immunosuppressant therapy, the portal zones are usually expanded by a mononuclear, primarily lymphocytic

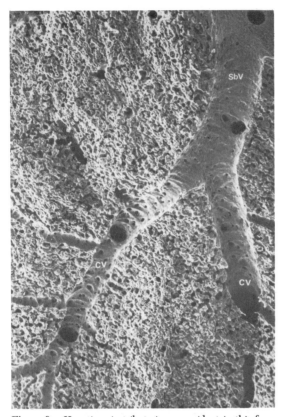

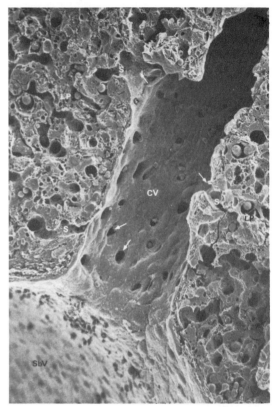

**Figure 8.** Hepatic vein tributaries are evident in this fractured feline liver preparation. The openings present on the wall of smaller and larger vessels are perforations due to sinusoids pouring into central (CV) and sublobular veins (SbV). These latter in turn are continous with larger hepatic vein tributaries. In the cat (as in other mammals but not in the human) the sinusoids empty directly not only into the central veins but also into larger branches of the hepatic veins. (X150.)

**Figure 9.** The luminal surface of this feline central vein (CV) is perforated by numerous openings (arrows) of sinusoids (S) running in the lobule along the hepatic plates (LP). On the bottom, the central vein, which represents the smallest hepatic vein tributary, enters a larger vessel corresponding to a sublobular vein (SbV). (X440.)

inflammatory infiltrate. The infiltrate may contain occasional eosinophils, neutrophils and plasma cells, but we have never seen epithelioid granulomas in a human patient with GVHD. There may be periportal acidophilic bodies with spotty piecemeal necrosis, but the limiting plates are generally intact (Fig. 15).

The altered bile ducts may have elongated or flattened shapes with small, compressed lumina but rarely contain inspissated bile (Figs. 13–17), quite the opposite of that seen in extrahepatic biliary obstruction. Epithelial alterations usually involve the entire duct circumference although some alterations may be segmental. Cytologic alterations include an increased N:C ratio, hyperchromatic enlarged nuclei, pyknotic or anucleate cells, and amphophilia. Cytoplasm has loss of su-

pranuclear PAS-positive material and occasionally is vacuolated (Fig. 16). In GVHD, some ducts contain cellular debris and papillary ingrowths of epithelium which project into the lumen (Fig. 15). On cross section, these projections appear as islands of epithelium within the lumen (Fig. 14B). Intraepithelial migration of lymphocytes into the duct wall and individual duct cell necrosis are uncommon, though these findings along with the degenerative appearance of the ducts may explain the pathogenesis of GVHD (Figs. 15–17a). We emphasize that the ductal alterations of GVHD are focal and not present in every triad, and that examination of serial sections or routine procurement of larger specimens will aid in identifying these changes.

The large-sized septal and intralobular ducts

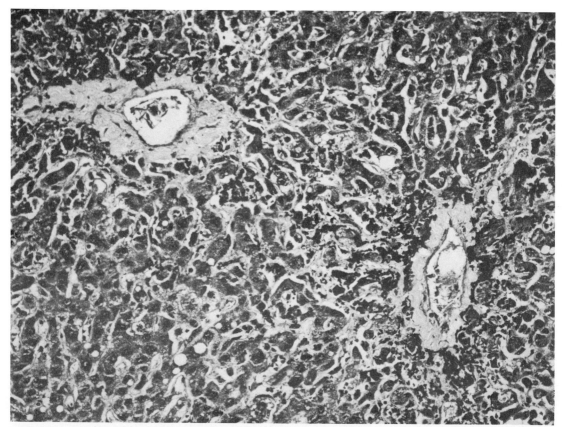

**Figures 10 (Low power) and 11 (High power).** (UPN 546 day 96) Centrilobular hepatotoxicity with persistent jaundice, hepatomegaly, and later encephalopathy developed during high-dose conditioning chemoradiation therapy with cytosine arabinoside, CY and TBI. Despite the clinical similarity to VOD, multiple sections at autopsy showed only phlebosclerosis, periadventitial and eccentric adventitial fibrous thickening around sublobular veins, hepatocellular degeneration and dropout, and sinusoidal fibrosis. Sometimes these findings coexist with VOD, indicating that both conditions originate from chemoradiation therapy. (Gomori's trichrome.)

are spared by GVHD although Sloane et al.[596] have described nuclear multilayering and lack of mucus accumulation in large-order bile ducts in patients with GVHD. In our histologic studies of severe canine GVHD, we have also noted that some of the large-order ducts show segmental loss of nuclei and cytoplasmic atypia.[23] We have examined the major extrahepatic biliary system in many patients with severe GVHD at autopsy and found no similar changes.

Beschorner et al.[51] semiquantitated the extent of bile duct injury in human GVHD by counting the number of triads containing injured bile ducts per 10 small triads. They found such bile duct injury to be significantly increased in patients with GVHD compared to those without GVHD. Most studies of liver GVHD have also emphasized that one of the frequent and characteristic features is the absolute reduction of small bile ducts (ductopenia), otherwise known as paucity of interlobular bile ducts.[494] However, assessment of ductopenia has several pitfalls. Autopsy specimens or large biopsies are most suitable since at least 20 triads are needed for an accurate assessment;[28,29] otherwise, some triads appearing to lack ducts may, in fact, represent tangentially sectioned triads. Studying serial sections may partially resolve this.

Nakanuma and Ohta devised a system for quantifying bile ducts per triad in primary biliary cirrhosis.[460] They point out that occasional triads contain two or three ducts. In normal liver, the small bile ducts lie adjacent to accompanying small arteries within a distance of three times the

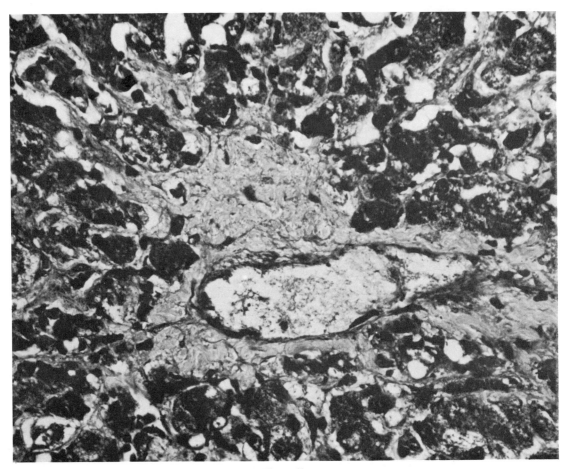

**Figure 11.**

external diameter of the artery. The extent of bile duct destruction can be expressed by the ratio of arteries to accompanying bile ducts. This relationship of artery:duct is especially important in GVHD in which small ductules commonly located at the margins of triads are, in fact, proliferated cholangioles rather than true bile ducts. In 1974, Lerner et al.[379] first proposed a histologic grading system for GVHD based on the quantity of injured ducts. In view of the difficulties in interpreting reactive versus degenerative changes in bile ducts and ductopenia, and because such reductions probably reflect duration of GVHD more than actual severity, we limit ourselves to a statement on the certainty of a diagnosis of liver GVHD based on an overall assessment of bile duct injury, ductopenia, and cholestatic changes.

When GVHD remains active over many weeks and months, the histological specimens often show profound panlobular cholestasis (Figs.

17–21). In zone 3 of the liver acinus the hepatocytes undergo extensive dropout and form liver cell rosettes around dilated bile canaliculi (Fig. 18). The remaining hepatocytes appear loosely attached and show extensive ballooning degeneration and heavy pigmentation with lipofuscins, iron and bile. Sinusoidal fibrosis and Kupffer cell hyperplasia may be prominent (Fig. 20b). Small central venules often have prominent endothelium with focal intimal thickening and subendothelial collections of debris, pigmented macrophages, and occasionally embolized hepatocytes. These nonspecific segmental changes are secondary to centrilobular injury and collapse. They should not be confused with the more specific concentric subendothelial thickening of VOD (Fig. 20b). Periportal alterations include bridging necrosis with portal-to-portal and portal-to-central bands, piecemeal necrosis and many dilated periportal cholangioles filled with

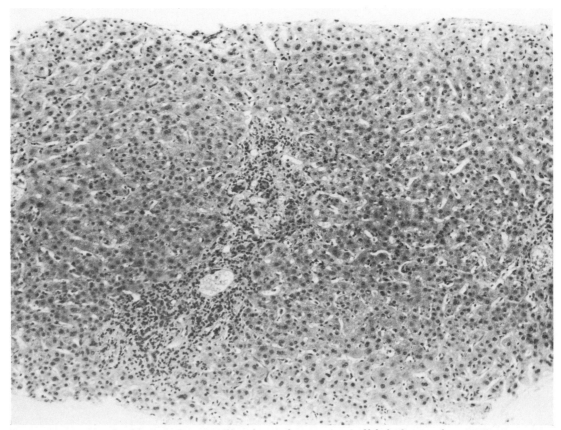

**Figure 12.** (UPN 882 day 72) Low-power view of liver biopsy showing pattern of lobular hepatitis from GVHD. Note parenchymal change and Kupffer cell hyperplasia are mild.

dense bile pigment (Figs. 18–20). The portal triads are moderately expanded by fibrous tissue admixed with mononuclear cells. Marginal bile ductule proliferation may be pronounced, while true interlobular bile ducts are often absent (Figs. 18, 19). In our coded study of 204 autopsied marrow recipients[583] we found that this histological constellation of periportal bile thrombi, triaditis, and severe lobular cholestasis was strongly associated with severe GVHD ($p < 0.0001$). Periportal bile thrombi may also develop in the presence of prolonged jaundice from VOD, but are much less frequent and usually occur as a single cholangiole. In some patients, these severe cholestatic changes were accompanied by little inflammatory response in the portal triads or lobules, presumably reflecting treatment with immunosuppressive agents (Fig. 19). Prolonged active liver GVHD is a potentially serious complication (with pericentral collapse

and sclerosis, sinusoidal fibrosis, and portal-to-portal bridging, producing a noncirrhotic portal hypertension) causing ascites, encephalopathy, frank hepatic failure, and hepatorenal syndrome. Such problems are compounded when severe GVHD is superimposed on VOD, producing submassive hepatic necrosis (Fig. 6).

*Chronic GVHD.* The histologic dichotomy between acute and chronic GVHD of the liver is not nearly as well-established as that for the cutaneous manifestations. As discussed elsewhere, patients with chronic GVHD may have three different modes of presentation: persistent acute liver GVHD becoming chronic, reexacerbation of GVHD after 100 days, or a *de novo* late onset with no preceding acute GVHD. The histologic findings are variable but largely dependent on the duration of active disease and the intervention with immunosuppressive therapy. Patients may have a picture of lobular hepatitis, chronic

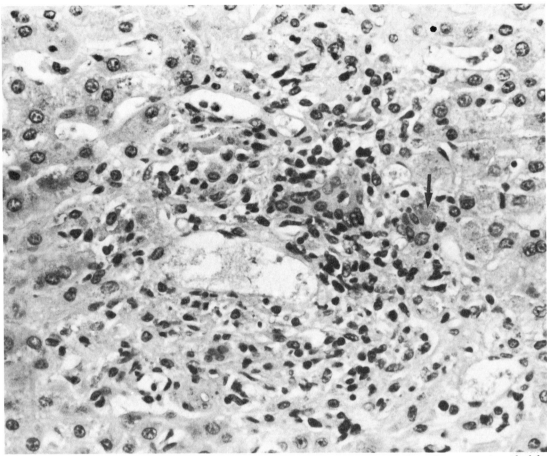

**Figure 13.**   (UPN 882 day 72) Elongated and atypical bile duct partially obscured by mononuclear inflammation. An acidophilic body lies along the limiting plate (arrow).

persistent, chronic septal, or chronic aggressive hepatitis (Figs. 21–23) with marked portal enlargement by inflammatory cells.[584] Usually, changes of occasional necrosis within the lobule are generally mild even when there is piecemeal necrosis or bridging necrosis. With chronic GVHD, the inflammatory response is sometimes more exuberant and often plasmacytic—a reflection, perhaps, of the patient's more complete immunological reconstitution or the cessation of methotrexate (MTX) after day 100 (Fig. 21b).

When absolute counts of bile ducts per portal triad are made as described above,[460] there is often a marked reduction or complete absence of small bile ducts (Fig. 23). We have seen only a few patients with chronic GVHD develop hepatic failure. The histology varied: one had extensive bridging fibrosis with early cirrhosis; another had an intact lobular architecture with canalicular bile plugs, portal fibrosis, and loss of all small bile

ducts. Autopsy histology from several patients with chronic GVHD, characterized by elevated alkaline phosphatase and normal to mild elevations of bilirubin, also varied. Some had a mild expansion of portal areas by dense fibrous tissue with little or no inflammation;[584] others had pronounced cholestasis with pseudoxanthomatous changes, particularly marked around the periportal and centrilobular zones, and dense plasmocytic infiltrates in the portal zones (Fig. 21). In all these patients, a paucity of small bile ducts was noted. The elevated alkaline phosphatase in some cases may represent residual damage to the intrahepatic biliary tree rather than active GVHD.

## Pathogenesis

Histologic studies of GVHD in monkeys, rodents, dogs, and horses all show alterations of small interlobular bile ducts, similar to those described in

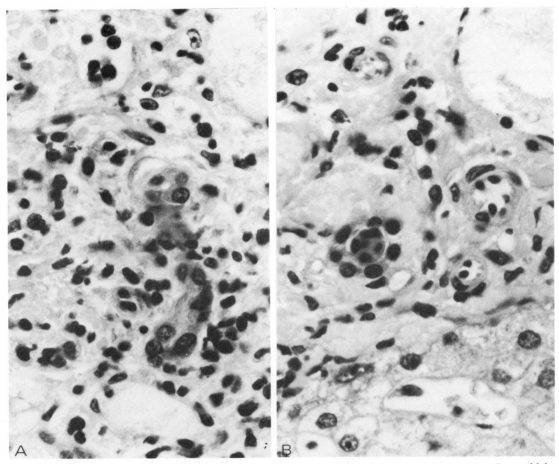

**Figure 14.** (UPN 504 day 25) Liver biopsy showing early stage GVHD. (A) Portal triad containing irregular, elongated bile duct with atypical ductal epithelial cells. Cells are flattened, nuclei are enlarged and reactive or absent on segments. Lymphoid cells are migrating into the duct wall. (B) High-power view of portal triad containing a cross section of a duct within a duct. This probably represents a papillary projection, a proliferative response to bile duct injury.

human GVHD.[23,54,352,496,519,546,708,709,759] There has been considerable controversy over the interpretation of these bile duct changes. Some investigators have suggested that perhaps they are merely reactive inflammatory changes from either bacterial or viral infections,[592] or to drug injury.[45,403] Others suggest they represent immunologically mediated injury.[46,51,584,596] Sale et al.[546] addressed this controversy in a coded histologic comparison in dogs. They analyzed the liver histology in irradiation controls and autografted and allografted dogs that receive mismatched marrow grafts without postgrafting MTX. All dogs had previously been immunized against canine hepatitis and distemper. As expected, nearly all the allografted dogs with hematopoietic engraftment developed severe GVHD, and only these dogs developed marked portal in-

flammation with injury and degeneration of the small interlobular bile ducts.

Why bile ducts might be the antigenic targets of GVHD and how such injury is immunologically mediated is not fully understood. MacFarlane et al.[402] have demonstrated a 790,000 dalton protein in bile duct epithelium which caused chronic, nonsuppurative, destructive cholangitis when injected into rabbits.[758] Interestingly, submaxillary gland ducts and bile ducts, both apparent targets of chronic GVHD, are derived from entoderm and bear Ia antigens,[373] a requisite for immunologic recognition. The findings of lymphocytes within the walls of damaged bile duct epithelium is interpreted as evidence of lymphocytotoxicity against antigens on the surface of the biliary cells. Bernuau et al.[46] have studied the electron microscopy of the liver in

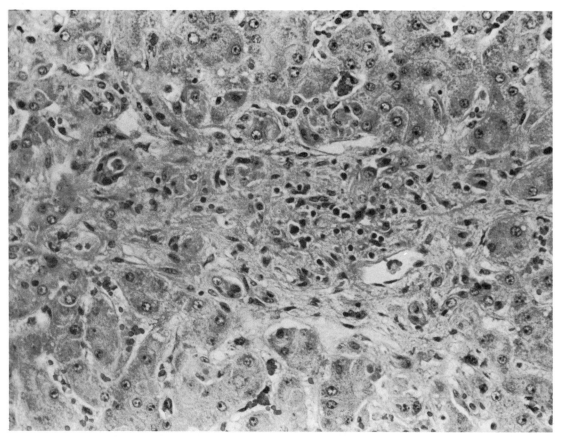

**Figure 15.** (UPN 640 day 18) One week after onset of hyperacute GVHD in patient receiving mismatched allogeneic graft, portal trial has a degenerative, partially necrotic small bile duct containing luminal debris (arrow). There is a slight mononuclear infiltrate and periportal acidophilic bodies.

GVHD. They found cells morphologically resembling killer lymphocytes with elongated lymphoid processes in close apposition to the membranes and bile duct epithelium. Damaged bile ducts demonstrated dilatation or swelling of the endoplastic reticulum, perinuclear space, and mitochondria, and necrosis and disruption of the basement membrane. The authors' observations resemble other ultrastructural reports of *in vitro* T-lymphocyte-mediated cytolysis,[383] chronic GVHD of the skin,[229] and rejection of pig liver allografts.[571] These similarities suggest that in GVHD the bile ducts are preferred antigenic targets injured by cell-mediated cytotoxicity. Using monoclonal antibodies in an avidin–biotin indicator system, Beschorner et al.[56] studied the immunological phenotype of the mononuclear cells infiltrating the liver triads in rat radiation chimeras with GVHD. In those with acute GVHD, 81–89% of the cells in the triads and sinusoids, and

60–74% of the cells infiltrating the bile ducts were nonhelper T-cells. In chronic GVHD, many of the cells in the triads had endogenous peroxidase. In the triads, 77–84% of the infiltrating cells were helper T-cells, as were 52–61% of the sinusoidal cells. No intraepithelial lymphocytic migration into bile ducts was present. Bernuau et al.[46] also noted hepatocyte necrosis and close contact between lymphocytes and hepatocytes in GVHD. Similar findings also reported in ultrastructural studies of chronic hepatitis[339] and alcoholic hepatitis[220] may represent nonspecific, antibody-dependent cytotoxicity between activated lymphocytes bearing Fc receptors for antibodies bound to hepatocyte membrane (see below).

Evidence for humoral immune mechanisms as opposed to cell-mediated cytotoxicity in the pathogenesis of liver GVHD is less striking. Patients with chronic GVHD have a variety of auto-antibodies, including occasional generation of

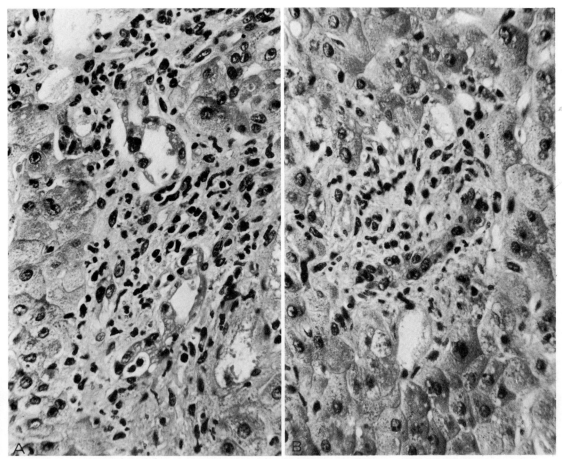

**Figure 16.** (UPN 1195 day 40) Liver biopsy 18 days after clinical onset of multisystem GVHD and progressive rise of liver function test. (*A*) Dilated, irregular bile ducts have cytoplasmic vacuolization and flattening. Note focal absence of epithelium and nuclei. (*B*) An elongated bile duct has nuclear irregularity and dropout. Lymphocytic migration into the duct wall is present in both photos.

antimitochondrial antibody,[584] a finding characteristic of primary biliary cirrhosis, but also found in a variety of other liver disorders.[347] It is also of interest that some patients with HBsAg-negative, autoimmune, chronic active hepatitis have linear deposits of autoantibody on hepatocellular membranes directed against liver membrane antigens.[298,433] Such autoantibodies to liver-specific hepatocytes and liver membrane antigens have not yet been investigated in liver GVHD.[154] Such antibodies directed against hepatocyte membrane antigens could be secondary epiphenomena. Lymphocyte reactivity to antigens derived from hepatocytes or bile ducts could be derived from a release of antigens from damaged tissue.[312] A direct effector role of these antibodies might include antibody-dependent cytotoxocity mediated by the binding of specific

Fc receptors on lymphocytes to the antibodies bound to the hepatocyte surface.

Other hepatotoxic effector mechanisms to be considered in the pathogenesis of liver GVHD are complement activation and circulating immune complexes.[729] We have performed direct immunofluorescence on eight liver biopsies from patients with chronic GVHD, looking for deposits of immunoglobulin (Ig) and complement (C'3) (Shulman unpub data). The study was unrevealing except for one patient with chronic GVHD who had diffuse cytoplasmic staining of bile ducts with C'3, blocked when these sections were first preincubated with unlabeled antibody. A similar unusual finding has been reported in primary biliary cirrhosis (PBC)[492] in which a chronically activated complement system may be involved with the pathogenesis.[310] Specifically, patients

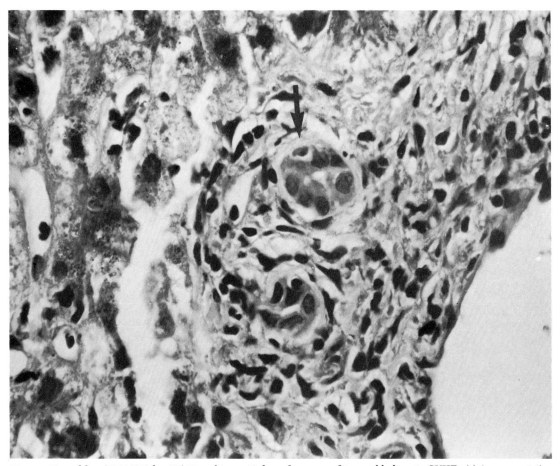

**Figures 17a and b.** (UPN 567 day 109) Liver biopsy 40 days after onset of intractable hepatic GVHD. (*a*) A representative portal triad contains two bile ducts with transepithelial lymphocytic migration and individual cell necrosis (arrow).

with PBC have a deficit of $C^{3b}$ receptors on Kupffer cells which might lead to delayed hepatic clearance of immune complexes, resulting in increased tissue deposition and injury.[323] Similar functional complement turnover studies have not been reported in GVHD. In our experience, the serum complement levels in patients with chronic GVHD are normal.[472]

### Comparison of GVHD with other immunologic liver disease

*Primary biliary cirrhosis (PBC).* The autoimmune liver disease, primary biliary cirrhosis, often occurs with scleroderma.[443] Many authors have pointed out the histologic similarities of PBC to chronic GVHD. Epstein et al.[186] have suggested that PBC may be part of delayed chronic GVHD arising from maternal-uterine transfusions causing a dry-gland (sicca) syndrome

resulting from damage to ductular epithelium in many organs, often associated with scleroderma. Ultrastructurally, damaged bile ducts in PBC resemble those in GVHD.[47]

Although the similarity between PBC and chronic GVHD has broad biologic implications, there are nevertheless differences between the two diseases. PBC characteristically affects middle-aged females and usually runs a protracted course over many years before death from liver failure. There is no propensity for increased viral or bacterial infection. PBC has a wide range of *in vivo* and *in vitro* immunological abnormalities as reviewed by James et al.[312] Serum levels of IgM antimitochondial antibodies and I-C are often elevated. Perhaps most important is the decreased numbers of suppressor T-cells generated in the autologous mixed leukocyte reaction using non-T-cells as stimulators, which may provide the

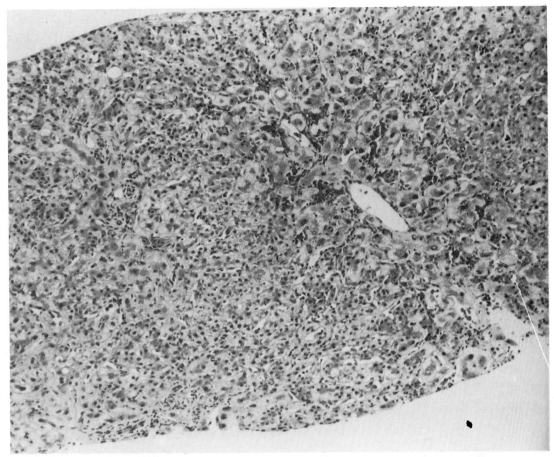

**Figure 17b.**   Marked hepatocellular cholestasis with ballooned centrilobular hepatocytes heavily laden with bile and lipofuscin pigment. The parenchymal inflammation and dropout are marked.

necessary immunologic environment for the various factors to cause PBC. Histologically portal areas often contain prominent lymphohistiocytic infiltrates with lymphoid follicles and granulomatous inflammation. Bile ducts are atypical and injured but these changes are often only segmental with the remaining ductal circumference appearing normal. Parenchymal copper is often increased while feathery degeneration is not striking.

In contrast to PBC, GVHD—whether acute or chronic—affects both sexes equally, and all ages. Chronic GVHD is associated with an increased propensity for bacterial and viral infections,[19,20] whereas serum levels of IgM and AMA are inconsistently elevated.[584,653] Elevation of circulating immune complexes in chronic GVHD has been reported by Graze and Gale.[263] However, we have not found immune-complex levels to be

consistently elevated or different from such levels found in healthy long-term survivors. The generation of suppressor T-cells in the autologous mixed leukocyte reaction is depressed in all long-term allogeneic recipients regardless of whether or not chronic GVHD is present (Chapter 5). Histologically, GVHD lacks portal lymphoid follicles or granulomatous inflammation. Small bile ducts are rapidly destroyed over a period of days to weeks while larger-sized bile ducts are spared. Cholestasis associated with GVHD begins in centrilobular areas with feathery degeneration, whereas in PBC, it is first evident in the periportal areas. We have found no increase of parenchymal copper in Rhodanine-stained sections from patients who have prolonged liver GVHD (Shulman, unpublished data). Unfortunately, an exact histologic comparison of PBC to chronic GVHD is hindered by the facts that both diseases

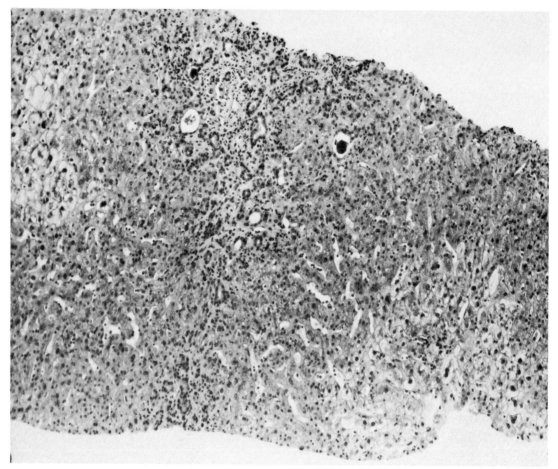

**Figure 18.** (UPN 341 day 88) Liver biopsy shows changes of prolonged GVHD: marked bile ductule proliferation, periportal bile lakes, portal–portal bridging, and centrilobular ballooning. At this stage, residual true ducts are destroyed or difficult to discern from the marked proliferation of bile ductules along the outer part of the triad. Diagnosis of GVHD relies on the overall appearance rather than on the finding of atypical or degenerative interlobular ducts.

have changing histology and samples in GVHD are obtained while patients are receiving immunosuppressive therapy.

*Liver allograft rejection.* Fennel et al.[202] have reviewed the histology of homografted liver transplants. The autopsy histology of many cases dying early after liver transplant was often that of vascular insufficiency or infection. However, in those patients dying later of apparent chronic rejection, there was marked atypia and destruction of the small bile ducts and profound hepatocellular cholestasis, while inflammation was variable and often mild. The typical changes of chronic liver rejection appeared virtually identical to those of GVHD, suggesting that in both condi-

tions the immunological targets include bile duct epithelium.

### DRUG-LIVER INJURY

Marrow transplant recipients are routinely exposed to other potentially hepatotoxic drugs, including: immunosuppressive agents; antibiotics, antifungal and antiviral drugs; sedatives; antiemetics; antipyretics; etc.[394,769] It is more difficult than usual to incriminate one particular drug in the face of concomitant drug use, VOD, GVHD, and viral hepatitis. Many drug-liver injuries cause a hepatitis clinically and histologically distinguishable from viral hepatitis. The

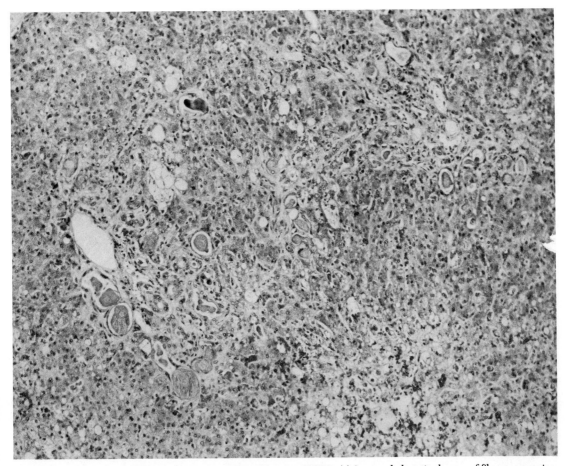

**Figures 19a and b.** (UPN 1195 day 71) Severe prolonged hepatic GVHD. (*a*) Severe cholestatic changes of fibrous expansion and bridging between triads, surrounded by dilated bile-filled cholangioles. Centrilobula hepatocyte ballooning.

question of whether either of these entities may be easily distinguished from acute GVHD remains unresolved. The following discussion emphasizes a few categories of drugs commonly used after marrow transplantation which may cause liver disease.

*Methotrexate (MTX)* is given intravenously on day 1 at 15mg/m², then on days 3,6,11, and thereafter at weekly intervals at 10 mg/m², up to day 100 as prophylaxis against the development of severe GVHD.[669] These doses are comparable to the divided intermittent oral doses of 10–75 mg/ m² every 1–4 weeks for treatment of psoriasis.[136,742] In contrast, high-dose MTX regimens for treatment of leukemia or sarcomas utilize 3–7 g/m² I.V. over 4–6 or 20–42 hours, followed by citrovorum factor rescue.[61,468] Occasionally, we have noted transient elevations of SGOT with el-

evated levels of blood MTX requiring citrovorum factor rescue in the days following prophylactic MTX doses. This is in agreement with literature on the hepatic consequences of high-dose MTX for malignancies after which elevations of transaminases are frequent.[506] After 4 months of high-dose MTX, the long-term consequences include fatty change, anisonucleosis, round-cell infiltration, hepatocyte necrosis, portal fibrosis, and cirrhosis.[468] Perhaps even more relevant are the reports of liver damage after long-term MTX use for psoriasis, where frequent, small doses are also associated with the same changes. When a cumulative dose exceeds 2–4 g, the prevalence of fibrosis increases, yet biochemical liver tests are unreliable in detecting this.[766] The duration of exposure to high blood levels of MTX seems to be the critical factor in liver toxicity.[61] Post-mar-

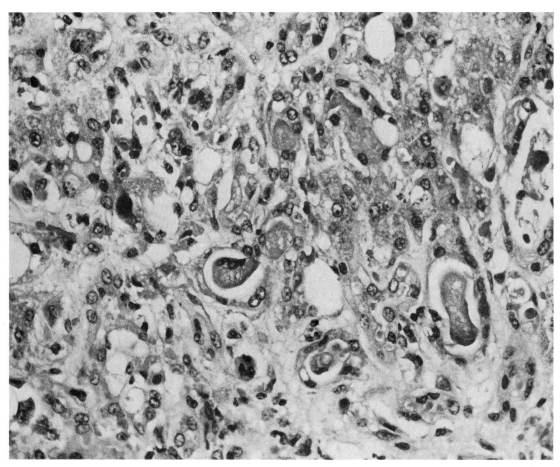

**Figure 19b.**    Higher-power view of periportal cholangioles. Interlobular bile ducts are not identifiable. The dark body (arrow) represents a CMV intranuclear inclusion, an infrequent finding in the liver despite many inclusions found elsewhere. These severe cholestatic changes are the consequence of severe prolonged liver GVHD and do not occur in patients dying with only systemic CMV infections.

row transplant MTX doses seem unlikely to produce long-term damage since weekly infusions are given for 3 months, blood levels of MTX are monitored and, if necessary, lowered by citrovorum rescue. In our coded histologic review of VOD in 204 autopsied marrow recipients, there was no obvious MTX effect on the liver.[583] Later, we specifically examined the necropsy histology of three patients who received additional higher doses of MTX in an attempt to treat severe acute GVHD. In these three patients, histology was not different from that of other patients with GVHD except for more pronounced enlargement and cytoplasmic clearing of periportal hepatocytes.

*Cyclosporine (Cyclosporin A) (CYA).* The fungal metabolite, cyclosporine, is a potent new immunosuppressive agent[450] reported to have great therapeutic potential for preventing or ameliorating rejection of kidney and liver allografts[90,349] and GVHD after allogeneic marrow transplantation.[511,513] Recently, Starzl has shown that the combination of CYA and prednisone markedly decreases rejection after orthotopic liver allograft.[614] Palacios and Moller have postulated that CYA may work on resting T-cells exposed to stimulating antigens by blocking HLA-DR receptors, thereby inhibiting the expression of receptors for T-cell growth factor interleukin 2.[486] Morris has reviewed studies of CYA suggesting that the generation of cytotoxic T-cells is inhibited, while there is a relative facilitation of suppressor T-cell activity.[450] Side effects of CYA include skin rashes, hirsutism, a capillary leak syndrome, and renal and hepatic toxicity.[585] Because of the prevalence of other liver disease, it is

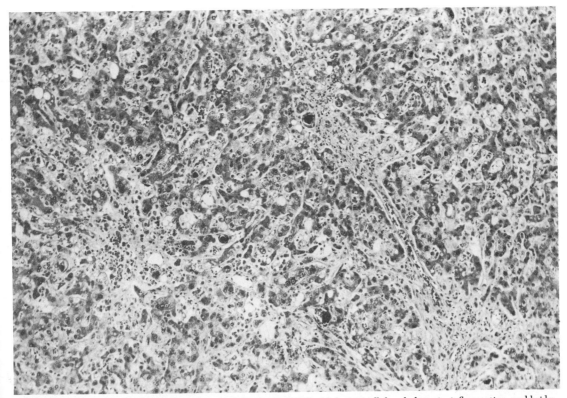

**Figures 20a and b.** (UPN 287 day 87) (*a*) Severe prolonged GVHD with hepatocellular cholestasis, inflammation, and bridging necrosis with periportal and pericentral bile plugs.

difficult to evaluate CYA hepatotoxicity in a setting of marrow transplantation. Studies of allogeneic marrow recipients given CYA suggest that this drug can cause a nonspecific centrilobular injury. In Powles' report,[511] several allogenic patients given CYA showed severe centrilobular hemorrhage. After receiving CYA in addition to CY/TBI conditioning, several of our patients developed hyperbilirubinemia (up to 50 mg/dl) and ascites. One such patient, with otherwise unexplained liver dysfunction, had spotty necrosis and atrophy of centrilobular hepatocytes and sinusoidal widening, consistent with a centrilobular hepatotoxicity (Fig. 24).

The route and timing of the adminstration of CYA, especially when given pretransplant along with conditioning therapy, may play an important role in the expression of such hepatotoxicity. We believe CYA may predispose or potentiate hepatotoxicity when patients are conditioned with only CY 200 mg/kg. Previously, we had found less than 1% of such patients have developed VOD. Yet, in 1981, we observed a cluster of three patients transplanted for aplastic anemia who received continuous administration of CYA before and after the CY conditioning, and who shortly after transplantation developed ascites and hepatorenal failure. VOD was strongly suspected in all and confirmed by liver biopsy in the single patient who had liver histology. Fortunately, the awareness of this problem, careful monitoring of cyclosporine blood levels, attention to the timing and route of administration, and the recent availability of an I.V. preparation have greatly reduced the potentiation. Although VOD is still very common (20%) among patients with leukemia conditioned with CY/TBI, CYA does not appear to increase their risk of developing it.

*Azathioprine.* An antimetabolite, azathioprine, is used as an immunosuppressant to control active chronic GVHD.[653] It is given in doses up to 1.5 mg/kg per day, usually in combination with prednisone, for months to years. Azathioprine hepatoxicity has been reported in animals and man; however, many of the reports

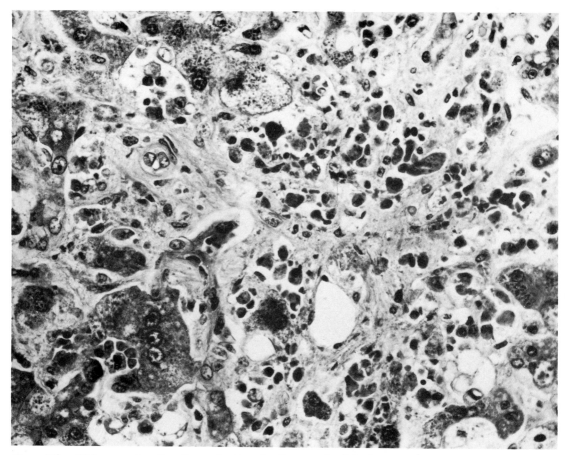

**Figure 20b.** High-power view of small central vein with collapse, multicellular hepatocyte dropout, foci of pigment-laden Kupffer cells, adn sinusoidal fibrosis. The wall of the sublobular vein is eccentrically thickened. Such changes must be distinguished from VOD. (Masson trichrome.)

in man involve renal transplant recipients in whom viral hepatitis is common.[428,604] Azathioprine hepatotoxicity produces jaundice and elevated alkaline phosphatase with moderate elevations of transaminases.[428] Histology is a nonspecific cholestasis with hepatocyte necrosis,[412] peliosis, and sporadic cases of VOD in renal transplant recipients.[147,606] In our experience with the above doses for chronic GVHD, both liver function tests and histology improve after azathioprine is begun, and toxicity does not occur. We observed one patients with chronic GVHD who accidentally received 3 mg/kg per day, twice the usual dose. Over 2 months, total bilirubin rose from 1.4 to 6.1 mg/dl, alkaline phosphatase fell from 6 times normal to normal, and SGOT remained moderately elevated at 3–4 times normal. Given the profiles of liver function tests with azathioprine toxicity, certainty in dis-

tinguishing such toxicity from chronic GVHD may be difficult. A liver biopsy would be useful since finding bile duct lesions or ductopenia is more consistent with GVHD. Other evidence of toxicity would require withdrawal of azathioprine and rechallenging of the patient at a later date.

*Parenteral Nutrition (PN).* Our marrow recipients generally receive PN with glucose, amino acids, and lipid emulsions during the first several weeks after transplantation. More prolonged PN is given or later reinstituted if intestinal GVHD interferes with appetite or absorption of nutrients. In infants, PN given for several weeks can cause severe but potentially reversible cholestasic hepatitis with bile ductule proliferation, triaditis, and bridging necrosis.[39,116] In adults, PN can cause hepatomegaly from fatty change and water accumulation; cholestatic hepatitis is rare. In the first weeks after marrow graft-

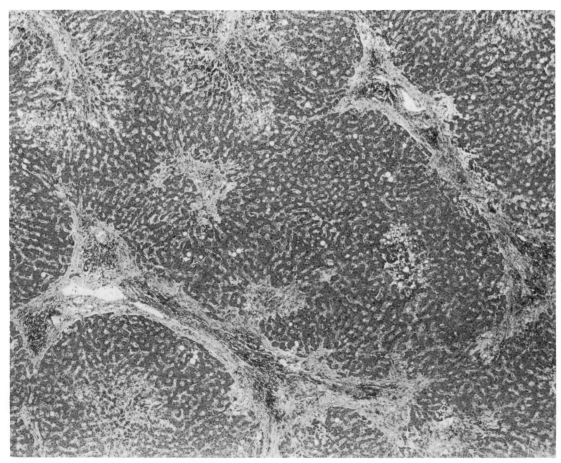

**Figures 21a and b.** (UPN 394 day 350) (*a*) Chronic GVHD with pattern of chronic septal hepatitis with bridging fibrosis and central and periportal hepatocellular cholestasis.

ing, PN-induced changes of hepatomegaly without jaundice or elevated liver tests can be confused with mild VOD, while GVHD would be very unlikely.

### INFECTIOUS LIVER DISEASE AFTER TRANSPLANTATION

Our data from serologic studies, liver histology, and cultures of nearly all liver biopsies and autopsies indicate the most common liver infections in marrow transplant recipients are viral, while the most serious are fungal.

### Viral hepatitis

Viral hepatitis remains a consideration throughout the transplant period. Four major groups of viruses cause hepatitis in the post-transplant setting: non-A–non-B (NANB); hepatitis B (HBV);

CMV; and much less often, other herpes viruses (simplex or varicella-zoster), adenovirus, or Papoviruses. Despite recent reports describing several histologic differences between Types A, B[1] and NANB,[500] the three types cannot be distinguished reliably using only morphologic criteria or length of incubation time. Even after serologic testing to exclude types A and B, the diagnosis of NANB viral hepatitis may actually represent a group of viruses,[295] including superimposition of the delta virus agent on HBV[531,598] or seronegative HBV in immunocompromised hosts in which the expression of antigen and antibody are temporarily suppressed.[717]

The marrow transplant recipient faces the jeopardy of viral hepatitis from several sources. Some acquire new viral infections from post-transplant exposure to blood products, granulocytes, or platelets as part of a systemic viral infec-

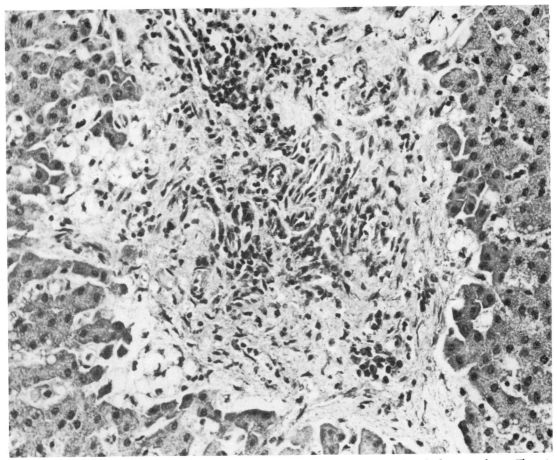

**Figure 21***b*.    Higher-power view of enlarged portal triad containing scattered plasma cells. Bile ducts are absent. There is pseudoxanthomatous transformation of periportal hepatocytes, but piecemeal necrosis is absent or minimal.

tion, or from reactivation of latent viral infections present before transplant.[297] A large number of our patients have hepatitis upon arrival at our Center, probably from prior transfusions.[418] Fortunately, the incidence of hepatitis from transfusions has been reduced by careful screening of blood donors and products, and by using family members or volunteer donors.

The diagnosis of viral hepatitis is often difficult in the marrow transplant setting due to the high prevalence of VOD and GVHD in these patients. Liver enzyme profiles of viral hepatitis are shared by other liver diseases. The histological distinction of early GVHD from viral hepatitis at times may be difficult to determine. Viral hepatitis has a broad morphological spectrum.[312,500] We previously have emphasized the great difficulty in distinguishing early phases of GVHD

from viral hepatitis. Even some apparent quantitative differences, such as more prominent acidophilic bodies and parenchymal inflammation in viral hepatitis, may actually reflect the degree of immunologic reconstitution or immunosuppressive treatment for GVHD, rather than true qualitative and pathogenic differences from viral hepatitis. Some acute hepatitides also have marked bile ductule proliferation and cholestatic features. Others have reported cholestasis and bile duct alterations in chronic active hepatitis consisting of hyperplasia, atypia, swelling, vacuolization, inflammatory cells within the duct wall, and necrosis.[509,581] The possibility of NANB hepatitis is also very worrisome since there are no serologic markers and 25–50% of infections may continue for at least 1 year.[45,295] Even patients developing acute hepatitis several

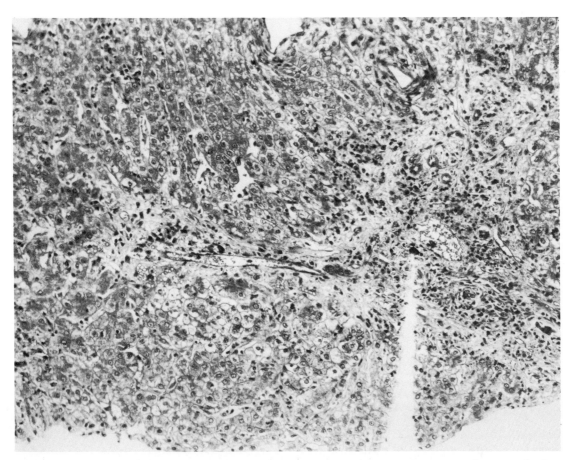

**Figure 22.** (UPN 773 day 200) Liver biopsy in patient with *de novo* late onset of extensive chronic GVHD beginning after day 100. Prominent portal-to-portal bridging, collapse, piecemeal necrosis, spotty parenchymal inflammation, and lobular unrest. Bile ductule proliferation with dropout of interlobular bile ducts adjacent to arterioles.

months after conditioning chemotherapy may be experienccng an acute exacerbation of chronic HBV infection.[297]

## CMV hepatitis

The histologic appearance of CMV hepatitis (i.e., multiple foci of hepatocellular necrosis, prominent parenchymal mononuclear cell inflammation, and portal inflammation with lymphocytes and immunoblasts) is little different from those of other viral hepatitides, including Epstein-Barr virus infection.[500] The sine qua non of CMV hepatitis is identifying the characteristic brick-red Cowdry type A, intranuclear and intracytoplasmic inclusion bodies on H&E-stained sections. The viral inclusions are usually found in bile duct epithelium or hepatocytes but may be in Kupffer cells or endothelium. The histologic

diagnosis of CMV hepatitis is usually difficult to prove after marrow transplantation; intranuclear inclusions are rarely found unless multiple blocks and levels are examined (Fig. 19*b*). Our impressions were confirmed by Hutton et al. who evaluated the utility of histology in the diagnosis of suspected CMV hepatitis in 43 patients with systemic CMV infections, 90% of whom had abnormal liver function tests. In fact, only 3 of 43 had histologic inclusions of CMV even though cultures were negative, while another 10 without inclusions did culture CMV.[301] CMV hepatitis has also been reported with massive hepatic necrosis with multiple intranuclear inclusions or as a granulomatous hepatitis.[69,108] We have never seen these features, however, in over 400 autopsies of marrow transplant recipients, all of whom had viral cultures of the liver.

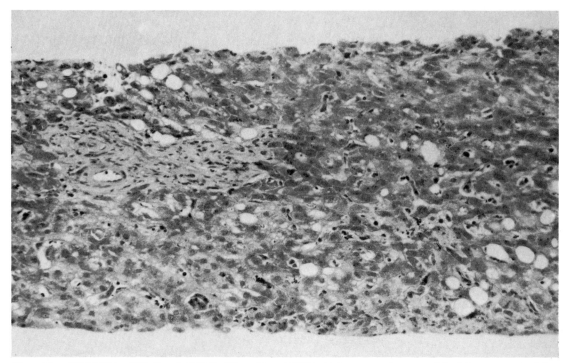

**Figure 23.** (UPN 567 day 324) Chronic GVHD of liver. Liver GVHD with hepatocyte disarray and focal dropout persisted for 10 months while receiving prednisone. Portal triad shows an artery and dropout of adjacent bile duct.

For several years, a controversy existed over whether the putative bile duct changes of GVHD were, in fact, secondary to CMV hepatitis. From an epidemiologic point of view, it has been difficult to exclude CMV as the cause of liver dysfunction or anicteric hepatitis due to the 50–60% frequency of systemic CMV infections among allogeneic recipients.[436] This is particularly true at autopsy, at which time a high percentage of patients dying as a result of systemic GVHD or CMV pneumonia frequently have the virus cultured from or identified in the lungs and other viscera. Finally, neonatal hepatitis from CMV[210] or reovirus infection[447] have been implicated as a cause of biliary atresia. Beschorner et al.[51] addressed the relationship of CMV and bile duct lesions in a coded study by quantifying the extent of hepatocytic necrosis and bile duct injury in four groups of patients: those with CMV with or without marrow transplants, those with marrow transplants with only GVHD, and those with marrow transplants with GVHD and CMV. As in any such study, the definitions of GVHD and CMV was somewhat problematic, since not all patients had multiple organ biopsies to document GVHD or had culture and histologic proof of

CMV. Nonetheless, this study demonstrated that the bile duct abnormalities occurred in all patients with either GVHD or CMV, or with both. More important, patients with GVHD had more extensive and qualitatively different bile duct lesions than those observed in patients with CMV infections.

Because of the profound state of immunosuppression in marrow transplant recipients, they are susceptible to unusual forms of hepatitis from varicella zoster, herpes simplex, and adenovirus. These latter hepatitides have enlarged, multilobular zones of coagulative necrosis and cytopathically altered cells containing enlarged, smudgy basophilic nuclei at the edge of the infarct (Fig. 25). Identification of the specific viral infection usually requires immunofluorescent studies and/or viral cultures. On occasion, we have seen a marked lymphoproliferative reaction in the portal triads of patients with systemic viral infections in whom liver viral cultures were negative and no inclusions were found. Similar histologic findings were noted in five of 43 patients with suspected CMV hepatitis reported by Hutton et al.[301]

One additional unusual form of viral hepatitis

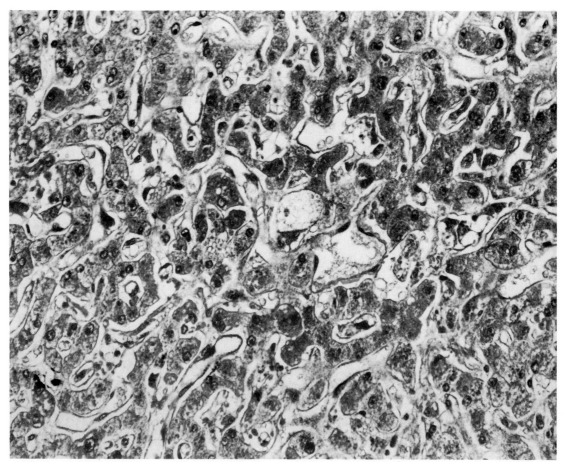

**Figure 24.** (UPN 1213 day 34) Case of suspected CYA hepatotoxicity with hyperbilirubinemia and no findings of VOD, GVHD, or hepatitis. Mild centrilobular disarray of individual hepatocyte degeneration and necrosis. (Gomori's trichrome.)

may be encountered with the Papoviruses, including the BK and JC groups belonging to the polyoma virus genus. O'Reilly et al.[483] have reported that otherwise unexplained transient hepatic dysfunction and elevations of SGOT, LDH, and alkaline phosphatase occurred between days 12–30 in seven of 16 patients with Papoviruria. Unfortunately, this does not exclude elevations of these tests secondary to septicemia, hyperalimentation, MTX, VOD, or drug-liver injury.

### Fungal disease

Disseminated fungal disease remains a problem in marrow transplant recipients, especially in the first month after grafting when there is profound granulocytopenia.[174,752] The incidence of fungal sepsis in these patients has declined in recent years, probably in relation to decontamination/ isolation protocols and early use of amphotericin

for unexplained fever. Many patients with deep fungal infections are without obvious signs or symptoms other than persistent fever unresponsive to antibiotics. The liver is commonly involved in such cases and may be the only organ infected.[323] Through 1981, fungal liver abscesses were found in 6% of Seattle autopsied marrow recipients. *Candida* organisms may populate the intestine, especially in patients treated with antibiotics, and probably seed the portal circulation, either by invasion of diseased intestine or by passsing through the normal intestine as yeast forms.[193,363,457,625]

Liver lesions range from microscopic granulomas to microabscesses to large cystic lesions to fungus balls in the biliary tree.[404] Persistent fever, liver tenderness, and alkaline phosphatase elevations are usually found. Ultrasound or CT scan imaging may show multiple lesions.[68,99]

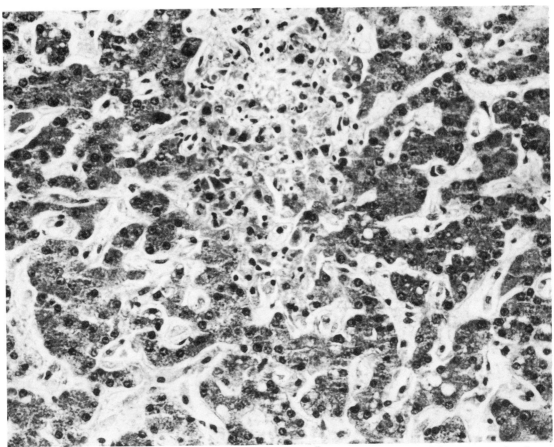

**Figure 25.** (UPN 1405 day 94) Adenovirus hepatitis confirmed by culture has randomly distributed discrete zones of confluent lytic necrosis. Cytopathically altered cells with enlarged hyperchromatic nuclei lie along edge of lesion. In contrast, hepatitis with herpes simplex or zoster produces more coagulative necrosis.

Percutaneous fine-needle aspiration, guided by imaging, may provide a diagnosis without resorting to laparotomy or high-risk liver biopsy.[68] The fungal organisms are usually *Candida* species, with *C. albicans* and *tropicalis* the most common. The other major fungal pathogen, *Aspergillus* species, runs a much more fulminant course, with the diagnosis of fungal liver disease often not made until autopsy.

**Bacterial infections**

Despite intestinal immunodeficiency and liver injury associated with GVHD, post-transplant bacterial infections (abscess, cholangitis) of the liver are surprisingly uncommon in our experience. The frequent use of broad-spectrum antibiotics for fever might explain this. However, a cholestatic jaundice due to remote bacterial infections, especially from Gram-negative organisms, may be occurring.[768] Elevations of serum alkaline phosphatase[196] and mild elevations of SGOT may also occur. This extrahepatic cause of liver dysfunction, though rarely serious, is of practical importance because of possible confusion with VOD, GVHD, or other drug-liver injury.

Fortunately, such infection-related jaundice can usually be distinguished from GVHD by clinical evidence of septicemia, positive blood cultures, and alkaline phosphatase less than two times normal. Likewise, the histology can usually be distinguished from GVHD since there is only a nonspecific reactive hepatitis with hepatocellular cholestasis, ballooning, patchy necrosis, and Kupffer-cell hyperplasia. Lefkowitz has reported that systemic infections may sometimes produce severe intrahepatic cholestasis with periportal bile thrombi resembling the picture of prolonged hepatic GVHD. However, unlike GVHD, such infection-related cholestasis has normal-appearing and normal numbers of small bile ducts, a moderate neutrophilic infiltrate in the triads, and less parenchymal canalicular cholestasis.[377]

## BILIARY DISEASE

Biliary disease, ascending cholangitis, or fungal infection of the gallbladder, in our experience, is rather rare in marrow transplant patients. However, two patients who received high-dose cytosine arabinoside (Ara-C) as part of the preconditioning therapy developed the picture of acalculus cholecystitis. Both had point tenderness in the RUQ, gallbladder enlargement, and hyperbilirubinemia. At laparotomy, the patients were found to have enlarged, congested gallbladders distended by inspissated bile (sludge). Histologic examination of the gallbladder revealed little inflammation but marked mucosal cytologic atypia, similar to the mucosal changes in the colon after high-dose Ara-C reported by Slavin et al.[594] It is possible that mucosal changes led to altered bile composition or to swelling and obstruction of the cystic duct. However, a number of other factors can also produce gallbladder dilatation and stasis and have been implicated in

acalculus cholecystitis.[101,327] These include multiple transfusions, dehydration, septicemia, gastrointestinal ileus, and analgesia-induced spasm of Oddi's sphincter. PN may be another factor since gallbladder dilatation and stasis occur when no stimuli for gallbladder contraction comes from the intestine, as when the patient receives all nutrition intravenously.[504]

## CONCLUSION

Many different liver diseases occur after bone marrow transplantation. Diagnosis depends on analysis of the clinical presentation, the timing and pattern of abnormalities of liver tests, serology for viruses, imaging tests, and liver histology. Table 1 summarizes the causes of transplant-related liver disease, organized by chronology and frequency of occurrence.

## ADDENDUM

Tutscka et al. have recently described centrilobular hemorrhagic necrosis after Cyclosporine A, confirming the observations of several other groups that Cyclosporine A can be a centrilobular hepatotoxin (see Drug-Liver Injury section above. (*Blood* **61**: 318–325, 1983.)

Snover et al. have recently published an important coded histologic study which reviewed 32 liver biopsies from patients felt to have hepatic acute or chronic GVHD and 64 nonbone marrow transplant biopsies. The latter included biopsies of patients with pretransplant liver dysfunction, viral hepatitis, extrahepatic obstruction, orthotopic liver allograft rejection, primary biliary cirrhosis, chronic hepatitis, CMV hepatitis, and inflammatory bowel disease.

The findings of extensive bile duct with minimal inflammatory changes were relatively specific for GVHD (91% positive predictive value, and 89% negative predictive value). However, there was considerable overlap of changes of GVHD and occasional cases of acute and chronic hepatic and extrahepatic obstruction with a 15% false-positive rate. Endotheliasis (luminal adherence of lymphocytes to central venous and/or portal vein endothelium) was highly specific for GVHD or liver allograft rejection, but present in only 40% of GVHD cases. (Snover et al.: *Hepatology* **4**: 127–130, 1984.)

**TABLE 1**

Frequency of Liver Diseases with Marrow Transplantation

|  | Common | Less Common |
|---|---|---|
| Pretransplant | Viral hepatitis<br>Malignancy | Drug-liver injury<br>VOD<br>Infection (fungal, bacterial) |
| Day 0–25 | VOD<br>Chemotherapy-related injury | GVHD<br>Viral hepatitis<br>Infection (fungal)<br>PN liver disease<br>Acalculous cholecystitis |
| Day 25–100 | Acute GVHD<br>Persistent VOD<br>Viral hepatitis<br>Drug-liver injury | Infection (fungal)<br>PN disease |
| After day 100 | Chronic GVHD | Viral hepatitis<br>Chronic active hepatitis<br>Cirrhosis<br>Drug-liver injury<br>Persistent VOD |

VOD = venocclusive disease.
GVHD = graft-vs.-host disease.
PN = parenteral nutrition.

# Chapter 8

# The sicca syndrome of GVHD

**George E. Sale, M.D.**

## Introduction

The emergence of a sicca syndrome as a clearly disease-specific feature of graft-vs.-host disease (GVHD) in humans is one of the most interesting developments in the description and pathogenetic understanding of this disease. Workers in the field had known for some time that animals with GVHD exhibited abnormalities of the oral and conjunctival mucosa, but some of these were not readily distinguished from acute or chronic sequellae of irradiation. "Mucositis" is ubiquitous after radiation and chemotherapy at doses commonly given marrow transplant recipients. However, patients with other signs of chronic GVHD rather commonly developed oral dryness, burning, changes in taste and dysphagia. Lichenoid lesions appeared on the palate, buccal mucosa, and tongue, and rather marked mucosal atrophy ensued. Many showed angular cheilitis. Nasal mucosa suffered similar dryness and atrophy with frequent epistaxis.

## ORAL PATHOLOGY

Histology of the oral structures revealed lesions in the stratified squamous epithelium in acute GVHD nearly identical to those in the epidermis. In the chronic phase, histology was that of a classical lichenoid reaction with moderately dense infiltrates of lymphocytes admixed with plasma cells. Minor and major salivary glands showed chronic periductular inflammatory reactions (Fig. 1–5).

The lip biopsy had previously been used extensively by many investigators to diagnose and follow Sjögren's syndrome. The application of this technique to chronic GVHD was a logical step and was first reported by Gratwohl et al.[262] and Lawley et al.[374] They reported four patients with chronic GVHD who had sicca syndrome and chronic inflammatory infiltrates of the minor salivary glands in biopsy tissue of the lip. The severity of the symptoms paralleled that of chronic GVHD, and the patients all had hypergammaglobulinemia.

The pathology of Sjögren's syndrome or Mikulicz' disease was systematically described in 1953 by Morgan and Castleman [448] who emphasized the lymphoplasmacytic infiltrates and the destruction of salivary ductules and acini. Islands of myoepithelial cells, which normally are in the basal layers of acini and ducts, were seen isolated in the connective tissues of the edematous and fibrotic interstitium of these major glands. The study of minor salivary glands in the lip and even nasal mucosa biopsy have been used to advantage in the diagnosis and follow-up of clinical disease.[134,510] Cummings reported a simple and reproducible 4-tiered histologic grading system for the salivary gland lesions of Sjögren's syndrome in 1971. This is based primarily on degree of lymphoid infiltrate, grade 4 being nearly total effacement and replacement of the glands with

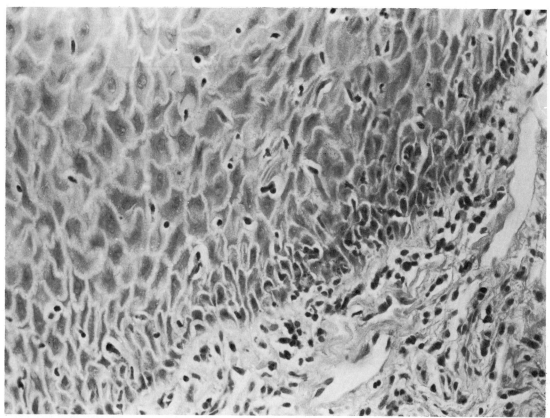

**Figure 1.** (UPN 877) Grade I–II borderline lesion in squamous epithelium of lip from a 20-year-old female allografted for aplastic anemia.

lymphoid infiltrates not uncommonly containing secondary lymphoid follicles (germinal centers). The grade 4 lesion is the histologic setting in which lymphoma is thought to develop, an event of significant frequency in Sjögren's syndrome. Chomette et al.[105] have studied the grading problem further and have discovered that myoepithelial islands, although common in the major salivary glands of patients with Sjögren's syndrome, are absent in minor salivary glands obtained from lip biopsy. They also suggest that lymphoid infiltrates are less consistently reliable in minor as opposed to major salivary glands as a grading criterion, and replace the system of Cummings with one based on the severity of damage and degree of fibrosis of the minor salivary glands.

Sjögren's syndrome is classically described as a triad of keratoconjunctivitis sicca, xerostomia, and rheumatoid arthritis.[63] Only a small percentage of patients with chronic GVHD have arthritis, and therefore these patients do not fit the classical syndrome perfectly. However, the sicca component in Sjögren's syndrome affects more than just the salivary and lacrimal glands. There is evidence that all levels of the respiratory tract, including even the eustachian tubes, are affected, as mucosal dryness and periglandular and periductular mononuclear cell infiltrates have been described at most levels of respiratory mucosa. This hyposecretion of mucus and the resulting increase in secretion viscosity probably contribute significantly to the ear and bronchial infection rates in both Sjögren's syndrome and chronic GVHD victims. Similarly, dryness of genital mucosa, probably also due to chronic inflammation of mucosal glands in both situations, results in an increased incidence of dyspareunia, web formation, and minor genitourinary tract infections.[63,129,584,653] The increased incidence of lymphoma in Sjögren's syndrome is paralleled by that in mice with GVHD[240] and possibly in hu-

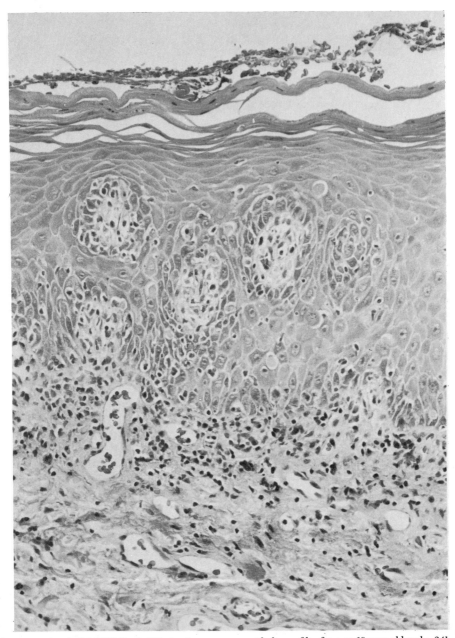

**Figure 2.** (UPN 1098) Grade II lesion in squamous epithelium of lip from an 18-year-old male, 341 days after allograft for acute nonlymphocytic leukemia. Note exocytosis, eosinophilic bodies, slight parakeratosis, and dilated vessels.

mans with GVHD, since some cases have already been reported after marrow transplantation. However, a clear relationship of the human cases to GVHD is not established.

To diagnose stomatitis and sialadenitis differentially after bone marrow transplantation re-

quires that the pathologist number radiation, chemotherapy, and superinfections, at the very least, among etiologic agents. As reported in many different animal models,[102,183–185,247,248] radiation at doses as low as 1200 rad produces damaging effects on salivary glands lasting many

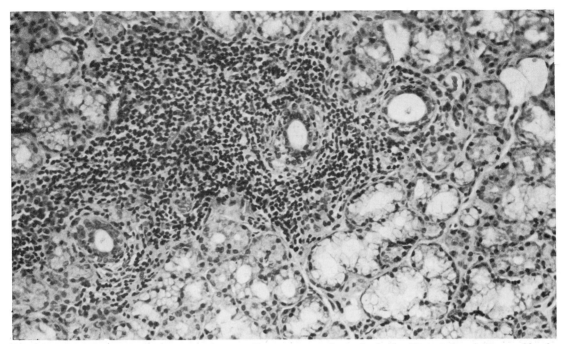

**Figure 3.** (UPN 815) Unusually intense lymphocytic infiltrate in minor salivary gland of lip. Biopsy is that of a 26-year-old male 4 years after allograft for aplastic anemia. Three ducts show varying degrees of invasion and destruction of epithelium by lymphoid cells.

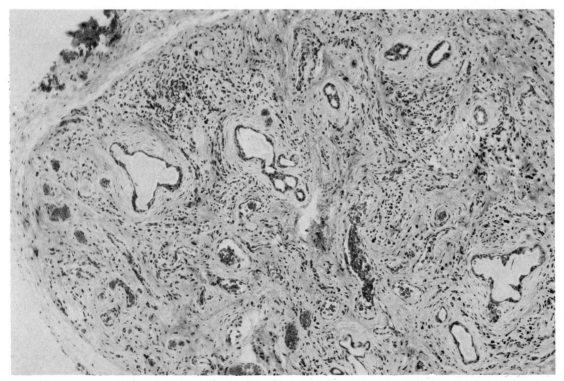

**Figure 4.** (UPN 568) Fibrotic lobule of minor salivary gland undergoing obliteration from a 28-year-old male transplanted for aplastic anemia. Ectatic ducts, interstitial fibrosis, residual lymphocytic infiltrates, and involvement of the entire lobule characterize specimen.

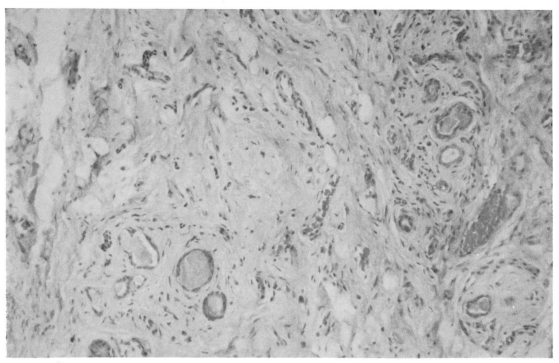

**Figure 5.**   (UPN 294) Dense fibrosis of minor salivary gland from lip of a 40-year-old, 4 years after graft for aplasia. (From Sale et al.[548]; reproduced with permission.)

weeks. The general pathology in the first week is that of acute destruction with inflammation. Total body irradiation (TBI) at doses of 600–1750 rad uniformly produces transient mucositis of the mouth and the entire gastrointestinal tract, as well as acute sialadenitis and pancreatitis manifested by amylasemia lasting 2 days or longer. Similar effects occur with most radiomimetic and other cytotoxic drugs, especially at high doses or in combination with radiation or with each other. Therefore, as with the skin and early liver changes, diagnostic acumen is low until the acute effects of such agents resolve. Furthermore, superinfection occurs frequently upon the compromised oral and conjunctival mucosa of these patients. Careful attention to data from viral, bacterial, and fungal cultures and smear morphology and serology will usually allow recognition of such superinfections.

Because of the above difficulties, and in order to devise better early diagnostic tests for chronic GVHD, our colleagues began systematically to study patients at about 100 days and 1 year after marrow transplantation, using multiple immunologic tests and studies of skin, oral, and other

biopsies, such as esophagus and liver when indicated by disease. The histological contribution to this effort was an attempt to devise criteria on lip and skin biopsies whose predictive value, sensitivity, and specificity for chronic GVHD, defined by eventual development of the recognizable systemic syndrome, could be described quantitatively. Sets of criteria were devised, tested in coded studies, and then analyzed using the predictive value statistical model as well as by means of statistical association of the various criteria with the disease.

Substratifications regarding such variables as radiation and time after transplant were also informative features of this analysis. The results of our first study of 115 lip biopsies from 84 patients, lacrimal tissue from 22 autopsies, and minor salivary glands from 31 patients with and without chronic GVHD were recently reported.[548] We devised two thresholds of severity, termed grade I and grade II, for the histology in mucosal and glandular tissues. It was evident early that Cummings' grading system for Sjögren's syndrome would not be appropriate since very few patients had more than grade I–II lymphoid infiltrates by that system, and since the primary lesion in the glands was lymphocytic infiltration and destruction of small ducts.

We used, therefore, a system very closely analogous to that which we have devised for the epidermal, esophageal, biliary duct, and colonic crypt epithelium, because the lesions are similar and the description aptly transfers between systems. Thus, we could use a grade I–II system for all four relevant epithelial targets: squamous oral mucosa, salivary duct, conjunctival epithelium, and lacrimal duct. Grade I was lymphocytic infiltration of the oral mucosa, conjunctiva, or ducts of salivary or lacrimal glands. Grade II required Grade I changes plus epithelial cell necrosis or "apoptosis" in each of these epithelia. Both grades were strongly associated with the development of chronic GVHD. Depending on the site and stratification of patient, the grade I criteria showed sensitivity of 80–86% and specificity ranging from 50 to 56%. Grade II criteria were 50–72% sensitive and 68–77% specific. Both acute and chronic GVHD showed strong statistical associations with grade II lesions in the surface ($p = 0.0002$) and salivary gland ($p = 0.0013$). A history of TBI showed no significant association with these lesions. Surface and gland involvement in the lip were 88–92% in agreement with each other. A slight clouding effect of a history of irradiation on the predictive value and association was suggested, which effect decreased over time. Subsequent detailed testing of these criteria on even larger numbers of patients has produced preliminary data lending strong support to the conclusions of our original histologic study.[654]

Studies of the saliva of human marrow transplant recipients with and without GVHD have been reported by Izutsu et al.[304–306] These show a significantly decreased salivary sodium and immunoglobulin A (IgA) in GVHD victims. Decreased flow rates and albumin concentrations were found in the patients with chronic GHVD. The data could not be explained by simple transudation across a damaged mucosal barrier. They instead suggest primary damage to the epithelial cells responsible for the handling of sodium and other electrolytes and are very similar to data reported in Sjögren's syndrome by Mandel and Baurmash.[407] The significant depression of salivary IgA may directly relate to the immunodefi-

ciency to bacteria exhibited by patients with chronic GVHD, particularly in the mouth, upper respiratory tract and bronchi. As in the case of scleroderma,[410] the incidence of dental disease, particularly caries and periodontitis, is high in chronic GVHD. A recent study showed a paucity of IgA-bearing plasma cells in the gut sections of allografted patients as compared to those of syngeneically grafted patients, with a further decrease in the allografted patients with GVHD.[53] These studies tend to support the idea that a general mucosal IgA deficiency is present in allograft recipients, which may be caused by the GVHR.

## OPHTHALMIC PATHOLOGY

Serious ocular sicca was also noticed in chronic GVHD patients.[582] An increase, then a gradual decrease, of lacrimation occurred, followed by profound dryness (xerophthalmia). Positive Schirmer's tests which measure decreased tear flow are very predictive for chronic GVHD. The usual sequellae of ophthalmic sicca occur, including keratoconjunctivitis sicca and herpes infections.[307–308] Cytomegalovirus infections of the conjunctiva also occur.

Our initial study also analyzed the predictive value, specificity, sensitivity, and statistical association of aggressor lymphocyte lesions of the lacrimal glands and conjunctiva (Figs. 6–12).[548] Grade II lacrimal lesions showed a strong association with GVHD ($p = 0.0013$) with 87% sensitivity, 88% specificity, and a 93% predictive value. The conjunctival lesions of grade II GVHD showed an 89% specificity, but the association with GVHD was not statistically significant based on 20 patients. An expanded study of 32 patients now shows a statistically significant association of grade II conjunctivitis with GVHD ($p = 0.01$) with sensitivity 61%, specificity 93%, and predictive value 92% (Table 1). Based on these studies, Table 2 lists grade I ("consistent") and grade II ("diagnostic") criteria for oral and ophthalmic GVHD.

In rats, the limbus but not the cornea appears to be involved in GVHD.[54] In humans, the cornea does not appear to be a primary target site for GVHD, although it can suffer severe secondary infections and damage due to the dryness.[307,308,548,584,656] Involvement of the limbus by GVHD has been minimal to absent in our

**TABLE 1**
Grade II Conjunctivitis versus Stage II GVHD
at Autopsy in 32 Patients Undergoing
Marrow Transplantation

|  | GVHD (Clinical grade II or greater) | |
|---|---|---|
|  | + | − |
| Conjunctivitis + | 11 | 1 |
| (Grade 2) − | 7 | 13 |

18  14  32
$p = 0.01$ by one-tailed $Chi^2$ test
Sensitivity 61%
Specificity 93%
Predictive value 92% (of positive test)

series so far, even in the presence of significant tarsal and conjunctival involvement. The tarsal plate becomes severely scarred in many of these patients. Evidence from our small study of complete tarsal plates obtained at autopsy seems to confirm the prediction[307] that the adenoid layer as well as the accessory lacrimal glands are damaged in GVHD. We have seen aggressor lymphocyte lesions of the meibomian glands, as well as the glands of Zeis, Moll, Wolfring, and Krause, all components of the tarsal plate (Figures 13–22).

### OTHER SITES

Involvement of other sites has been noted in our studies in small percentages of cases (Fig. 23). We reported bronchopulmonary sicca involvement in tracheal and bronchial tissues from chronic GVHD victims in 1980,[584] but we have not been able to confirm a statistical association of aggressor lymphocyte lesions with acute GVHD in either canine or human patients (Chapter 10).

We have seen involvement of the larger radicles of the biliary tree and of pancreatic ducts in only a few cases of very severe acute GVHD in dogs and humans. The severe chronic pancreatic fibrosis seen in a significant number of canines is almost certainly radiation-induced, as its prevalence and incidence are identical in autografted and allografted dogs. We have also seen involvement of breast glandular epithelium in three patients with GVHD (Figs. 24–29). Breast involvement has been reported in Sjögren's syndrome but can be difficult to distinguish from the common inflammatory lesions of fibrocystic disease of the breast. Our cases show clear evidence, however, of invasion and destruction of epithelial cells, as illustrated. Furthermore, one of the cases occurred in a prepubertal male. However, cellular distortion and some degree of naturally occurring apoptosis may occur in fibrocystic disease, fibroadenoma, and gynecomastia.[3] Therefore, the differentiation of a lesion caused by a GVHR from these entities may be impossible on purely histologic grounds.

### PATHOGENESIS

The unexplained propensity of GVHD to attack epithelial targets, particularly those involving small ductal structures (i.e., those in the eccrine and salivary glands, biliary tree, colonic crypts, breast, lacrimal, pancreatic, and bronchopulmonary mucosal glands) has stimulated the imaginations of many authors. It is important to distinguish analogies from identities, however, and speculation should be read with this in mind. For example, Epstein et al.[186] have drawn an analogy between chronic GVHD and primary biliary cirrhosis (PBC), which they term a "dry

**TABLE 2**
Oral and Ophthalmic Histologic Criteria for GVHD

|  | Squamous Mucosa of Lip or Mouth | Ducts of Salivary or Lacrimal Gland | Conjunctiva and Tarsal Plate |
|---|---|---|---|
| "Consistent" lesion: | Basal vacuolar degeneration with mononuclear infiltrates | Abnormal periductal mononuclear infiltrates | Mononuclear cell infiltration |
| "Diagnostic" lesion: | Eosinophilic bodies as in skin | Ductal epithelial cell necrosis, often with dilatation and attenuation or obliteration | Basal cell necrosis in epithelium of conjunctiva or tarsal plate |

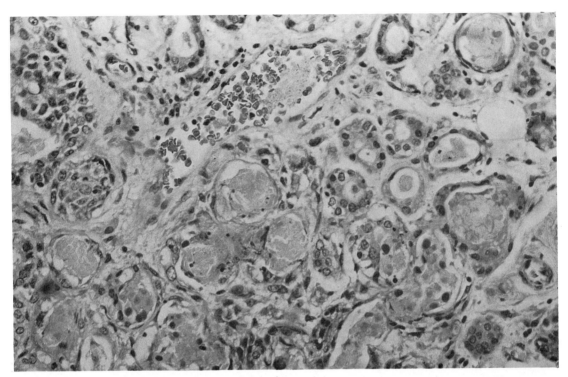

**Figure 6.** Acute lacrimal gland destruction in an 18-year-old white female victim of mismatched lymphoid allograft due to unirradiated transfusions, 23 days following last transfusion and 12 days since onset of severe actue GVHD. Although ducts are most involved, some damage to acini is also present.

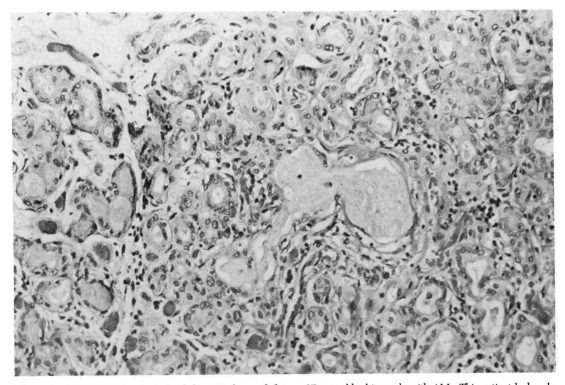

**Figure 7.** (UPN 1547) Lacrimal gland day 102 after graft from a 27-year-old white male with ALL. This patient had early profound sicca syndrome. Note prominent destruction and dilation of ducts.

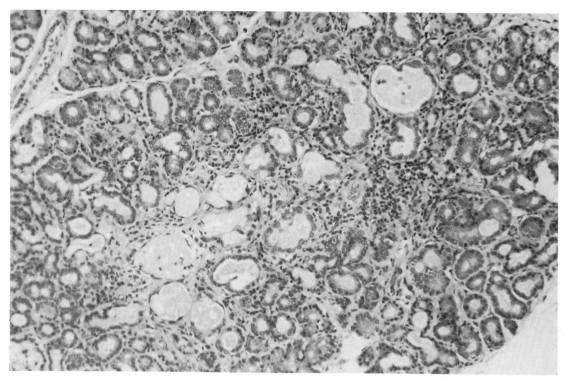

**Figure 8.** (UPN 996) Lacrimal damage in a 15-year-old male, 120 days after first transplant and 54 days after second transplant for aplasia following rejection of first transplant.

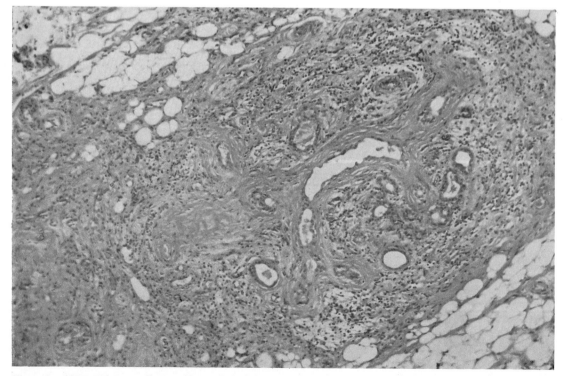

**Figure 9.** (UPN 677) Dense fibrosis of lacrimal gland from a 30-year-old male with chronic GVHD who died 4 years after allograft for lymphoid lymphoma–leukemia.

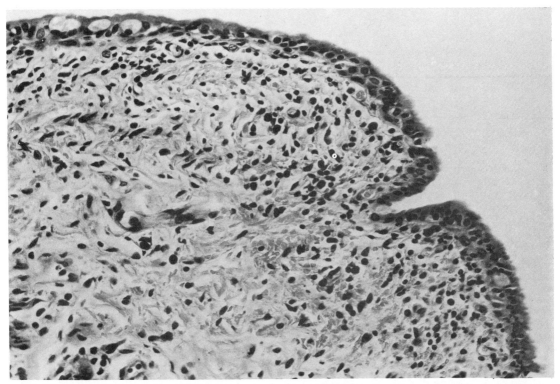

**Figures 10 and 11.** Low-power view of palpebral conjunctiva, day 95 after allograft in 20-year-old male patient with ALL. Prominent lymphoid infiltrate penetrates epithelium; grade I, focal II GVHD.

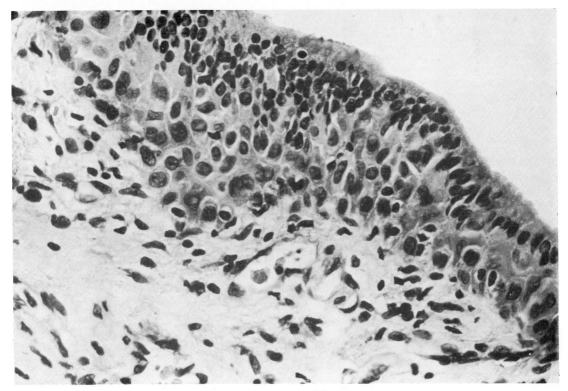

**Figure 11.** Higher power view of the same specimen.

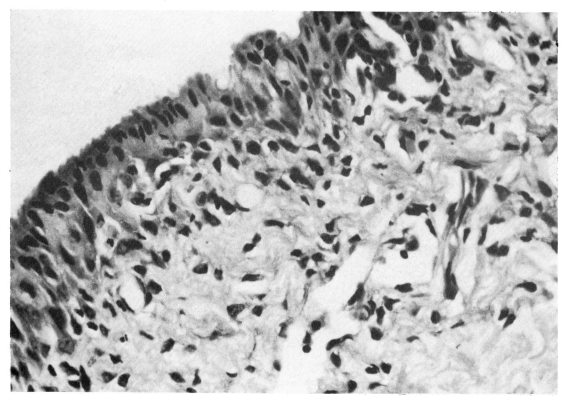

**Figure 12.**   Grade II lesions of conjuctiva in a 28-year-old female day 27 after allograft for CML. Eosinophilic body at left near basal layer of epithelium.

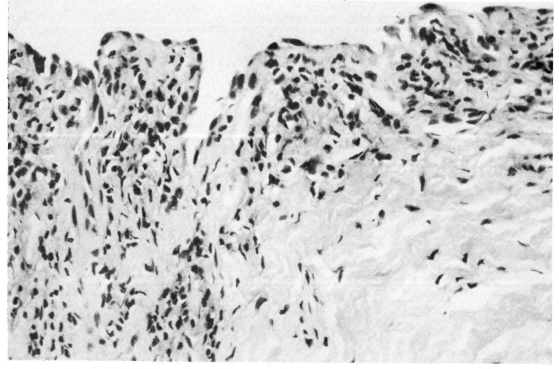

**Figure 13.**   Grade III–IV damage in tarsal plate region of conjunctiva. Specimen from same patient as Figure 12.

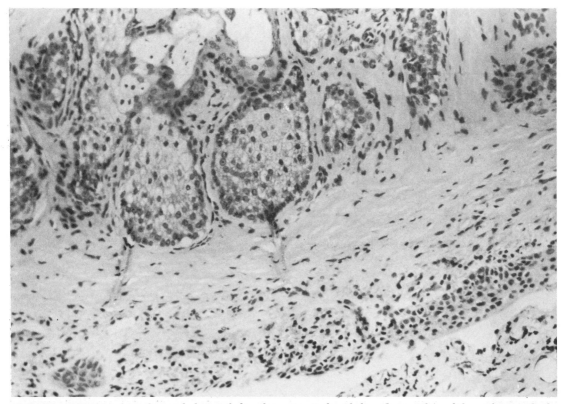

**Figure 14.** GVHD involving the tarsal plate, including the conjunctival epithelium (lower right) and the meibomian glands (upper portion of photo), in white male who died 95 days post allograft for ALL. Specimen from patient UPN 1568.

gland syndrome." Major histocompatibility antigenic differences are emphasized in this hypothesis, whereas most human chronic GVHD patients have received HLA-matched, MLC-compatible bone marrow. The hypothesis would remain tenable if minor histocompatibility differences were invoked, however. The etiologic hypothesis is also advanced here that a GVHR, due to an *in utero* infusion of incompatible maternal lymphoid cells, might be responsible for the development of PBC in later life. This is similar to the etiologic hypothesis of Seemayer for SCID.[575] Unexplained by Epstein's hypothesis are the latency period of two to four decades and the female preponderance of PBC. Resemblances of the hepatic histology in the two have been reported both in animals and humans.[47,519,584]

Cystic fibrosis is another disease bearing some resemblances to chronic GVHD, particularly relating to the abnormalities in mucus secretion and sodium transport in small ducts, but the resemblance is quite superficial. Abnormalities of sodium and mucus secretion in GVHD are clearly secondary to damage induced by the inflammatory processes in these organs. In cystic fibrosis, no initial inflammation of these glandular structures exists, and they are histologically normal before the onset of infection. Examples of involvement of various organs with acute and chronic GVHD analogous to the lesions of natural Sjögren's syndrome in man are illustrated.

## CONCLUSION

Evidence in humans and animals suggests that a sicca syndrome with features quite analogous to those of naturally occurring Sjögren's syndrome are a part of GVHD. Evidence available to date suggests that these lesions are separable from secondary effects of irradiation, chemotherapy, or infection, and that there is an immunologically mediated attack on the epithelium of the small ducts of the salivary, lacrimal, and minor seromucous glands of the respiratory tree. Suggestive additional evidence is presented for involvement of the breast, tarsal plate structures, and genitourinary tract.[129]

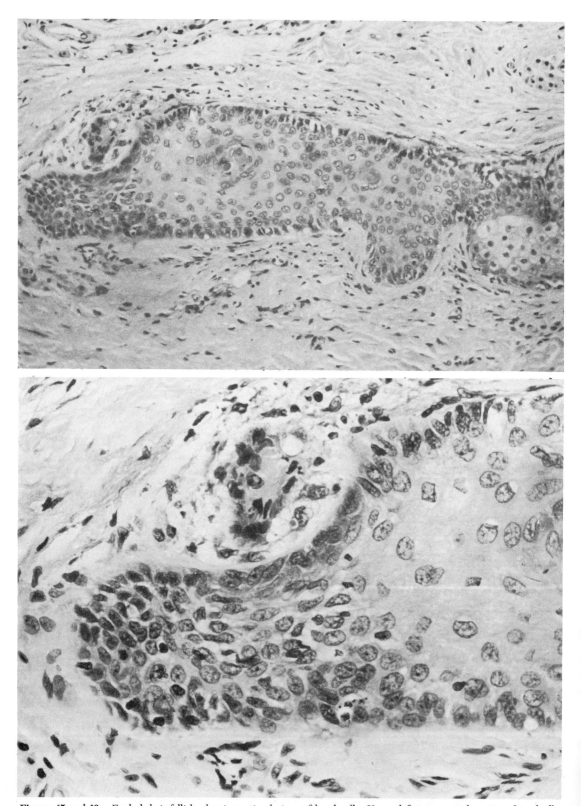

**Figures 15 and 16.** Eyelash hair follicle showing active lesions of basal cells. Upper left is tangential section of markedly involved bulb base. Higher-power view of same eyelash bulb showing active necrosis. Specimen from patient UPN 1568.

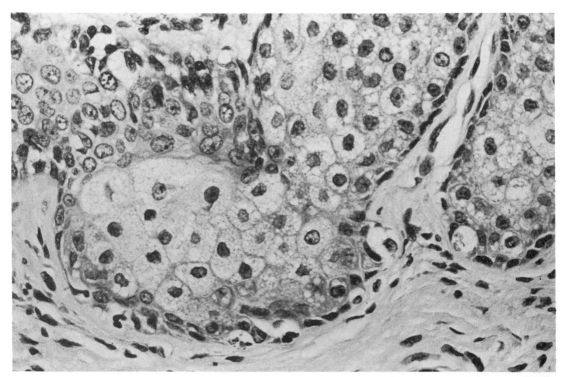

**Figure 17.** Focus of basal cell sebaceous (meibomian) gland involvement showing necrosis of individual cells (lower middle, right middle). Specimen from patient UPN 1568.

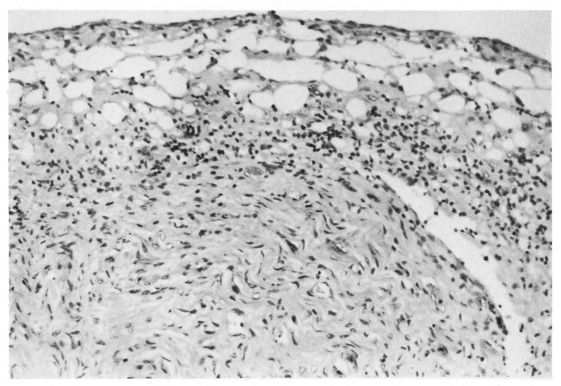

**Figure 18.** Severe meibomian gland involvement with blurring of border between sebaceous epithelium and connective tissue. Specimen from patient UPN 1568.

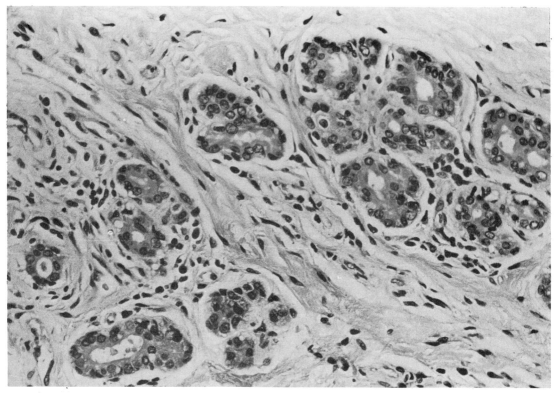

**Figure 19.**    Accessory lacrimal gland (of Krause) in tarsal plate showing invasive and destructive lesions of the ducts. Specimen from patient UPN 1568.

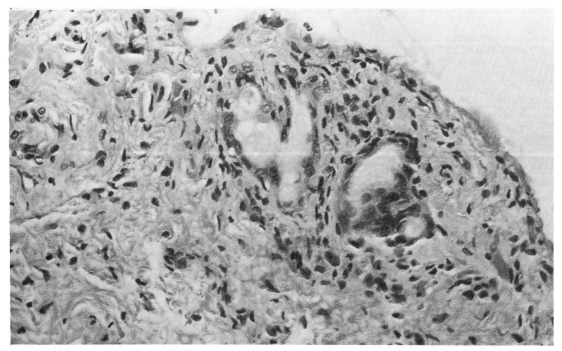

**Figure 20.**    Severe sicca in 27-year-old male on day 101. Glands of Moll (accessory sweat glands near eyelash follicle of tarsal plate) are involved with invasive destructive lesions of GVHD as were other areas in this patient's tarsal plate, mouth, skin, and liver. Specimen from patient UPN 1547.

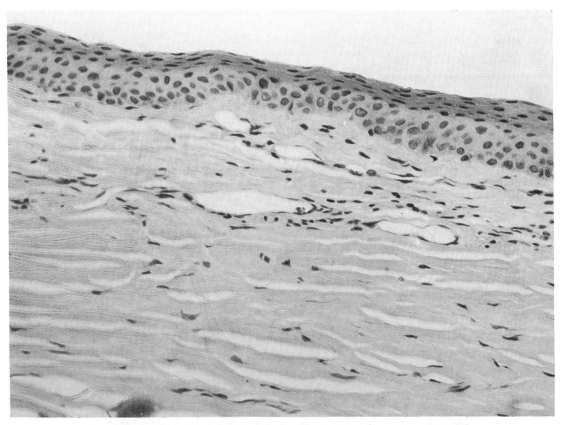

**Figure 21.** Limbus without significant abnormality. Specimen from patient UPN 1547.

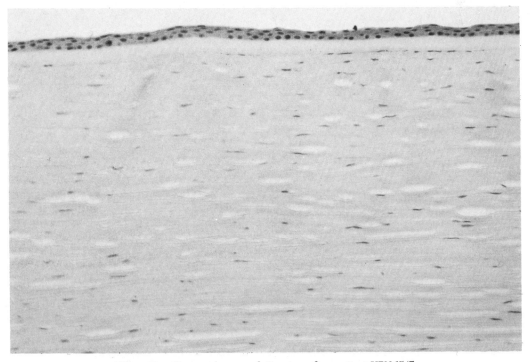

**Figure 22.** Cornea, also normal. Specimen from patient UPN 1547.

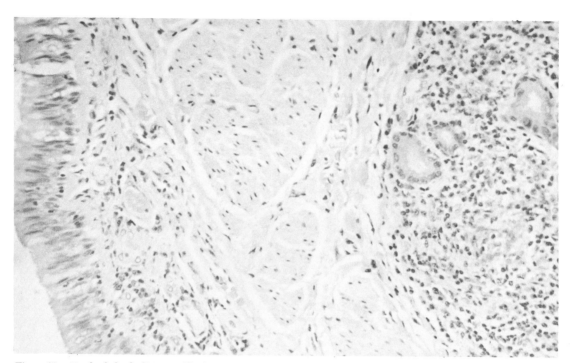

**Figure 23.**    Tracheal gland of 14-year-old white male dying with chronic GVHD, 18 months after allograft for aplastic anemia. The surface epithelium is nearly undisturbed, but there is intense lymphoplasmacytic infiltrate of the mucosal gland and ductal destruction. Specimen from patient UPN 717.

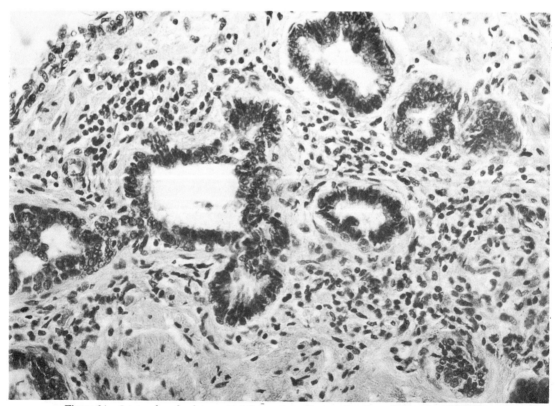

**Figure 24.**    Intense lymphoplasmacytic inflammation of breast. Specimen from patient UPN 717.

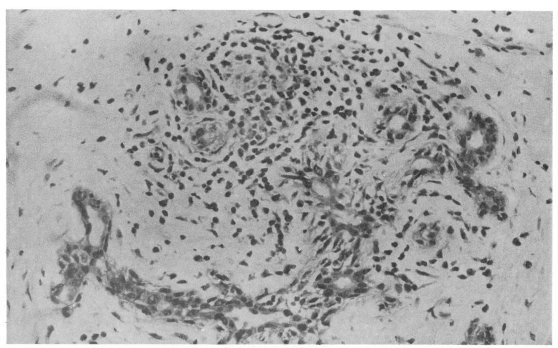

**Figure 25.** A 19-year-old female allografted for AML exhibited invasive and destructive breast epithelial lesions. Ductular epithelium invaded by lymphocytes. Specimen from patient UPN 717.

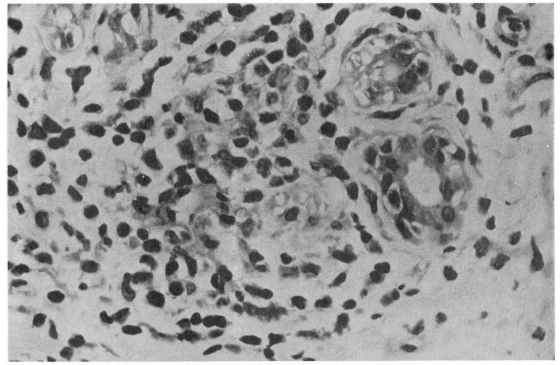

**Figure 26.** Higher-power view of breast lesion in same patient. These observations suggest that breast epithelium is a target in GVHD. Similar changes have been reported in Sjögren's syndrome. Differential diagnosis includes ordinary fibrocystic disease. Specimen from patient UPN 717.

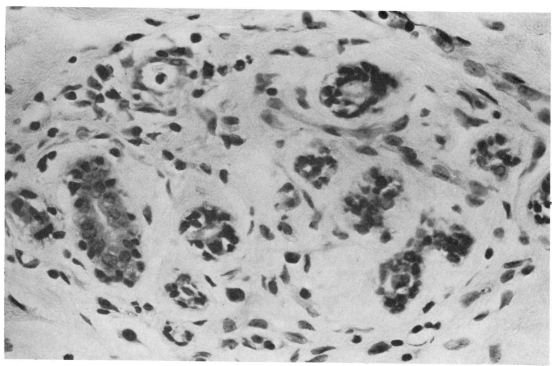

**Figure 27.**   Breast lesion from a 28-year-old female allografted for ANL. Lymphocytes invade and destroy epithelium. Specimen from patient UPN 1114.

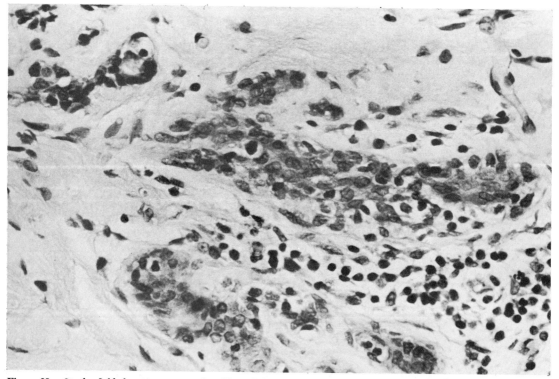

**Figure 28.**   Similar field showing an intensely infiltrated duct, sectioned longitudinally, adjacent to a similar one sectioned transversely. Specimen from patient UPN 1114.

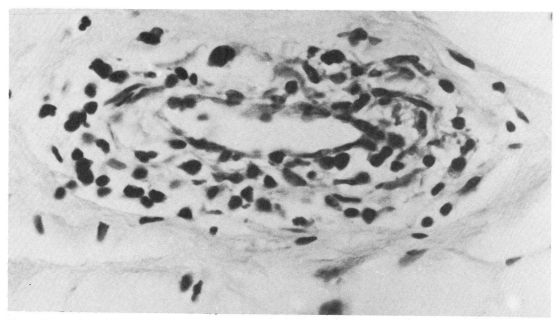

**Figure 29.** Higher-power view of similar breast duct with marked infiltration and destruction of ductal epithelium. There is edema and attenuation of the duct epithelium. Specimen from patient UPN 1114.

# Chapter 9

# Lower respiratory tract

Robert C. Hackman, M.D.

## Introduction

Pneumonia continues to be one of the major complications of bone marrow transplantation. Clinical bacterial pneumonia, defined as a new pulmonary infiltrate accompanied by positive blood or transtracheal cultures, is uncommon. Likewise, the lung biopsy rarely displays acute pneumonia with a significant neutrophilic infiltrate or is culture-positive for bacterial pathogens. In contrast, clinical interstitial pneumonia develops in more than 40% of allograft recipients and has a staggering 75% mortality rate.[440] Histologically, interstitial pneumonia is our most common diagnosis in lung obtained at biopsy and autopsy.

Post-transplant pneumonia may be associated with any commonly pathogenic or opportunistic infectious agent, may consist of pulmonary hemorrhage or neoplastic infiltration, or may be an idiopathic interstitial process. Its treatment should be based on a pathologist's examination of an adequate sample of lung parenchyma, preferably obtained by open lung biopsy. This chapter focuses on idiopathic interstitial pneumonia (IIP) and will include discussion of the possible roles of chemotherapy, irradiation, and GVHD in the development of post-transplant pneumonia. The role of infectious agents will be discussed in Chapter 12.

## OPEN VERSUS TRANSBRONCHIAL LUNG BIOPSY

Techniques of pneumonia diagnosis in immunocompromised patients vary in different centers.[15,311,338,588] It is difficult to make satisfactory comparisons of the published data because of variations in patient populations, in study designs, and in definitions of "diagnosis."

Open lung biopsy has come to be our preferred diagnostic approach despite theoretical disadvantages of general anesthesia and thoracotomy. During the past 12 years, we have performed over 200 open lung biopsies as part of the management of more than 1200 allogeneic and syngeneic graft recipients. Biopsies are performed when possible within 24 hours of the clinical diagnosis of pneumonia manifested by respiratory symptoms and signs, arterial blood gas abnormalities, and radiographic pulmonary infiltrates.

By comparing simultaneous fiberoptic bronchoscopy and transbronchial biopsy (TBB) with thoracotomy and open lung biopsy in 24 patients with diffuse post-transplant pneumonia, we clearly demonstrated the relative insensitivity of TBB. Had it been used alone, we would have missed the diagnoses in two of five patients with Pneumocystis pneumonia and in all of five patients with CMV pneumonia. There were no complications following open lung biopsy. In contrast, three patients developed significant intrabronchial bleeding associated with TBB despite transfusion maintenance of platelet counts above 50,000/mm³.[611] It is true, however, that on rare occasions pneumothorax and life-threatening hemorrhage have developed following open biopsy.

Open biopsy is superior in several ways to operative techniques which do not allow direct examination of the lung and also obtain only small fragments of pulmonary tissue. The specimen can be selected from an area of focal abnormality which may not be appreciated radiographically. The tip of the lingula is avoided. In addition, open biopsy allows the surgeon to obtain definite hemostasis under direct vision, a distinct advantage in patients who are often severely thrombocytopenic.

For the pathologist, the larger open biopsy specimen (approximately 5–6 cm³) greatly increases the opportunity to histologically identify scattered foci of infection with microorganisms such as *Pneumocystis carinii* and CMV. There is also adequate tissue for frozen sections and touch imprints, which often provide us with a diagnosis of CMV pneumonia within 2 or 3 hours of surgery.[585a] Sufficient cultures may be obtained to allow isolation of the many infectious agents which threaten immunocompromised patients. Finally, tissue is available for possible immunohistological studies of infection or immune-mediated damage as well as for ultrastructural analysis.

## PROCESSING OF THE OPEN LUNG BIOPSY SPECIMEN

Studies of the tissue obtained at biopsy focus initially on identification of infectious agents. Techniques must be rapid, sensitive, and specific in order to benefit the patient immediately. The fresh specimen is delivered directly from the surgeon to the pathology laboratory in order to minimize handling artifacts.[94] At any hour of the day, processing by a technician and analysis by a pathologist begin immediately. The specimen is not inflated with fixative because imprints, cultures, a frozen section, and samples for different fixatives are obtained in the laboratory. Frozen sections and touch imprints are fixed in 95% ethanol and stained with hematoxylin and eosin (H&E),

rapid methenamine silver,[405] and Papanicolaou (PAP) stains. PAP fixation and staining are especially helpful for identification of CMV intranuclear inclusions.[585a] In addition, air-dried touch imprints are stained with H&E, rapid methenamine silver, Wright-Giemsa, and Gram stains. This preliminary evaluation indicates the histology and often demonstrates a microorganism. We are now studying the impact of immediate fluorescent antibody staining of lung frozen sections with a panel of mouse monoclonal antibodies to CMV,[251] herpes simplex virus (HSV) types 1 and 2,[252] varicella-zoster virus (VZV), and Chlamydia[623] on the rapidity, sensitivity, and specificity of our preliminary and final pneumonia diagnoses. Additional stains on the permanent sections include PAS, stains for acid-fast organisms, Steiner and Steiner for Legionella, and a Brown and Hopps gram stain. Bacterial, fungal, acid-fast, Pneumocystis and Legionella controls are included. The choice of fixation and staining techniques in different laboratories is influenced by personal preference and experience as well as the nature of the patient population. In an individual case, the number of imprints and sections analyzed with various stains is also a reflection of tissue alterations, such as granulomata and focal necrosis. Tissue is distributed for viral, bacterial, fungal, Mycoplasma and Chlamydia cultures.

An important aspect of the study of pneumonia in these complex cases is the need not only to be comprehensive in the search for multiple microorganisms, but also to anticipate later retrospective studies of possible mechanisms of injury. Small segments of lung parenchyma taken through preliminary processing steps and properly stored have become remarkably valuable as part of a consecutive series of cases which later can be analyzed simultaneously. For instance, we store two specimens in viral transport media and the frozen section block at -70°C, and also begin processing tissue for electron microscopy and for embedding in methacrylate. Examples of such retrospective studies are nucleic acid hybridization to detect viral genetic material, immunopathology studies of immune complex involvement, and both culture and microscopic searches for previously undetected microorganisms. Some of these studies may be unanticipated or technically unfeasible at the time of biopsy.

## BRONCHOPNEUMONIA

We have identified acute pneumonia with a predominantly neutrophilic infiltrate in only 2% of approximately 200 open lung biopsies. This small proportion reflects the effect of multiple influences, including reduced exposure to bacterial pathogens in a protective environment which often includes a laminar airflow facility; use of broad-spectrum antibiotics, both prophylactically and in response to unexplained fever; activation of latent viruses associated with interstitial pneumonia; granulocytopenia with decreased neutrophils available for infiltration but increased susceptibility to bacterial infection; and the capacity of radiation and chemotherapeutic agents to produce interstitial pneumonia. Occasionally, acute bacterial or fungal pneumonia is present at autopsy in a patient with interstitial pneumonia at the time of prior open biopsy. While the underlying interstitial alterations are usually still detectable, the fact that they reflect earlier damage which probably predisposed the lung to a terminal acute inflammation would probably not be appreciated from studying only the autopsy lung. The extensive use of open biopsy diagnosis by the Seattle group may therefore partially account for the high proportion of our pneumonia cases classified as interstitial.

## INTERSTITIAL PNEUMONIA

Clinically, the term "interstitial pneumonia" refers broadly to a syndrome of fever, a poorly productive cough, tachypnea, dyspnea, and hypoxia associated with an infiltrate which is generally diffuse, but in some cases, nodular or segmental. Histologically, interstitial pneumonia emphasizes the predominance of inflammatory alterations in the lung's loose internal supporting tissue, in contrast to the primarily intra-alveolar changes present in acute bacterial pneumonia. The interstitium is a thin, continuous, fibrocellular meshwork surrounding the pulmonary alveolar capillaries, thereby forming the internal substance of the alveolar septa, and also enveloping larger vessels and airways. In normal lung, this narrow zone readily allows diffusion of dissolved gases. In interstitial pneumonia, it is diffusely or focally widened, edematous, infiltrated by inflammatory cells, and sometimes hemor-

rhagic. There may be patchy interstitial fibrosis. The infiltrating cells are predominantly lymphocytes and plasma cells. Smaller numbers of polymorphonuclear leukocytes and eosinophils may be present.

## PATHOLOGY OF ADULT RESPIRATORY DISTRESS SYNDROME

Interstitial pneumonia probably develops from damage to epithelial as well as to endothelial cells. Thus, the alveoli are not spared. Within the same specimen, there may be different stages of injury and various combinations of alveolar epithelial necrosis, intra-alveolar edema and often hemorrhage, hyaline membranes composed of degenerating cells and fibrin, alveolar epithelial hyperplasia as type 2 pneumocytes regenerate, intra-alveolar accumulation of macrophages, and intra-alveolar as well as interstitial fibrosis. These features of interstitial pneumonia are very similar to those of diffuse alveolar damage (DAD). This term has been applied to the pulmonary alterations seen in the adult respiratory distress syndrome (ARDS) and a variety of very similar clinical syndromes characterized by the acute onset of dyspnea associated with diffuse pulmonary infiltrates, decreased lung compliance, severe hypoxemia, and a rapid and often fatal course.[529] The histological features of DAD are nonspecific reflections of pulmonary injury. They can be divided into an early exudative stage with edema and hyaline membranes and a later, often overlapping, proliferative stage with fibrosis.[337,338]

In a high proportion of our cases of interstitial pneumonia, the predominant histological changes are those of DAD. Figure 1 illustrates severe interstitial edema expanding a lobular septum in a patient with IIP biopsied on day 9. The inflammatory infiltrate in these early post-transplant cases is often mild and perivascular in location (Fig. 2). There may also be alveolar exudation and hemorrhage, changes which are often adjacent to blood vessels, as in Figure 3 from another early (day 10) interstitial pneumonia case. Methacrylate sections demonstrated evidence of injury to small- and medium-sized vessels in this lung (Figs. 4 and 5). We have not seen vascular damage or alveolar inflammation associated with the intravascular bone fragments occasionally pres-

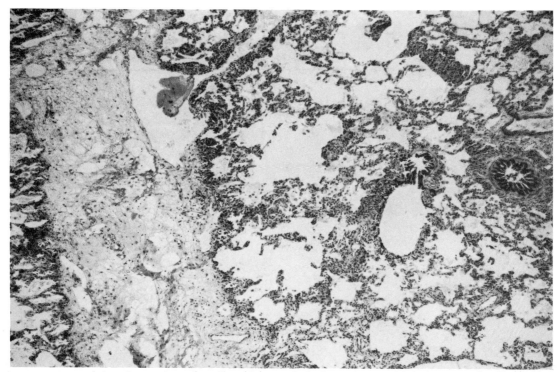

**Figure 1.** An open-lung biopsy obtained on day 9 shows marked edema of an interlobular septum and mild interstitial inflammatory infiltration around vessels and bronchioles. This interstitial pneumonia was idiopathic (IIP).

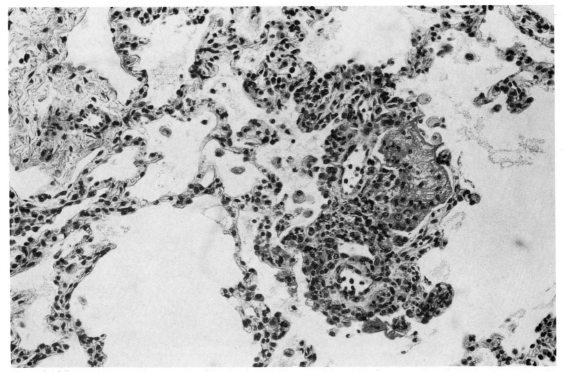

**Figure 2.** The bronchovascular association of the interstitial infiltrate and alveolar exudate is evident in the same biopsy shown in Fig. 1.

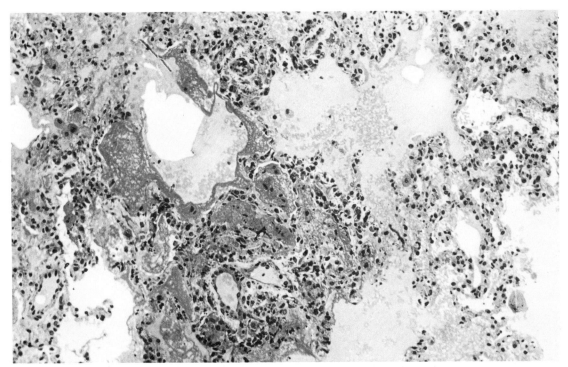

**Figure 3.**    In this day 10 biopsy of IIP, there is a focal interstitial and alveolar exudate associated with vessels and more diffuse pulmonary edema and hemorrhage. Early hyaline membranes were present elsewhere.

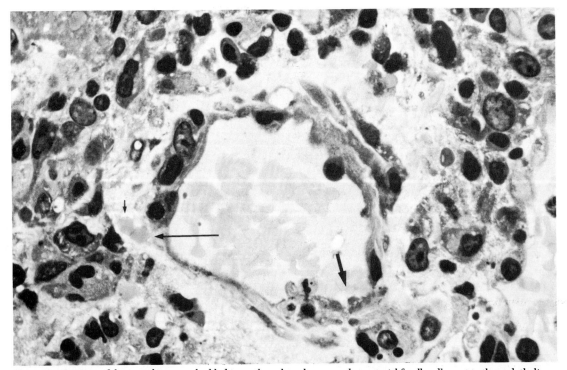

**Figure 4.**    Sections of the same biopsy embedded in methacrylate show granular material focally adherent to the endothelium (large arrow). This may represent endothelial degeneration or early formation of a platelet–fibrin thrombus. On the opposite side of the vessel, there is a subendothelial cluster of mononuclear cells resembling lymphocytes. Erythrocytes (small arrows) extravasate through the edematous vessel wall. (Hematoxylin with Lee, oil-immersion, ×128.)

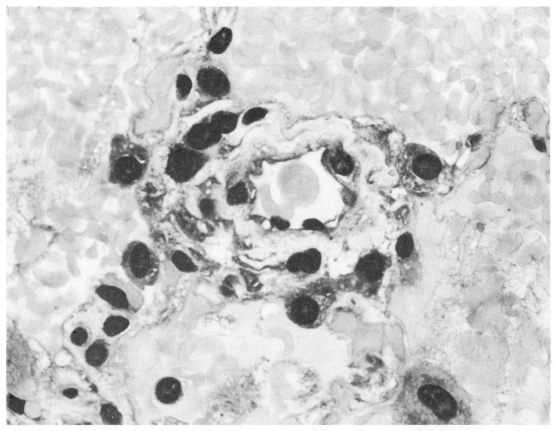

**Figure 5.** Vascular damage in the same biopsy includes endothelial irregularity with lymphocytic infiltration and edema of the vessel wall. Inflammation and edema extend into adjacent alveolar septa (lower left). There is severe hemorrhage. (Hematoxylin with Lee, oil immersion, ×128.)

ent in the lungs of transplant recipients (Fig. 6). In interstitial pneumonia, pulmonary decompensation may be fulminant and rapidly fatal, with the terminal pneumonitis consisting of severe exudative DAD (Fig. 7). With more prolonged inflammation, interstitial and alveolar fibrosis may develop to create a proliferative stage (Figs. 8 and 9).

Because interstitial involvement is the common element associated with the above alterations, and because their various combinations are nonspecific, we use the general descriptive term "interstitial pneumonia." Katzenstein and Askin[338] refer to DAD as an acute interstitial pneumonia in contrast to usual interstitial pneumonitis (UIP), which they describe as chronic. Using their formulation, the typically rapid onset and progression of pneumonia in marrow transplant recipients would be more consistent with an

"acute" process than with a "chronic" pneumonia, such as UIP, which usually begins insidiously and progresses over a period of years.

### IDIOPATHIC INTERSTITIAL PNEUMONIA (IIP)

Our criterion for this diagnosis is the presence of interstitial pneumonia, as described above, without histologic or culture evidence of bacterial, fungal, protozoan, or viral involvement. These cases do not differ significantly from CMV-associated pneumonia clinically, radiographically, or in their time of onset or relationship to conditioning regimens and GVHD. The case-fatality rate is 65%, somewhat lower than the 90% for CMV pneumonia.[440] These similarities with CMV pneumonia suggest an infectious etiology, possibly involving a known microorganism such as polyoma virus, Chlamydia, Epstein-Barr virus

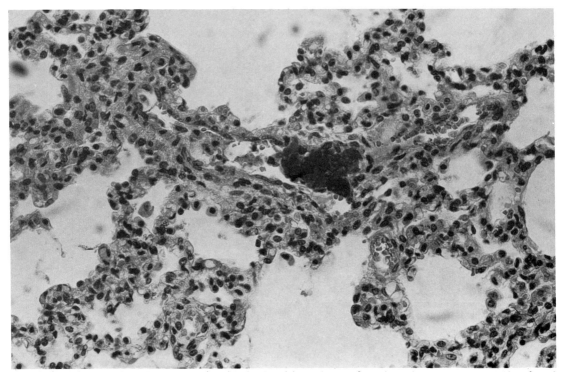

**Figure 6.**    Intravascular bone fragments (center) from the marrow infusion are occasionally present in the lungs as incidental findings. They are unassociated with histological or clinical evidence of pulmonary damage.

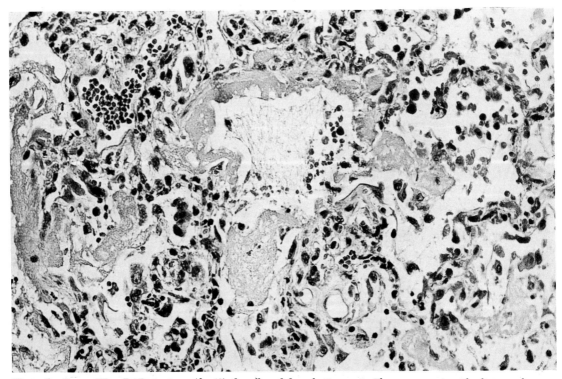

**Figure 7.**    Severe IIP or DAD at autopsy (day 18) after allograft for aplastic anemia. There are prominent hyaline membranes, interstitial infiltration and edema, alveolar epithelial damage, and alveolar exudation.

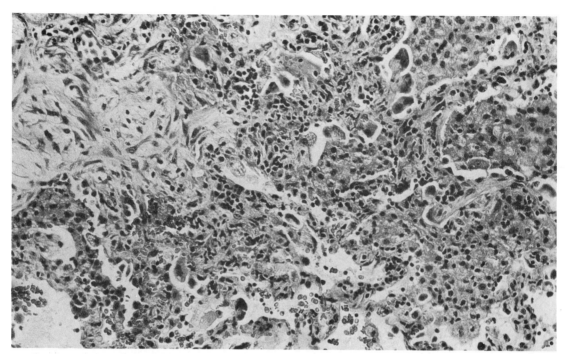

**Figure 8.** In this biopsy from day 54, interstitial and intra-alveolar fibrosis (upper left) is one feature of IIP. Viral inclusions are not present in the scattered large cells. There are many intra-alveolar macrophages. During the subsequent 2 years, this patient intermittently has developed pulmonary infiltrates which then subside.

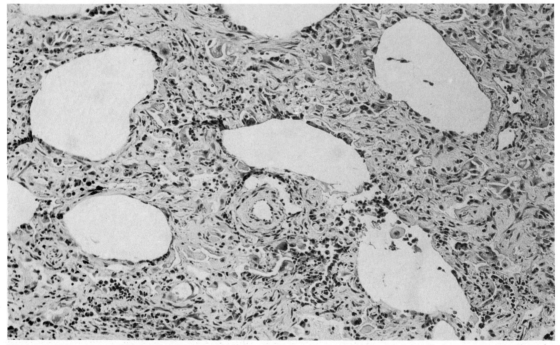

**Figure 9.** More severe fibrosis imparts a honeycomb appearance to this day 75 biopsy of IIP. This patient developed a bilateral interstitial infiltrate on day 49. Serum IgG and IgM microimmunofluorescence titers of antibody to *Chlamydia trachomatis* were negative until day 64, when both converted and remained at 1:32. However, Chlamydia could not be implicated more directly. Cultures as well as fluorescent antibody and routine histological studies of biopsy and autopsy lung demonstrated no organisms.[437]

(EBV), or an unidentified agent analogous to Legionella prior to its characterization. On the other hand, the likelihood of an infectious etiology for IIP is decreased by its lack of association with severe GVHD, since the latter disorder and its treatment are immunosuppressive and associated with a general increase of infectious complications.[439] In addition, we have no direct evidence to implicate infection in the pathogenesis of IIP. The high prevalence of CMV in marrow transplant recipients, as well as the sometimes scanty numbers of diagnostic inclusion-bearing cells in lung biopsy and slow viral growth in cell culture, raises the question of CMV involvement undetected by these conventional techniques. Through use of *in situ* hybridization analysis to detect CMV RNA, we have not found significant differences in lung tissue from marrow recipients with IIP when compared with either transplant recipients without pneumonia or nontransplant controls. In contrast, viral RNA levels are significantly higher in CMV-associated pneumonia in which the virus has been cultured and/or characteristic intranuclear and intracytoplasmic viral inclusions are present.[467] With regard to other known infectious agents, lung cultures for Chlamydia, Mycoplasma, *Legionella pneumophila*, and BK virus as well as cocultivation studies for EBV have been negative.

Inflammatory mechanisms of pulmonary damage are being extensively studied both clinically and in several animal systems[321,563,730] and will not be reviewed here. It is quite possible that pulmonary reactions involving cytotoxic antibody, immune complexes, or cell-mediated drug hypersensitivity may develop in the post-transplant setting. For instance, damage from irradiation may initiate reparative processes such as fibroblast proliferation. These may tend to become irreversible because of imbalances in normal regulatory influences mediated by alveolar macrophages and other cells undergoing replacement from the marrow donor.

We have been unable to document significant pulmonary patterns of immunoglobulin and complement deposition following transplantation (Shulman, unpublished observations). Regarding the current evidence that complement activation and neutrophil aggregation may help initiate ARDS,[321,529,730] it is interesting that several patients have developed characteristic clinical and histological ARDS while profoundly neutropenic (Maunder, Riff, Hackman, Albert, and Springmeyer, unpublished observations). The numbers of circulating granulocytes in these patients were below those described as protective in the prevention of ARDS in experimental animals.[286]

## ROLE OF RADIATION AND CHEMOTHERAPY IN DEVELOPMENT OF PNEUMONIA

The similarities of IIP and CMV-associated interstitial pneumonia mentioned above may actually reflect the common causal influence of physical agents, specifically radiation and cytotoxic drugs, rather than biological ones. Although the etiology of interstitial pneumonia in this complex clinical setting is multifactorial, some of our data implicate the preparative regimen. For example, patients with aplastic anemia conditioned with CY+TBI had a higher incidence than those who received only CY.[439,640] Appelbaum et al.[11] studied IIP in patients transplanted for leukemia by comparing its prevalence in 100 recipients of syngeneic marrow (11%) with that in 351 allogeneic marrow recipients (13%). The preparative regimens of both groups were comparable, usually consisting of CY+TBI. The similar prevalences suggested that IIP is the result of pulmonary toxicity. This evidence was strengthened by the finding that additional chemotherapy given with the standard CY+TBI regimen was an independent risk factor. The only other risk factor in twins was older age, suggesting an age-related increase in susceptibility to pulmonary damage or decrease in reparative capacity.

Experimental animal studies as well as clinical experience in humans have clearly established not only the potential pulmonary toxicity of radiation,[194,270] and many chemotherapeutic agents,[236,747] but also their enhanced combined effects.[169,282,502] Most marrow allograft recipients are given CY in their preparative regimen and methotrexate for subsequent control of GVHD, both drugs with clinically reported pulmonary complications.[109,607] Murine studies have demonstrated an increase in radiation pulmonary toxicity with use of CY.[502] A dose relationship has been described between radiation and fatal pneumonitis in patients given single-dose, half-body, palliative radiotherapy for metastatic carcinoma.[716] The prediction from these data of a 50 and 95% incidence at 930 and 1060 rad, respectively, is much higher than the 11 and 13% incidence of IIP which we have observed in recipients of twin and allograft marrow. This difference probably reflects the toxicity of dose rates of 50–400 rad/minute in comparison to the 7.5 rad/minute of the transplantation regimen.[11] Data pooled from different marrow transplantation centers which use a dose rate of less than 15 rad/minute indicate a dose–response relationship between estimated absorbed lung radiation and incidence of IIP.[341] There is evidence that the incidence is decreased by fractionation of TBI as well as by lung shielding.[503] It must be remembered that the incidence of IIP is probably an underestimate of pulmonary toxicity from radiation and chemotherapy, since it excludes cases associated with a microorganism. Cases with an

associated infectious agent may have been initiated by damage from these physical agents with subsequent proliferation of a latent, dormant, or environmental microbe.

There are no specific histological features characteristic of pulmonary damage by radiation or chemotherapeutic agents. The alterations are generally those of DAD. Thus, there are various combinations of interstitial edema, congestion, hemorrhage and inflammatory infiltration; alveolar epithelial degeneration and hyperplasia; and intra-alveolar edema, hemorrhage, and hyaline membranes. Interstitial and intra-alveolar fibrosis may be present, reflecting the organizing stage of pulmonary damage.[194,335,338] We occasionally document epithelial atypia similar to that ascribed to cytotoxic drugs such as bleomycin, busulfan, and CY (Fig. 10).[283,607] These epi-

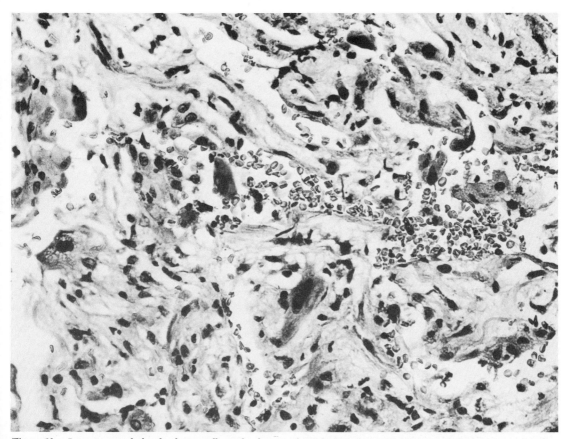

**Figure 10.** Large, atypical alveolar lining cells in this biopsy of IIP from a twin marrow recipient display bizarre shapes, multinucleation, and hyperchromatic staining. Although such cytological features are nonspecific, they may reflect chemoradiation toxicity. This 60-year-old male was transplanted for AMML in relapse and received a 5-day cytoreduction course of daunomycin, cytosine arabinoside, and 6-thioguanine followed by CY (60 mg/kg × 2) and 1000 rad TBI. He died of pneumonia 3 days after the above biopsy (day 61).

thelial alterations, as well as the fibroblast atypia sometimes ascribed to radiation damage (Fig. 11), may be present without exposure to such agents and, in turn, may be absent when these factors have probably had a causal influence in pneumonia development.

## ASSOCIATION OF GVHD WITH PNEUMONIA

The incidence and lethality of pneumonia increase in association with the severity of acute GVHD.[466,671] Until recently, this relationship has been generally attributed to the immunosuppressive effects of GVHD and its treatment while, at the same time, it was recognized that a direct effect of GVHD on the lung was possible.[466] The Johns Hopkins' marrow transplant group has presented data in support of the hypothesis that acute GVHD may develop in the large airways and give rise to a clinicopathological entity referred to as "lymphocytic bronchitis." Histologically (Fig. 12), this consists of lymphocytic infiltration of bronchial epithelium associated with necrosis of individual epithelial cells. In addition, there is subepithelial inflammation which may involve mucous glands. It has been suggested that this destructive inflammatory process impairs mucociliary function and leads to bronchopneumonia.[50]

We have been unable to confirm these data in either of two large autopsy reviews, one involving human[272] and the other canine[476] marrow recipients. In each study, we identified the histological alterations described as lymphocytic bronchitis in a significant number of subjects. This was done in a coded fashion to avoid possible bias arising from other information about the subjects. In 84 human allograft recipients, there was no correlation between the airway lesion and the presence of acute GVHD of other organs. Of further interest was the presence of lymphocytic bronchitis in four of 14 (30%) trauma victims maintained with mechanical ventilatory support for at least 48 hours before death, and in three of eight (38%) nontransplant patients who died with viral pneumonia (Fig. 13). We concluded that the inflammatory alterations are nonspecific and apparently not a reflection of acute GVHD.

Other clinical centers for marrow transplantation have been unable to implicate lymphocytic bronchitis as a GVH process; e.g., Connor[123]

and Blume, cited by Tutschka.[696] The presence at autopsy of chronic inflammation of airway mucosal glands in several patients with the sicca syndrome of chronic GVHD has suggested to us that involvement with sicca may occasionally extend to the trachea and bronchi (Fig. 14).[584] A patient with chronic GVHD who developed obstructive pulmonary disease with widespread obliteration of small airways at autopsy has been described.[532] We have four similar patients with clinical obstructive airway disease and chronic GVHD. An open-lung biopsy from one patient demonstrated bronchiolitis obliterans (Fig. 15).[258] It is possible that some combination of chronic sinusitis with resulting purulent secretions, esophageal dysfunction with aspiration, and the immune impairment of GVHD may adequately account for this airway damage.

Pulmonary studies of GVHD have been carried out in experimental animals. In order to reduce the number of factors, such as mechanical ventilatory support, which might give rise to the histologic features of lymphocytic bronchitis, we studied 46 canine allograft recipients and 25 autograft recipients. Coded autopsy sections of airways, skin, liver, and gastrointestinal tract were evaluated for lymphocytic bronchitis and acute GVHD. The presence of the airway inflammation did not correlate with receipt of a marrow allograft, with acute GVHD of other systems, or with the presence of acute pneumonia. In addition, it was present in autograft recipients (Fig. 16). We concluded that lymphocytic bronchitis is a reflection of nonspecific airway inflammation.[476] Stein-Streilein et al.[622] produced a local pulmonary GVHR in $F_1$ hybrid hamsters by airway inoculation of parental lymph node cells. This consisted of intra-alveolar and interstitial lymphocytic infiltration without airway epithelial inflammation or necrosis. Of greater interest in the present context is their inability to produce any histologic alterations in the lungs of animals which developed systemic GVHD following intravenous or intracutaneous inoculation of hyperimmune parental cells.

## CONCLUSION

Interstitial pneumonia is a frequent and serious complication of marrow transplantation. The idiopathic form appears to reflect chemoradiation

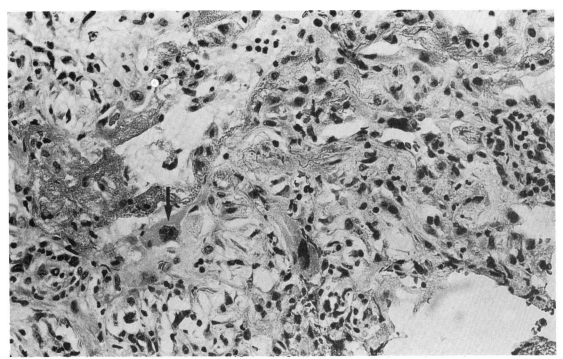

**Figure 11.** Atypical cells resembling "radiation fibroblasts" are nonspecific, but may be related to chemotherapy and irradiation. This IIP which developed in a twin marrow recipient was biopsied on day 141. Prominent nucleoli in atypical cells (arrow) may display clear halos and lead to mistaken diagnosis of viral infection. The patient is now free of pulmonary problems 2½ years later.

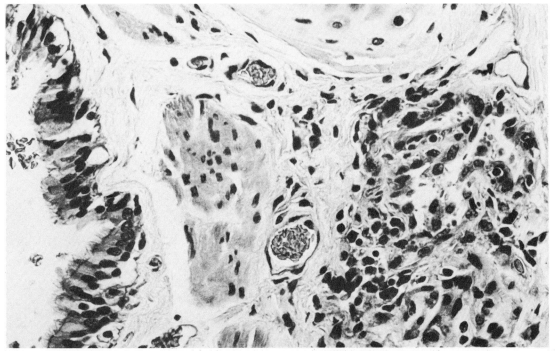

**Figure 12.** A section of canine mainstem bronchus from an allograft recipient shows lymphocytic infiltration of mucosal epithelium and submucosal gland. There is associated epithelial necrosis. Although ascribed to acute pulmonary GVHD, this "lymphocytic bronchitis" is nonspecific in coded histological studies of humans and dogs.

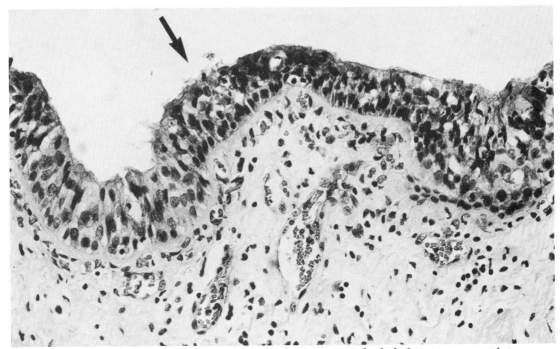

**Figure 13.** This section of bronchus is from an infant with pulmonary atresia who died of respiratory syncytial virus pneumonia. Although lymphocytic mucosal infiltration associated with epithelial necrosis ("lymphocytic bronchitis") is present (arrow), the patient was not a marrow recipient.

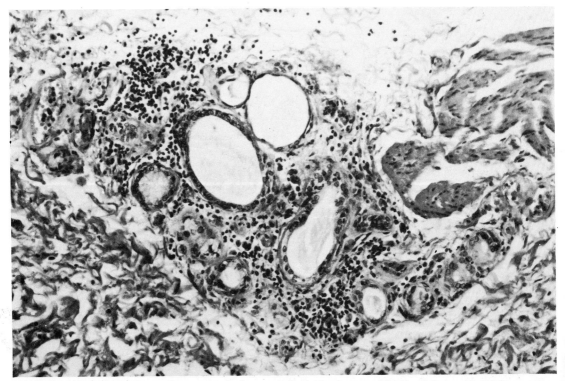

**Figure 14.** Trachea with chronic inflammation of submucosal gland. The ducts are dilated and show epithelial degeneration and lymphocytic infiltration. Chronic GVHD affects the lacrimal and salivary glands in a similar fashion, producing a sicca syndrome. This tissue was obtained at autopsy (day 458) from a patient with severe chronic GVHD.

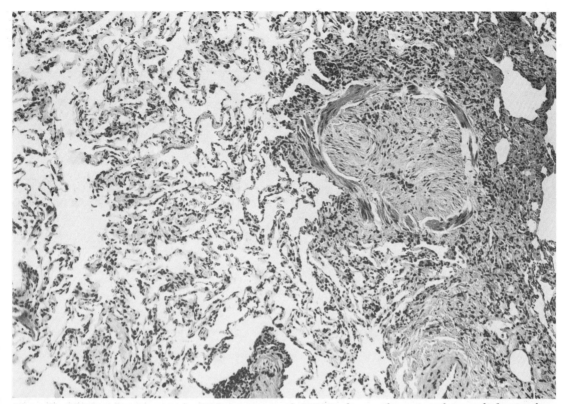

**Figure 15.** This open-lung biopsy on day 396 from a patient with GVHD and severe obstructive pulmonary dysfunction shows a constrictive type of bronchiolitis obliterans[258] which affected some bronchioles. A very mild lymphocytic interstitial infiltrate was present only in peribronchial areas. It is unclear whether this inflammatory bronchiolar damage reflects a direct immunological GVH reaction or a secondary complication.

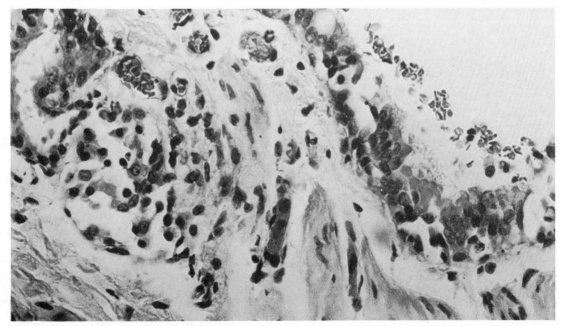

**Figure 16.** This section of bronchus from a canine autologous marrow recipient illustrates the nonspecific nature of mucosal lymphocytic infiltration associated with epithelial necrosis ("lymphocytic bronchitis").

toxicity and must now be diagnosed by ruling out infection. Development of CMV pneumonia is apparently related to immunosuppression in patients with latent infection or with exogenous infection from contaminated blood products. Other infectious etiologies include herpes simplex (HSV), varicella, adenovirus, and *Pneumocystis carinii*. The major influence of acute GVHD appears to be immunosuppression.

It is important to obtain rapid and specific pneumonia diagnosis in marrow recipients for the following reasons: 1) they are very susceptible to a large number of infectious agents; 2) therapy is becoming available for increasing numbers of these organisms (e.g., trimethoprim-sulfa for *Pneumocystis*, acyclovir for HSV); 3) empiric therapy in the absence of a specific diagnosis may produce significant toxicity; and 4) the use of corticosteroids for pneumonia is probably inappropriate if infection is actually present. Currently, open-lung biopsy is required to establish a diagnosis firmly, since pulmonary involvement may be patchy and many studies are required to rule out the multiple infectious agents.

Evaluation of a monoclonal antibody to CMV in pneumonia diagnosis by open-lung biopsy has demonstrated that immunofluorescent analysis with it is more sensitive than routine histological techniques, equal in sensitivity to *in situ* viral nucleic acid hybridization, and more rapid than viral culture. In addition, it allows the identification of individual CMV-infected cells in bronchoalveolar lavage specimens from some patients, indicating that the need for thoracotomy and open-lung biopsy in pneumonia diagnosis may decrease.[275] Such advances will not only reduce diagnostic delay and morbidity but will also increase sensitivity and specificity. This will provide a firm basis for the treatment of individual patients as well as pathogenetic data for the possible reduction of pulmonary complications in subsequent individuals.

# Chapter 10

# Pathology of the lymphoreticular system

George E. Sale, M.D.

## Introduction

The reactions which occur within the lymphoid tissues in GVHD are often loosely referred to as the GVH *reaction*: the *in vivo* counterpart of the mixed lymphocyte reaction (Figs. 1–3). The subsequent events are said to constitute GVH *disease*. This initial lymphoid tissue destruction is considered a main cause of the profound immunodeficiency which occurs in such hosts. However, it seems important to stress that these assertions are known to be certain only in non-radiated host, in certain $F_1$ hybrid combinations. In radiation chimeras, on the other hand, the host lymphoid system has been dealt a lethal blow and only some of the hardier cell types within that system (plasma cells and some macrophages, for example) will survive to interact with donor cells. Interpretations of the morphologic changes which fail to take into account these important caveats, therefore, will be of little value. The published literature on this subject is quite limited, both in animals and in humans.

GVHD, especially in lymphoid tissue, may be compared to a black box. We have some knowledge of what goes in, in terms of the need for donor T-cells and for initial alloantigenic stimulation, and we have phenomenological data about what comes out (GVHR/D syndrome in the target tissue or target cell lesions), but we have an opacified view of the mechanisms. Furthermore,

we do not fully understand the relevance of the various *in vitro* and local models of GVHR, such as the epopliteal lymph node assay, to the systemic syndromes. Before we will, one hazards, a great deal more research on normal lymphoid physiology and traffic *in vivo* must be productive. Such research is difficult because of the complexity of *in vivo* models. New approaches to these problems are now available, however, in the form of markers permitting the localization of immunoregulatory cell subsets, particularly monoclonal antibodies identifying immunologically relevant lymphocyte and natural killer (NK) cells. Application of these techniques to the problem has a bright future.

It is almost certain that the study of lymphoid cell traffic in the lymph nodes, spleen, Peyer's patches, bone marrow, and thymus will yield more important and revealing information than will study of the peripheral blood compartment. The latter is extensively studied, not because it is likely to be particularly significant, but because it is so accessible. Because the number of variables impinging on the lymphoreticular tissues in a radiation chimera of any species is so large, systematic study of these tissues *in vivo* is problematic. Van Bekkum[708] points out that among these variables are host species, host/donor combinations, radiation dose, and graft-cell dose. Therefore, even when one is comparing models that closely parallel each other in methodology and

Figures 1–3 are from a woman given conventional chemotherapy for ALL followed by unirradiated granulocyte transfusions.

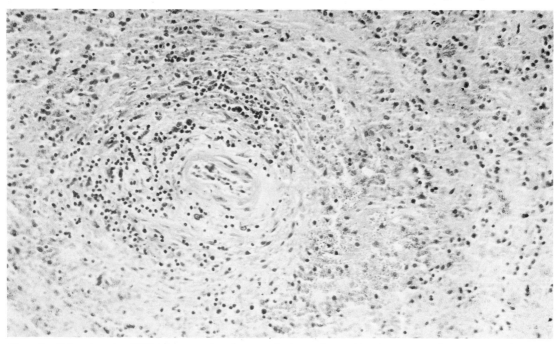

**Figure 1.**    Spleen in severe GVHD due to accidental, mismatched, transfusion-induced allograft.[739] Twelve days after onset of GVHD and 23 days after last normal granulocyte transfusion, this patient's spleen shows profound lymphoid atrophy near splenic arteriole. Fine particles at lower right are masses of microorganisms, largely Gram-negative rods. This is, unfortunately, another characteristic feature of fulminant acute GVHD associated with denudation of ileal and colonic epithelium.

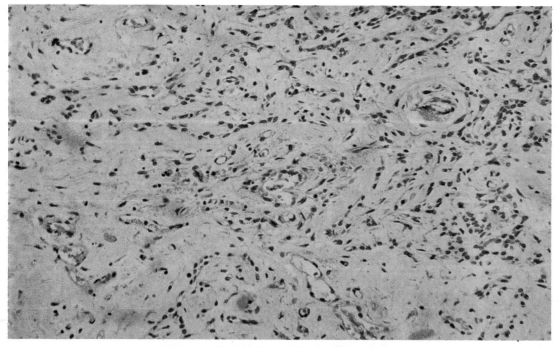

**Figure 2.**    Thymus shows profound cellular depletion.

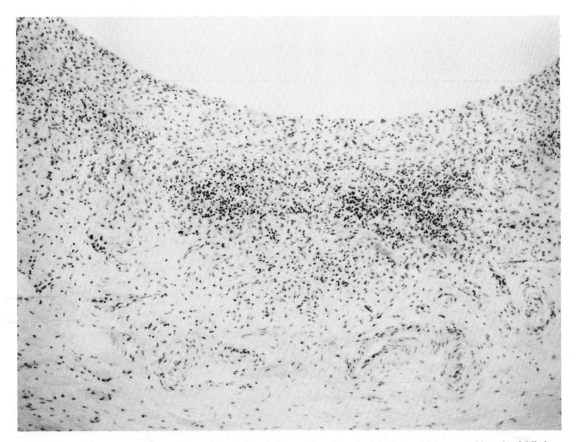

**Figure 3.** Low-power view of appendix with loss of epithelium and with marked depletion of the normal lymphoid follicles.

genetics (comparing, for example, a DLA-matched dog radiation chimera to an H-2-matched mouse radiation chimera), one cannot make even simple assumptions about the identity of lymphoid tissue reactions in the two. To this must be added consideration of the additional chemotherapy-induced damage, superinfections of all kinds, stress, and other drugs. It is not so much surprising, therefore, that the literature reveals discrepancies, as that it reveals any agreement. Before attempting a description of the effects of GVHR, damage by such important agents as radiation and chemotherapy will be considered. Then the more complex situation of GVHR or GVHD in nodal and other tissues can be discussed against this background.

## RADIATION HISTOPATHOLOGY OF THE LYMPH NODES, SPLEEN, AND THYMUS

Local irradiation produces quite different effects than does total body irradiation (TBI). Local irradiation at 3000 rad to a lymph node produces rapid death of all its lymphocytes within 12 hours, beginning as early as a few minutes after irradiation. By 2 days later, cellular replacement of the lymph nodes has occurred, and within a few more days the germinal centers have returned. This is presumably due to rapid replacement by the normal lymphocytes outside the irradiation field. A second wave of atrophy occurs 2 weeks later, presumably a result of vascular damage. There follows a gradual process of vascular, interstitial, and capsular fibrosis over the next year. Total obliteration and fibrosis of the node is complete by that time. These late atrophic changes are thought by most to be due to the damage to arterioles, veins, lymphatics, and capillaries produced by the radiation.[95]

The response to TBI differs because all the lymphocytes in the body are targets. According to Casarett,[95] the changes induced by doses of TBI in the mid-lethal range in mice are as follows. Within an hour, destruction of lymphocytes begins and continues for several more hours, and by 1 day, there is marked depletion. Regeneration begins in the nodes and spleen by the end of the first week and in the thymus by the end of the second. The lymph node regeneration is a diffuse cortical process without germinal center formation until the third week. The spleen lags about 2 weeks behind the nodes in regeneration, and the thymus lags a week or two behind the spleen. The thymic regeneration is said to be evident at first in the medulla and then spreads through the cortex. There are no late fibrotic changes described in these animals.

It is important to note that syngeneic or autogeneic bone marrow or spleen cell transplantation is a near equivalent to these TBI experiments, except that one can use larger than midlethal doses of TBI. There are important species differences in sensitivity of lymphoreticular tissues to TBI, however. Syngeneically grafted mice and rats recover normal lymph node and thymic morphology almost as rapidly as do those given midlethal irradiation. But the data on

lower primates from van Bekkum and others[708] and our studies of dogs[352] and humans[164] clearly show that the tempo of recovery of normal lymph node structure, particularly as evidenced by the return of normal germinal center morphology, is long delayed (Fig. 4). In fact, we were able to show few differences between recipients of syngeneic and of allogeneic marrow grafts in either dogs or humans for the first 100 days after transplantation. This was recently confirmed for human mesenteric nodes.[53] This fact remains unexplained and is also a clear caveat to the attribution of any putative superimposed changes to GVHR.

The thymus gland is at least as dynamic a freeway for lymphocyte traffic as the lymph node. Understanding of this structure has only begun. It is regarded as very difficult to study in human adults because it undergoes significant atrophy by age 20–40. Autografted canine radiation chimeras sacrificed after 264 days have completely reconstituted and normal thymus morphology, as illustrated in Figures 5–7. That the

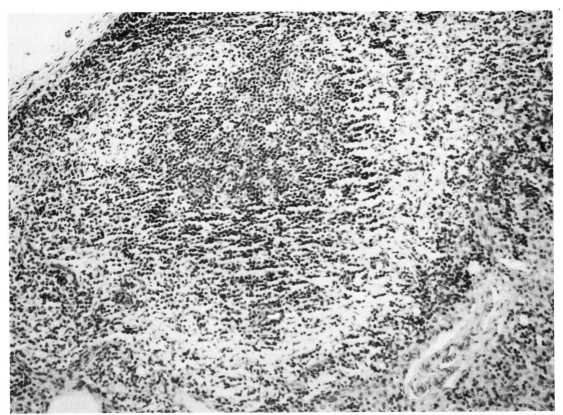

**Figure 4.** Lymph node cortex of canine autograft recipient 294 days after graft showing complete recovery of normal lymphoid germinal center structure.

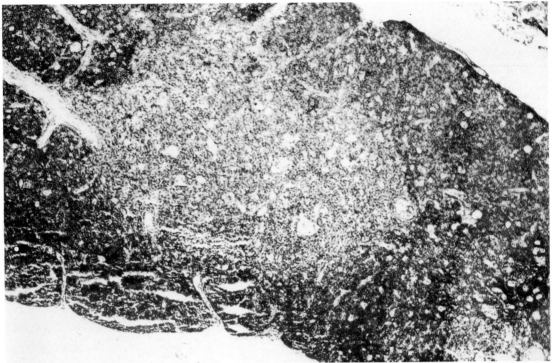

**Figure 5.** Thymus of marrow autograft 294 days after infusion. Structure and cellularity of both cortex and medulla are completely normal. Specimen from Dog A370.

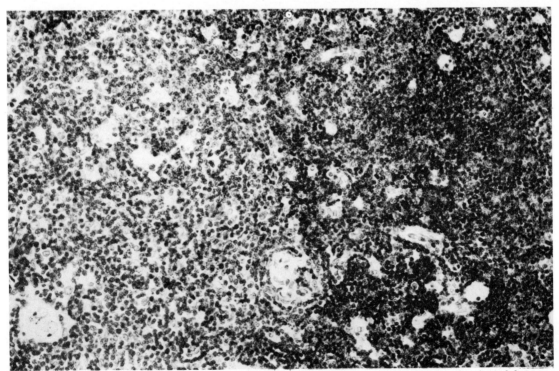

**Figure 6.** Thymus showing cellular cortex with normal medulla and well-differentiated Hassal's corpuscle at lower left. Specimen from Dog A370.

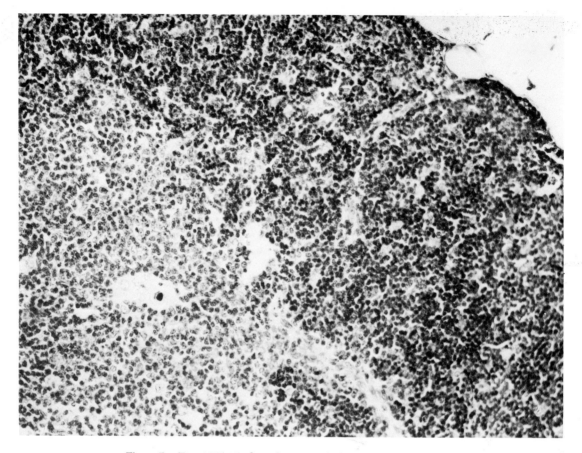

**Figure 7.** (Dog A259) 354 days after autograft also shows normal thymus.

thymus is extremely sensitive to irradiation is clearly evident in cases sacrificed earlier (Figs. 8–10). We have observed the early changes in dogs (at intervals of from 1 to 6 weeks after transplantation) due to irradiation alone and have found minimal evidence of regeneration at day 14. At 6 weeks after autograft, one of two dogs revealed nearly normal lymphoid cellularity and sufficient repair of medullary damage to exhibit differentiating epithelial cells that were beginning to form Hassal's corpuscles (Fig. 11). In the rat, the thymus repairs itself by 2–3 weeks after syngeneic marrow transplantation.[54,55,455]

Total lymphoid irradiation (TLI) including the thymus within the field was introduced clinically in the course of the treatment of Hodgkin's disease and other lymphomas[233] and was found to be profoundly immunosuppressive. Slavin and colleagues have studied TLI extensively as a pre-conditioning modality for marrow transplantation in mice, especially for the prevention of rejection or GVHD. Although the histopathologic events in lymph node and thymus are again rather nonspecific, the immunodeficiency state has been described in considerable detail.[595] The response in mice of T-cells to sheep erythrocytes (SRBC) is depressed for a month. The IgM response to SRBC returns in 46 days, but the IgG response is suppressed for 200 days. Long-term studies show prolonged depression of peripheral blood T-lymphocytes as well as hypertrophy of the B-cell compartment. The responses in mixed lymphocyte culture are depressed for only a month but responsiveness to phytohemagglutinin (PHA) and concanavalin A is subnormal for many months. Prolonged survival of incompatible skin grafts is produced, and a decreased GVHD mortality after murine allogeneic spleen grafts is seen. The presence of nonspecific as well as antigen-specific suppressor cells has been

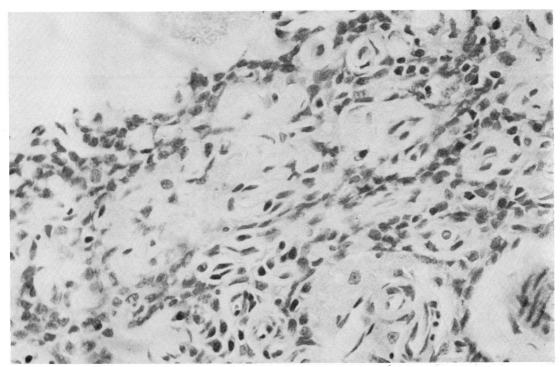

**Figure 8.** (Dog B353) Thymus gland 14 days after autograft following 1200 rad TBI (= 12 Gy). The parenchyma is markedly depleted of lymphocytes. Residuum displays a loosely distributed stroma containing scattered plasma cells, fibroblasts, macrophages, and degenerating epithelial and other cells. Such thymuses cannot be distinguished histologically from those in dogs undergoing acute GVHD.

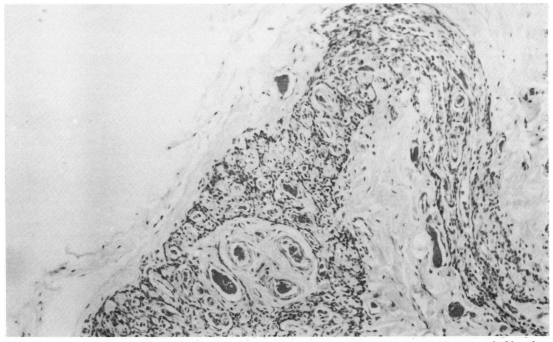

**Figure 9.** Low-power view of thymus with severe acute GVHD at autopsy, 18 days after allograft. There is marked lymphocyte depletion. Specimen from Dog B275.

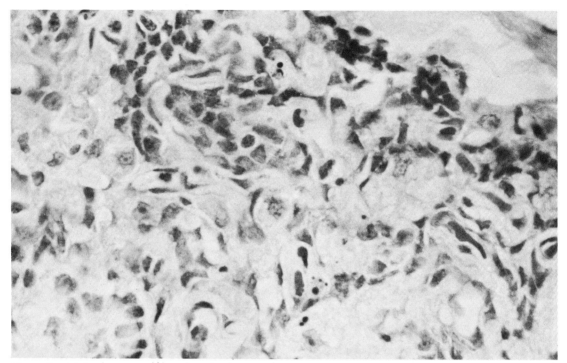

**Figure 10.** Medium-power view. Note foci of necrosis manifested by degeneration of individual cell nuclei (upper and lower middle). Such features suggest the epithelial features of GVHD but are difficult to distinguish from necrosis caused by the stress, radiation, and infectious processes occurring within the same time periods. (Compare to Fig. 14, Dog B353.) Specimen from Dog B275.

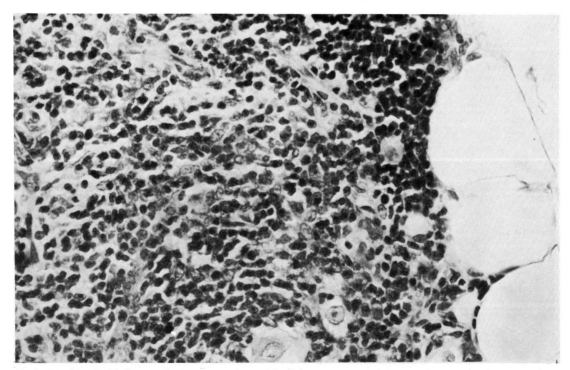

**Figure 11.** (Dog B340) Thymus of marrow autograit 42 days after autograft. Repopulation of cortex proceeds well. Viable-appearing epithelial cells can be seen at the lower right, and at lower middle a young Hassal's corpuscle is forming.

shown and is suspected as a mechanism for the tolerance of the host by the graft. The important point here is that some changes in immune function which could be attributed to GVHR can be induced with TBI or TLI alone. Therefore, caution is necessary when discussing the role of GVHR in immunodeficiency after marrow grafting with irradiation.

## EFFECTS OF CHEMOTHERAPY ON LYMPHOID TISSUES

Alkylating and other agents used to treat tumors or to suppress immunity profoundly alter lymphoid tissue in animals and humans. An illustrative prototype is cyclophosphamide (CY).[291,594,761] Stockman et al.[624] studied the differential effects of sublethal doses of CY on B- and T-cell zones in mouse spleen and lymph node. B-cell zones were found to show earlier and more prolonged depletion. Responses of spleen cells to pokeweed mitogen were more markedly depressed by CY than were responses to PHA. Furthermore, CY blocked the ability of the animals to form primary antibody against keyhole limpet hemocyanin without blocking this antigen's ability to induce splenic lymphocyte transformation. The conclusion was that CY preferentially kills B-cells. The reason, however, may be that in normal lymphoid tissues, the B-cell compartment is more actively dividing, which would be only an incidentally distinguishing feature between B- and T-cells. In humans, large doses of CY produce severe lymphoid depletion in 3–10 days. Nearly total lymphoid depeletion develops in 10–20 days. Erythrophagocytosis by prominent medullary and sinusoidal macrophages occurs between days 0 and 20. Splenic white pulp is nearly obliterated for 20 to 30 days, but by about 5 weeks is regenerated. These data were based on a study of 39 patients given high doses of CY.[594]

## GRAFT-VS.-HOST REACTION AND DISEASE

It is evident that the situation in the lymphoid tissues of the allogeneic radiation chimera is complex and is superimposed upon the background of primary radiation and chemotherapy damage. As reviewed by van Bekkum, primates, rabbits, and some parent-to-$F_1$ mouse transplant combinations will show profound nodal destruction during the first week and rapid regeneration in the second week, but then a very profound necrosis and destruction of lymphocytes in the nodes at the end of the second week. This is referred to as an "allergic suicide" reaction attributed to the reactions of donor lymphoid cells to a large excess of host antigens. The brisk reaction kills donor and host cells alike. Profound lymphoid atrophy ensues for 3 months. In syngeneic mice and some other parent-to-$F_1$ combinations, only acute radiation damage occurs, with nearly total recovery in 3 weeks. Other combinations, such as transplants from C57 B1 to CBA mice, produce a much less marked early regeneration and "suicide" reaction but still show 3 months of profound atrophy.[713]

It is possible to study the GVHR alone without radiation effects in some $F_1$ hybrid transplants. An example is that described by Seemayer et al.[573] Here, the reaction was produced by injecting parental spleen cells from mice of the A($H$-$2^a$) strain into $F_1$ hybrids, designated CBA($H$-$2^k$)XA($H$-$2^a$), and sacrificing the animals between days 4–42 after grafting. The spleen showed early enlargement with increased lymphoblasts and megakaryocytes in the red pulp. Hemorrhage, necrosis, and late fibrosis followed the disappearance of malpighian corpuscles and reduction in spleen size. The lymph nodes enlarged and their germinal centers progressively disappeared. The structure was replaced by immunoblasts and histiocytes. Other examples of unirradiated recipients include the restorations attempted in severe combined immune deficiency (SCID) in humans and Arabian foals, but sufficient sequential data are not available to follow the precise sequence of events in their lymph nodes.

The profound nodal enlargement reaction followed by massive "allergic suicide" is found, therefore, only in some of the GVHR models and cannot be regarded as an obligatory event. To our knowledge, clinical adenopathy as a part of the systemic GVHR is unusual in either human or canine marrow transplant recipients. Few of the animals and none of the humans have had frequent sequential lymph node histologic studies. Severe GVHRs are often accompanied by nonspecific granulomatous reactions in lymphoreticular structures, as are many other kinds of destructive reactions in such tissue. Among the most thoroughly studied models is the rat radiation chimera.[54,55] The syngeneically grafted control animals in this model began to recover evidence of primary and of even secondary germinal center formation in their lymph nodes by day 28. The allogeneic chimeras, on the other hand, showed at best only primary follicle regeneration by this time, and there was more delayed recovery in the animals that had received both bone marrow cells and spleen cells from their donors.

In 1976, Drenguis[164] summarized the results of our study of lymphoid reconstitution based on autopsies of 29 allografted patients who received matched-sibling donor-marrow transplants (27 for leukemia and two for aplasia) and 11 syngeneic graft recipients (all leukemia). Semiquantitative estimates of lymph node cellularity, percent of lymphocytes, plasma cells, and macrophages, as well as the time course of the return of cortical nodules and primary and secondary germinal centers were made. Plasma cell immunoglobulin light- and heavy-chain production were also studied using immunoperoxidase methods (PAP) on paraffin-embedded tissues. The 29 allografted patients survived from 7 to 458 days post transplant, and the 11 syngeneic graft recipients (five identical twins, six autografts) survived 5–364 days. Only patients who had good grafts and no relapse were studied. The two aplastic anemia patients had received CY preconditioning, whereas all the leukemia patients received CY, 1000 rad TBI and, in some cases, additional chemotherapy.

The results showed a marked uniformity among all cases and an unexpected similarity between the findings in syngeneic as compared to allogeneic graft recipients. The cellularity of the lymph node cortices was variable, but on the average was moderately depressed in all groups between days 1–30 (17 autopsies). There was no additional recovery between days 30–70 in 13 autopsies. In 10 autopsies between days 70–458, the cellularity of the cortex recovered further but was still slightly below normal in all cases. The only discernible difference between the allogeneic and syngeneic graft recipients was that, during the first four weeks, four of four syngeneic graft recipients showed a marked decrease in lymphoid cellularity, whereas of the

allograft recipients, four showed slight and eight showed moderate lymphoid cortical cellularity decreases. It is uncertain whether this difference is meaningful; if so, it may indicate an early reaction between donor lymphoid cells and some radioresistant residual host cell types in the allograft patients. However, other causes such as infection cannot be ruled out.

Table 1 shows the differences between syngeneic and allogeneic graft recipients with respect to cortical cellularity, early and late after grafting. In this entire series only two patients showed the return of normal secondary germinal centers (at days 73 and 94 post grafting) and both were allograft recipients. Nearly all patients showed poorly defined, loose fibrosis in the sites of previously existing germinal centers. Most also showed the return of poorly defined, round nodules of lymphoid cells resembling primary follicles, as early as day 12 in allografts, and day 5 in syngeneic grafts. However, plasmacytoid cells admixed with occasional immunoblasts constituted the majority of the repopulating cells in the cortical regions as the post-transplant intervals increased.

Thirty-three cases were evaluated in successful experiments for cytoplasmic immunoglobulins G, A, M, and for kappa and lambda light chains, using an indirect immunoperoxidase technique on paraffin-embedded lymph node sections. Results indicated that of these cases, 10 failed to show staining; that was usually associated with low plasma cell counts. Failure to stain was commonest in specimens obtained at days 0–14 after grafting. After day 14, five of five syngeneic cases showed staining and 14 of 20 allografted cases showed stainable Ig by the method. There was no decrease in the rate of failure to stain with increasing post-transplant interval in the allografted patients. We had predicted that IgM staining might return faster than IgG staining. Before day 50 five of 10 (50%) cases showed predominance of IgM staining, whereas after day 50, only three of 13 cases were IgM predominant (23%). This shows a trend toward predominance of IgM staining in the early cases but is not statistically significant ($p$ value greater than 0.05 by Fisher's exact test). Interpretation of these data should be tempered by the knowledge that plasma cells are extremely radioresistant and,

**TABLE 1**

Cortical Cellularity and Total Cortical Lymphoid Cell Counts in Syngeneic versus Allogeneic Marrow Recipients[164]

| Day after Graft | Syngeneic Graft Recipients (11) | | Allograft Recipients (27) | |
|---|---|---|---|---|
| | Cortical Cellularity[a] | Lymphoid Cells[b] | Cortical Cellularity[a] | Lymphoid Cells[b] |
| 0 – 14 | −3 | 30% | −2 | 45% |
| 80 – 100 | −1.5 | 75% | −1 | 65% |

[a]Mean cellularity expressed as: 0 = normal, −1 = slight decrease, −2 = moderate decrease, −3 = severe decrease, by the method of Cottier et al.[130]

[b]Lymphoid cells here are lymphocytes plus plasma cells plus immunoblasts in *cortex*.

therefore, a significant contribution of host plasma cells to the results is likely, at least in the earlier post-transplant periods.

All cases showed a polyclonal pattern. Most showed an IgG predominance and about an equal frequency of kappa- and lambda-positive cells. One case, UPN 170, showed a strongly IgG kappa predominance although IgM, IgA, and lambda-positive cells were also present. There was a pronounced polymorphous immunoblastic plasmacytosis of lymph nodes without any evidence of monomorphous immunoblastic nodule formation or "cloning" similar to that often used by Lukes as evidence of impending monoclonality in immunoblastic sarcoma. Furthermore, the case had no evidence of splenic, hepatic, or gastrointestinal immunoproliferation similar to that reported in immunoblastic sarcomas after bone marrow or thymic transplantations.[259,521,569]

Beschorner et al.[53] studied the intestinal B-cell compartment as a reflection of intestinal immunity in human marrow graft recipients. Their study used semiquantitative grading of plasma cells bearing IgA, IgM, and IgG as labeled by immunoperoxidase methods in paraffin sections of autopsied small bowel (Fig. 12). Patients with allograft had greater mucosal injury and greater depletion of lamina propia plasma cells bearing IgM and IgA than did syngeneically grafted patients or patients with graft rejection. The injury and depletion were somewhat more severe in patients with GVHD. Mesenteric nodes before day 133 showed no germinal centers in any patient. Germinal centers reappeared between days 133 and 607 but these longer-term survivors included

no autografted patients, no GVHD patients, and no rejecting patients, so they reflect only patients without GVHD dying late of other causes.

Study of the thymus gland in GVHD has led Seemayer, Lapp, and Bolande[573] to suggest that *in utero* thymic GVHD, mediated by maternal T-lymphocytes passing through a compromised placental barrier, may be etiologic for SCID or for primary biliary atresia. They have evidence in $F_1$ hybrid murine transplant studies that thymic epithelium is directly damaged by lymphocytes and that this is independent of the adrenocortical influences on the thymic cortex that occur during severe stress. The target cells appear to be epithelial cells and Hassal's corpuscles in the thymic medulla. Seddick et al.[572] have been able to induce a T-cell functional defect in mice undergoing GVHR and attribute this to thymic epithelial cell damage.

The thymic changes in human marrow transplant recipients have been difficult to interpret due to the large number of variables and to the normal thymic atrophy in adults.[49] We have seen that profound thymic atrophy persists for months to years in dog radiation chimeras, independent of detectable GVHD. Yet, as mentioned above, complete restoration of normal thymic cortical and medullary morphology will occur in autografted dogs by about 6 weeks after grafting. This suggest that a long-lasting but subclinical GVHR occurs in the thymus of all of the allografted animals, independent of any clinical evidence of the disease. Figures 13–15 show thymus from dogs surviving more than 126 days after allografting from DLA-matched littermate donors. There is profound atrophy and destruction

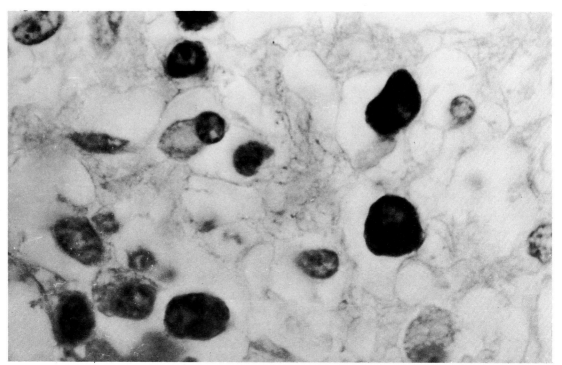

**Figure 12.** (UPN 358) Fifty-year-old male day 57 post allograft for AML who died of CMV infection disseminating to lungs and gut. Oil immersion field of immunoperoxidase reaction for lambda light chain of human immunoglobulin. Polyclonal return of rectal plasma cell population, indicated by negative staining of elongated plasma cell at upper middle. Two plasma cells at right show dense cytoplasmic staining for lambda light chain.

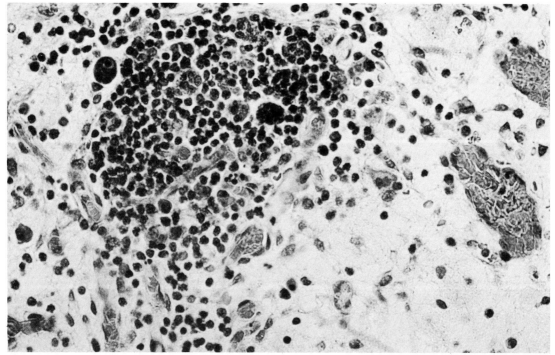

**Figure 13.** Profound thymic atrophy in dog euthanized day 126 because of chronic GVHD. Similar atrophy is found, however, in all long-term surviving *allografted* dogs in our series regardless of their GVHD status. Specimen from Dog A292.

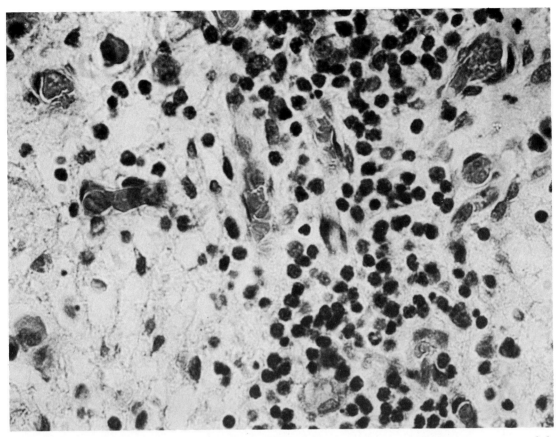

**Figure 14.** Higher-power views shows two damaged Hassal's corpuscles (upper and lower middle). The upper one is invaded by mononuclear cells similar to those illustrated by Seemayer et al.[573,574]

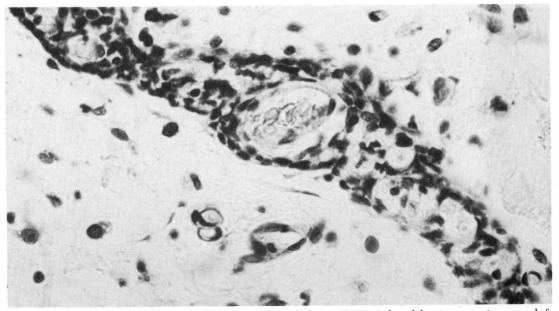

**Figure 15.** (Dog A983) Second example of a thymus from a dog with chronic GVHD. S-shaped thymic remnant is composed of epithelial and macrophage debris among small numbers of mononuclear cells.

of epithelium. The thymus of a comparable auto-graft is shown in Figures 5–7. Earlier after graft-ing, all dogs showed severe thymic damage (Figs. 8–10). Only the autografts showed complete mor-phologic reconstitution, however. No differences have so far been detected between thymic struc-ture of allografted dogs with or without clinical GVHD.

Some very interesting deductions about lym-phoid structure in GVHD can be drawn from the elegant studies of Muller-Ruchholtz and col-leagues[455,665] using antibody pretreatment of marrow-and spleen-transplanted rats. Not only were they able to modify or prevent clinical GVHD in these models using antilymphocyte and antithymocyte antibodies, but they also modified the tempo and character of the mor-phologic reconstitution of the recipients' lymph nodes and thymuses. The tissues of treated ani-mals generally showed a much more rapid recon-stitution toward normal structure, whereas the tissues of recipients of untreated bone marrow did not reconstitute. Kolb et al. showed similar results in dogs.[665] Such work has stimulated active interest in pretreatment of human bone marrow, particularly with monoclonal antibodies, for the purpose of removing T-cells and their pre-cursors from the marrow graft. Potential applica-tions also include removing residual tumor cells from marrow prior to autografting for leukemia and other tumors.

### HOST-VS.-HOST REACTION:

### LYMPH NODE PATHOLOGY OF BONE MARROW GRAFT FAILURE AND REJECTION

Figures 16–19 illustrate two cases which sharply emphasize the difficulties of lymph node histol-ogy after grafting. Case UPN 755 is a primary graft failure in aplastic anemia 34 days after trans-plant, and UPN 514 is that of rejection after defi-nite engraftment. Both show diffuse plasma-cytoid immunoblastic hyperplasia, indistin-guishable from the pattern in most allografted dogs and humans after lymph node regeneration within the first 100 days. In the successfully allo-grafted dogs and humans, donor cells populate the nodes. In UPN 514, however, the cells were of host origin. The histology seems identical in the three types of situations.

### LYMPHORETICULAR NEOPLASIA AND MARROW TRANSPLANTATION

The immune surveillance theory of Burnett pre-dicted that increased numbers of neoplasms would develop in immunodeficient hosts.[89] Gatti and Good reported such an increase in con-genital immunodeficiency.[231] Starzl et al. noted greatly increased lymphoma incidence after renal transplantation.[613] The work of the Gleichmanns and their colleagues in F$_1$ hybrid GVHD[16] and the studies of Cornelius[128] in rapid viral induc-tion of murine lymphomas in GVHD added sup-port for the theory. The lack of an increased incidence of tumors in nude mice, which are T-cell deficient, raised doubts about the concept, but it was rescued by the discovery of NK cells and a slight broadening of the definition of the term "immune" to include the natural resistance phenomenon. The X-linked lymphoproliferative syndrome in humans, discovered and elucidated by Purtilo and colleagues, represents a genetic immunodeficiency state highly conducive to lym-phomagenesis, particularly that associated with the Epstein-Barr (EBV) virus.[348] The lymphomas of renal transplant recipients comprise a good ex-ample of the problems associated with diagnosis of these lymphoproliferative entities. Five patients studied by Frizzera et al.[222] showed a polymor-phic and polyclonal lymphoid hyperplasia with atypia, chromosomal abnormalities, and necrosis suggestive of the incipient development of a monoclonal malignant process. The authors dis-tinguish these cases from both immunoblastic sarcomas and immunoblastic lymphadenopathy (or angioimmunoblastic lymphadenitis). Clearly, however, there is a continuum among these en-tities, sometimes resulting in a monoclonal im-munoblastic sarcoma.

As noted above, a clearly benign polyclonal plasmacytoid hyperplasia occurs routinely in the lymph nodes of canine and human transplant re-cipients.[352,584] We had observed this frequently in humans (Fig. 20) and had noted one par-ticularly striking case involving the portal triads as well as the nodes (Figs. 21, 22). Gossett and Gale[259] reported a case of immunoblastic sar-coma of the gut occurring about 60 days post grafting in a marrow transplant recipient who had been treated for acute myelogenous leukemia. The proliferation was of monoclonal B-cells ac-

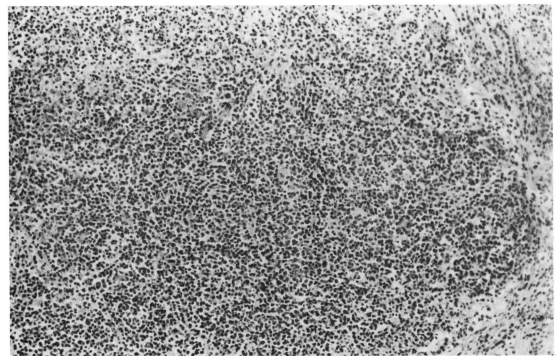

**Figure 16.** Low-power view of lymphoplasmacytic hyperplasia of lymph node in 32-year-old male allograft recipient 34 days after allograft for aplastic anemia. Note diffuse replacement of node without germinal centers. Specimen from patient UPN 755.

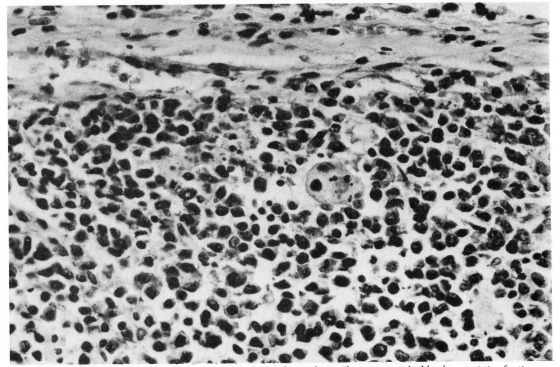

**Figure 17.** Higher-power view showing immunoplasmacytic hyperplasia. This pattern is highly characteristic of active repopulation of allograft lymph nodes and seems independent of the presence of GVHD in our experience. In this case, however, the patient had just undergone a primary marrow graft failure and died of infection. Specimen from patient UPN 755.

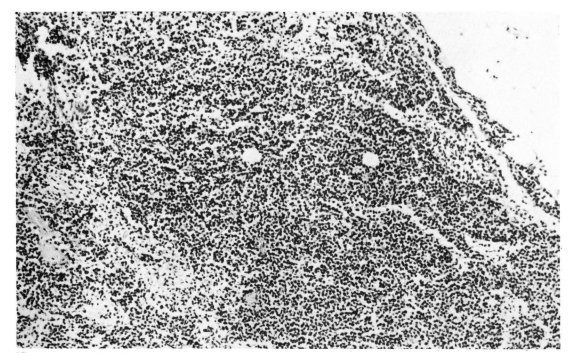

**Figure 18.**  Lymph node from 10-year-old female dying 72 days after allograft for aplastic anemia, shows diffuse immunoplasmacytoid hyperplasia just as in many successful allografts. However, this is a case of immune marrow graft rejection after a well-proven marrow graft. Specimen from patient UPN 514.

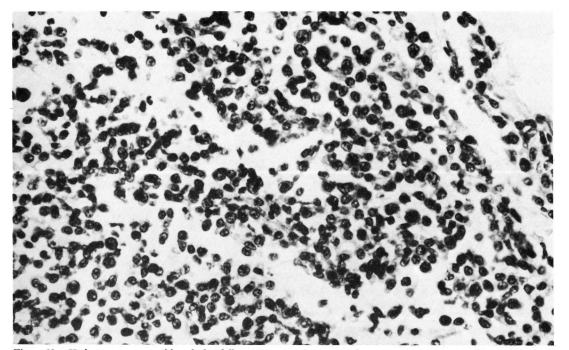

**Figure 19.**  Higher-power view. Although this diffuse pattern is a common finding in successful canine and human allografts with donor cells populating the nodes, cytogenetic data in this case clearly indicated the cells to be of host origin. This may, therefore, represent the lymph node pattern seen in immune marrow graft rejection. However, it is not histologically distinguishable from the picture of repopulation in successfully engrafted human or canine radiation chimeras with or without GVHD. Specimen from patient UPN 514.

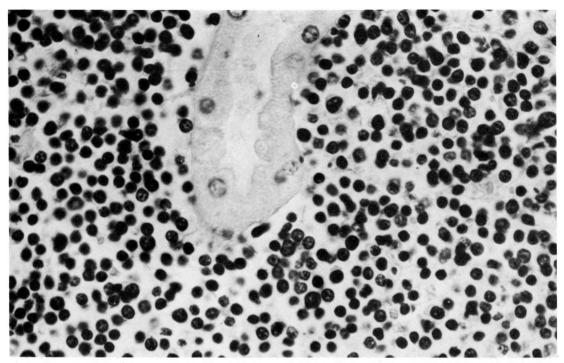

**Figure 20.**   (UPN 304) A 12-year-old male allografted for ALL in relapse developed active GVHD of skin, gut, and liver and died of CMV pneumonia on day 102. At autopsy, he had a 1.5-cm diameter intrarenal mass composed of plasmacytoid cells as shown. Immunoperoxidase indirect (PAP) technique revealed that the proliferation was positive for both lambda and kappa light chains, indicating its polyclonality.

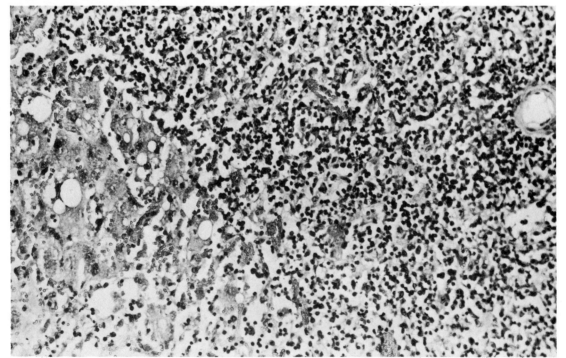

**Figure 21.**   Pronounced immunoblastic hyperplasia of portal tracts in a 21-year-old female allografted for aplastic anemia. This patient had GVHD and disseminated herpes infection. Specimen from patient UPN 657.

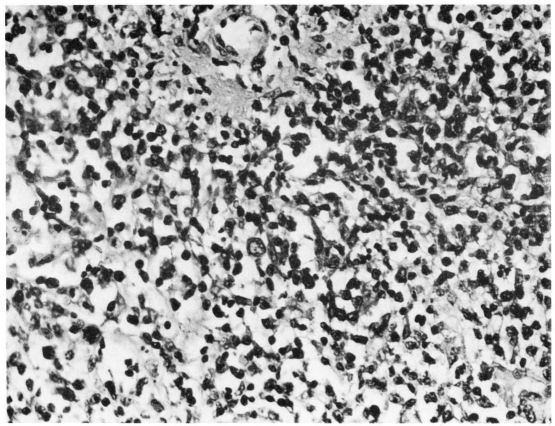

**Figure 22.**    Medium-power view illustrating that the proliferation consists of lymphocytes, plasmacytoid cells, and immunoblasts. Specimen from patient UPN 657.

cording to immunoglobulin light-chain production labeled by Taylor's immunoperoxidase method. The donor origin of this tumor was suggested by chromatin analysis. Donor-cell leukemia recurrence proven by cytogenetics in opposite-sex-donor combinations had been reported several years previously and the phenomenon has been confirmed at other centers.[77] Until recently, it had occurred in our series only in patients given TBI alone without CY and only in a leukemic form. Our group instituted careful studies of all recurrent leukemias as well as solid-tumor cases, and we found two tumors, which were monoclonal B-cell immunoblastic sarcomas. So far, one of these has been shown to contain EBV genome in the chromosomes of tumor cells.[273,569] This was composed of donor cells, whereas the other was of host cells (Fig. 23). Borzy et al.[75] had recently reported a polyclonal proliferation resembling immunoblastic sarcoma

in the gut of a thymic transplant recipient, but neither the donor–host nor the EBV aspects were investigated. Reece et al.[521] reported evidence of EBV genome in a fatal disseminated polyclonal malignant B-cell immunoblastic sarcoma developing after thymic transplantation in a 5-year-old girl with combined immunodeficiency. The general pathology associated with this group of diseases is well discussed in a recent symposium.[348] Radiation alone may explain an overall increase of malignancies in marrow transplant recipients, as emphasized in our recent study in canine radiation chimeras.[144]

Careful study of any new or seemingly recurrent tumor in a marrow transplant recipient is important and requires preparation well beforehand. Determination should be made of donor-vs.-host cell type, cytogenetic abnormalities, immunological markers, EBV genotypic and phenotypic markers (EBNA, viral capsular anti-

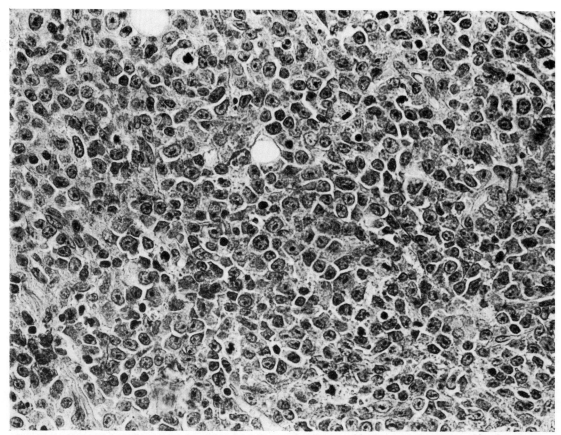

**Figure 23.** (UPN 1134) Medium-power histology of B-cell monoclonal immunoblastic sarcoma. A 26-year-old male with acute myelosclerosis developed this 5-cm, paraspinal mass several months after allograft. Cytogenetics revealed host origin of tumor cells.

gens, early antigens), and morphology. An attempt should be made to co-culture tumor cells with umbilical cord lymphoid cells to detect transformation of B-lymphocytes by EBV. Fresh tissue should be obtained in order to attempt DNA hybridization studies as well.[348,569] The pathologist is the central figure in assuring that the tissue is properly processed. Such work will add to the knowledge of the relationship of EBV to tumors as well as contribute to proper evaluation and care of marrow transplant recipients. Some of the clinically apparent adenopathies will not only be polyclonal, but will be totally unrelated to the tumor recurrence, so that one can make no assumptions about a single episode and each must be carefully studied in detail. For example, one of our recent cases of suspected lymphoma occurred about 49 days after allograft in a teenage male with null-cell acute lymphoblastic leukemia (null-ALL). This patient suddenly developed

unilateral neck adenopathy. A biopsy showed a polymorphous proliferation composed of 90% donor T-lymphocytes, no null cells, and very few B-cells (Fig. 24). There was no evidence of EBV, and no host cells were found. Nodal proliferation rapidly and spontaneously regressed over 1 week's time, and the patient returned home clinically well. Since there was a local herpes mouth infection, the adenopathy was tentatively attributed to this. Three weeks later, the marrow showed 40% null-ALL blasts, indicating a recurrence of the patient's original tumor. The adenopathy might be alternatively explained as transient evidence of a graft-vs.-tumor effect heralding the recurrence.

### CONCLUSION

The lymphoreticular tissues are assumed to be a very important way station in both the afferent

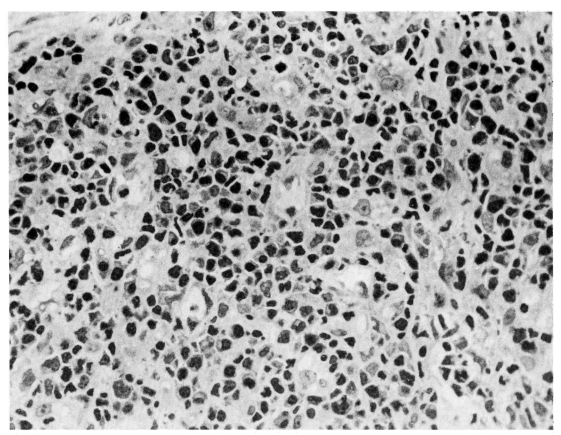

**Figure 24.** (UPN 1437) Methacrylate-embedded section of cervical lymph node from 22-year-old male with transient uni-lateral cervical lymphadenopathy developing about 100 days post allograft for null-cell ALL, transplanted in remission. These cells were shown to be 90% erythrocyte rosette-positive T-cells expressing the Ia antigen as measured by the monoclonal antibody designated 7.2. This adenopathy spontaneously regressed, but 4 weeks later the original null-cell ALL with completely different cytologic features recurred in bone marrow and peripheral blood. (See text for additional history.)

and efferent limbs of the immune response in general and the GVHR in particular. Yet, little of what occurs there is understood, in part because the morphology of lymphoid tissues is affected by multiple variables. It is the combined task of cellular immunologists and immunopathologists to elucidate this situation, and the increasing sophistication of the available methods makes this likely. Careful study of the sequellae of radiation, chemotherapy, and GVHR in the immune system may provide fundamental new insights into the structure and function of both the lymphoid organs and their associated epithelia. In some of these immunosuppressed hosts, tumors occur with a frequency greater than in the general population and require alert, careful, and detailed study. The pathologist who is willing to exploit new molecular methods in their elucidation will

make major contributions directly from the cutting board.

### ADDENDUM

We recently reviewed the thymus gland of a 13-year-old boy who died more than 1700 days after marrow allograft for ALL with no evidence of tumor. This boy had grade III GVHD of the skin at day 37 and later developed chronic GVHD of the skin. This gradually resolved without treatment. At over 5 years postgrafting, the patient was killed instantly in an automobile accident. The thymus showed normal cortex, medulla, and Hassal's corpuscles, upon coroner's autopsy. Because of the total lack of stress effect, this represents a unique case which provides strong evidence that thymus gland can recover in patients who recover clinically even from chronic GVHD, and that these patients can become stable long-term chimeras. It is strong evidence in favor of the hypothesis of Seemayer and Lapp that thymus damage is fundamental to the immunodeficiency of GVHD[575] and also strongly supports the hypothesis of Müller-Ruchholtz and Müller-Hermelink that thymic morphology and function should return to normal in tolerant allograft recipients.[455] (Manuscript in preparation.)

# Chapter 11

# Pathology of other organ systems

George E. Sale, M.D.
Howard M. Shulman, M.D.

## Introduction

Most postgrafting histologic alterations in organ systems other than those discussed in specific chapters are manifestations of infection or chemoradiation therapy. However, processes which resemble GVHD occur sporadically in "nonclassical" target organs. Lesions reported in some organs have been attributed to GVHD without statistically convincing support. Some can be produced only in certain strain or species combinations. Others are defined as graft-vs.-host reaction (GVHR) using loose operational or nonspecific criteria. Evaluating the association of certain histologic changes (for example, perivascular infiltrates and arterial lesions in the kidney) with GVHD requires the repeated stratification of histologic data to control for concurrent variables, such as age, pretransplant conditioning regimen, duration of survival post transplantation, and viral infections. Appropriate stratification is difficult and often results in groups containing only small numbers.

Some of these tissues are not available in every autopsy, making comparisons difficult. Furthermore, the same differential diagnostic problems exist for these lesions as for the better established ones. We hypothesize that certain changes, even when present in as few as 25% of patients, may be due to GVHD when the changes resemble those in autoimmune diseases or GVHD in other organs, when cultures exclude an infectious etiol-

ogy, and when comparisons render assigning such changes to chemoradiation therapy alone unlikely. This chapter discusses general pathology in systems outside the accepted targets of GVHD and critically reviews the attribution of lesions in them to GVHD.

### CENTRAL NERVOUS SYSTEM

Significant problems in humans after marrow transplantation relate primarily to bleeding and infection in the first 2 months postgrafting, and to recurrent tumor or complications of therapy in the later postgrafting period. The problem of bleeding is almost entirely a function of inadequate platelet counts in both the aplastic anemia patients pretransplantation, and in all patients between days 0–30 post-transplantation. New problems may arise later in two groups of patients. The first are those who reject their grafts. Second attempts at engraftment from the same or new donors usually fail due to the intervention of infection or bleeding before the second graft can "take." The second group develops poor megakaryocyte engraftment, or platelet consumption. Catastrophic brain or spinal cord hemorrhages have been mercifully infrequent in our experience due to the support provided by a large regional blood bank with a very able coagulation laboratory. However, massive fatal intracerebral hemorrhage, as well as transecting spinal cord hemorrhage, has occurred occasionally, even when platelet counts were above levels usually accepted as dangerous.

The range of infectious problems affecting the central nervous system (CNS) parallels that of disseminated infections in general, but the order is reversed. The most frequent problems are fungal. When disseminated aspergillosis is diagnosed, the brain is often involved with one or multiple lesions, most frequently exhibiting vascular invasion and distally infarcted brain. Zygomycetes infecting the paranasal and frontal sinuses invade vessels similarly, as do some originating in other sites, such as arteriovenous shunts. Bacterial infections occur less frequently, often in patients with severe gastrointestinal GVHD who develop disseminated Gram-negative bacillary infections. One case of *Nocardia caviae* infection originating in a lung abscess was found at autopsy to have disseminated into the pons and basal ganglia, forming multiple microabscesses containing the organisms. Viral infections seem much less frequent, as we are only rarely able to culture viruses from brain tissue. Of the eight cases of toxoplasmosis we have diagnosed, three involved the brain.

Recurrence of leukemia cells in the cerebrospinal fluid (CSF) occasionally occurs, especially in patients transplanted while in relapse. It is primarily a phenomenon in patients with ALL who have previously had CNS involvement with leukemia, and is markedly decreased by the use of post-transplant MTX. A positive CSF prior to transplantation is a strong predictor of recurrence of leukemia.[281] If this happens to patients transplanted while in remission, however, it is a late event. Malignant glial tumors have been reported outside the marrow transplantation setting in leukemic children treated with CNS irradiation and intrathecal chemotherapy, usually methotrexate (MTX).[106] We have seen two and reported one such case after marrow transplantation.[553] One canine radiation chimera in our laboratory also recently developed a malignant glioma.[146b] Careful observation of all transplantation patients will be needed to determine the epidemiologic and etiologic implications of these tumors.

Of particular concern is the problem of toxicity from chemotherapy after exposure of the CNS to chemoradiotherapy,[62,250,334] particularly leukoencephalopathy, whose pathology has been well described.[541] Sanders et al. (unpublished data) studied our experience with leukoencephalopathy in relation to the problems of relapse and intrathecal MTX. Patients at highest risk for leukoencephalopathy were those with a history of CNS leukemia who received at least six doses of post-transplant intrathecal MTX. The incidence is low, but clearly the management of patients transplanted for leukemia must balance the risk of recurrent leukemia against the potential risk of developing leukoencephalopathy.

Other antineoplastic drugs have been implicated in neurotoxicity. Sullivan et al.[655] report an association between the use of nitrogen mustard in combination with cyclophosphamide conditioning, and an acute, delayed neurotoxicity syndrome consisting of seizures, confusion, dementia, and hydrocephalus. Many of the histologic changes are relatively nonspecific and include an increase of corpora amylacea, subcortical gliosis, leptomeningeal thickening, satellitosis around cortical neurons, and an increase of thickened vessels in the subcortical white matter. Other neurotoxic agents used in marrow recipients include cytosine arabinoside, interferon, and acyclovir, as used for the treatment of viral pneumonia. Knowledge of the neuropathology accompanying the clinical signs is very sparse.

There are no clinical findings to suggest a GVHR in the brain although a series of reports suggests a GVHR in neonatal rat brain.[141,267,268] Findings included decreased cellularity in the external germinal layer in the developing cerebellum of neonatal $F_1$ rat chimeras. This was associated with significant decreases in cerebellar weight, DNA, RNA, and protein content, as well as incorporation of tritiated thymidine into DNA. The authors suggest that malnutrition alone cannot be the explanation since it causes a different set of histologic changes. They postulate humoral mediators and exclude cellular immune attack because of a lack of inflammatory infiltrate. There are no data suggesting that adult brain cells in any species show similar changes.

## CARDIOVASCULAR SYSTEM

Hemorrhage, infection, and toxicity comprise the complications in the heart and vessels of transplant recipients. The clinically significant bleeding is usually the result of pericardial tamponade from viral, fungal, or uremic pericarditis in the presence of thrombocytopenia. Those deep-seated and disseminated fungal infections which produce multiple emboli to other viscera will often involve the myocardium, with *Candida albicans* and *Aspergillus* leading the list. Rarely, bacterial infections disseminating from the gut will seed the myocardium with microabscesses containing *Pseudomonas* or even *Clostridia*. Bacterial and nonbacterial (marantic) endocarditis have occurred in only a few instances, one associated with a (subclavian vein) Hickman catheter infection. Viral infections occasionally encountered in combination with cardiac failure include Coxsackie myocarditis, which can be mistaken for failure due to direct toxicity of such drugs as daunomycin, cyclophosphamide (CY), or adriamycin. Toxoplasmosis occurs occasionally.

Myocardial infarction is unusual, probably because the young population has a low prevalence of severe atherosclerosis. However, severe hypoxia is common in patients with interstitial pneumonia. These patients frequently exhibit cardiomegaly with ventricular dilation and occasionally have small infarcts of such watershed areas as papillary muscles and upper interventricular septum.

Evidence for GVHD involving the myocardium is conflicting. The early rodent studies of chronic GVHD by Stastny et al.[615] showed chronic inflammatory reaction involving the valves and, in rare instances, the myocardium and the coronary arteries. In the more recent rat model of GVHD of Beschorner et al.[54,55] myocardial abnormalities were present in half the animals but consisted only of interstitial edema and sparse lymphocytic infiltration. The relationship of myocardial findings to GVHD in man remains controversial. Graze and Gale[262] illustrated concentric intimal sclerosis of the major coronary artery in a young patient with chronic GVHD and likened these changes to those occurring in scleroderma. Shulman et al.[584] found perivascular chronic inflammatory cell infiltrates, focal dropout of myocytes and fibrosis, and eccentric coronary artery intimal sclerosis in patients with chronic GVHD. Certainly, these findings, which resemble those in progressive systemic sclerosis, should encourage further controlled observations. However, the etiology of these changes could as well relate to viral infections or late toxic effects from conditioning.

## GENITOURINARY SYSTEM

### Hemorrhage

Hemorrhagic cystitis is a well-known complication of therapy with CY. This troublesome complication can often be avoided by hydration and diuresis to prevent toxic injury by the renal excretion of the activated metabolites. Hemorrhagic cystitis occurs immediately after conditioning regimen or after a delay. It produces marked bleeding and can later lead to a small fibrotic bladder. Histologically, the bladder mucosa is partially or completely ulcerated and the remaining epithelium displays cytologic atypia. The edematous submucosa contains vessels with fibrinoid necrosis of their walls, similar to those found in the myocardium. Some smooth muscle cells of the bladder wall may also be necrotic.[592] Similar changes may occasionally be found in the ureters and renal pelvis.

### Infection

About 7% of autopsied marrow recipients have evidence of disseminated fungal infection that usually includes subclinical involvement of the kidney. The most frequent organism is *Candida*, which grows within the tubules and also produces miliary abscesses. Less frequently, vascular invasion occurs with disseminated aspergillosis. Occasionally, bacterial septicemia, especially with such organisms as *Pseudomonas*, produces abscesses. In adult patients dying with systemic cytomegalovirus (CMV) infection, involvement of the kidney can usually be demonstrated if enough sections are reviewed. CMV produces inclusions in the tubular epithelium and the glomeruli, but only rarely produces foci of necrosis. Two groups have reported CMV-associated glomerulopathy in renal allograft recipients.[280a,526a] The changes, however, lack prognostic significance and are nonspecific. They include glomerular enlargement, endothelial necrosis, and accumulation within glomerular tufts of mononuclear cells and fibrils. In our transplant population, CMV viremia and renal failure frequently coexist, but we have never demonstrated an association between the two phenomena.

CMV viremia and system infection frequently occur without any accompanying change in renal function. We have seen changes identical to those reported in CMV glomerulopathy in patients who, at autopsy, have no cultural or histologic evidence of CMV. We have seen one case of a disseminated adenovirus infection producing renal failure secondary to large areas of cortical necrosis accompanied by many inclusion-bearing cells.

## GVHD

In animal and clinical studies, GVHD has had no consistent association with renal insufficiency. An immune complex glomerulonephritis with proteinuria has been clearly demonstrated in mice with chronic GVHD.[238,381] These authors present convincing evidence that: 1) immune complexes are present in dense, lumpy subepithelial deposits, demonstrable by immunofluorescence and electron microscopy; 2) the antigen is of host origin; and 3) the antibody is of donor origin. The ability to produce this requires an $H_2$-locus-dependent antigen in the host which is recognized as incompatible by the donor. In other words, a major histoincompatibility is needed. Furthermore, not all $H_2$ incompatible combinations exhibit the lesion. If analogy exists between mice and other species, such as humans, one might expect the probability of developing glomerulonephritis to be maximal in some HLA-mismatched combinations.

Other murine studies of GVHD have reported varied findings in renal pathology. Rappaport et al.[519] studied radiation chimeric rodents undergoing lethal GVHR across $H_2$ and non-$H_2$ histocompatibility barriers. They described a progressive, proliferative glomerulonephritis with mesangial widening, hypercellularity, thickened basement membranes, flattening of foot processes, and lymphocytic infiltration of glomerular tufts, eventuating in glomerulosclerosis and arteriolosclerosis. Morton et al.[451] also examined renal histology in radiation-chimeric DBA/2 mice receiving syngeneic and allogeneic marrow grafts from BALB/C2 mice after TBI. At 10 months post transplant, both the syngeneic and allogeneic graft recipients had glomerular hypercellularity with variable nuclear size and injured capillary (mesangial) sclerosis. Stastny et al.[615] described

mild focal thickening of glomerular basement membranes and unassociated perivascular inflammation. Beschorner et al.[53,54] studied chronic GVHD in the rat radiation chimera and found no specific histologic changes in the kidneys.

Involvement of the human kidney in GVHD remains unlikely. Graze and Gale[263] have described a lobular glomerulonephritis and arteriosclerosis in patients with chronic GVHD. We found that patients dying with chronic GVHD had a variety of glomerular and vascular changes.[584] Glomeruli frequently had moderate to marked mesangial expansion and sclerosis and variable hypercellularity. The peripheral basal lamina was irregularly thickened and split, and occasionally contained subendothelial dense bodies. Arterioles had a local distribution of eccentric intimal thickening with degeneration and loss of media smooth muscle and an increase of interstitial matrix. However, these observations cannot be taken as evidence for immunologically mediated injury caused by GVHD without adequate controls.

Some relevant antineoplastic agents have known renal toxicity.[563a] *Cis*-platin and streptozoticin have been shown to cause marked tubular injury in man and *cis*-platin has been associated with systemic hypertension. Chronic renal failure with glomerular sclerosis and extensive tubular injury was reported after treatment with methyl CCNU. Mitomycin has caused glomerular necrosis and a microangiopathic hemolytic anemia. Fajardo[195] has reported that rabbits receiving adriamycin develop severe glomerular vacuolization, dilatation of tubules, and interstitial fibrosis. The effects of irradiation on the kidney have been studied in man and animals.[194,328,342] After 2000 rad of fractionated irradiation, radiation-induced renal disease may develop. The initial lesion probably involves injury to the vascular endothelium with the subsequent changes of tubular atrophy and glomerular sclerosis—secondary phenomena.[194]

On rare occasions, we have found fibrin within the loops of some glomeruli consistent with a disseminated intravascular coagulation. Spruce et al.[612] reported one case of hemolytic–uremic syndrome 9 months after marrow transplantation. A hemolytic–uremic syndrome with renal insufficiency has also been reported after treatment with cyclosporine (CYA) by several authors.[513,585] We reported hypertension, thrombocytopenia, and a microangiopathic anemia associated with microthrombi composed of thrombin and platelets at the hili of glomeruli. The mechanism of the hemolytic–uremic-like syndrome developing after CYA is unknown, but may be secondary to drug-induced endothelial injury. The tubular injury thought to be caused by CYA is more common and usually reversible.

### ENDOCRINE AND OTHER SYSTEMS

### Pituitary

To date, complications involving the pituitary gland have been confined to edema and infarction secondary to cerebral edema after respirator therapy, and to involvement of the meninges by recurrent leukemia or lymphoma.

### Adrenals

Congestion and subtotal hemorrhage are relatively frequent, especially in Gram-negative bacteremia. The adrenal gland appears to be even more frequently involved in disseminated CMV infection than is the liver. Typical lesions at the corticomedullary junction will show foci of necrosis surrounded by moderate infiltrates of lymphocytes and plasma cells. A search of several sections will often reveal typical CMV inclusion bodies (Figs. 1 and 2). No evidence of involvement with GVHD has been found.

### Thyroid

This gland is the occasional site for disseminated fungal infection. Interstitial fibrosis has been reported both in systemic sclerosis and in one case of chronic GVHD.[584] No lesions resembling autoimmune thyroiditis are reported.

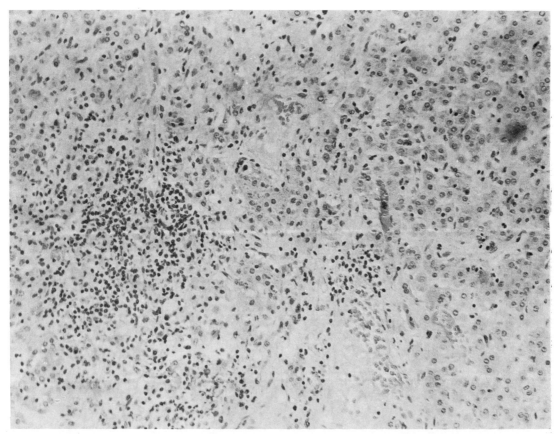

**Figure 1.** Cytomegalovirus infection of the adrenal gland at medium power. There are two focal lymphocytic infiltrates accompanied by necrosis. Identification of cytomegalovirus inclusion bodies may require a few serial sections. An infected cell is visible on the right. Specimen from patient UPN 600.

## Parathyroid

In our autopsy experience, chief cell hyperplasia is relatively common after marrow transplantation. Secondary hyperparathyroidism may be the explanation. Abnormal bone resorption by osteoclasts is not uncommon in marrow biopsies or autopsies and further study may confirm this impression (Muller-Hermelink, personal communication).

## Gonads

Testicular aspermia and ovarian atrophy are constant sequellae of the chemoradiotherapy that is given marrow graft recipients. The sterility is not always permanent, but the genetic consequences of reproduction after such therapy are unknown.

## Pancreas

GVHD involving the beta cells of the pancreatic islets has been reported in semiallogeneic $F_1$ hybrid mice by Kolb et al.[353,583] but does not seem to occur in humans or in other species. In our experience, the pancreatic and larger biliary ducts may rarely be involved by particularly severe GVHD in dogs and humans, but usually only the smaller interlobular hepatic bile ducts are affected. About 10% of our autopsies exhibit interstitial pancreatitis ranging from slight to severe, but there is no evidence that this is related to GVHD. Shock, septicemia, viral infections, and other secondary problems in these severely ill patients are more likely causes.

In 1977, we reported multiple hepatic adenomas and pancreatic islet cell tumors in a transplant patient with aplastic anemia who had been treated for about 5 years with androgens and glucocorticoids.[544] Since that time, a number of other patients with similar findings have been reported. Androgen and oral contraceptive therapy had already been associated with liver tumors, but the syndrome of both hepatic and islet adenomas had not. Novak et al.[474] reported three

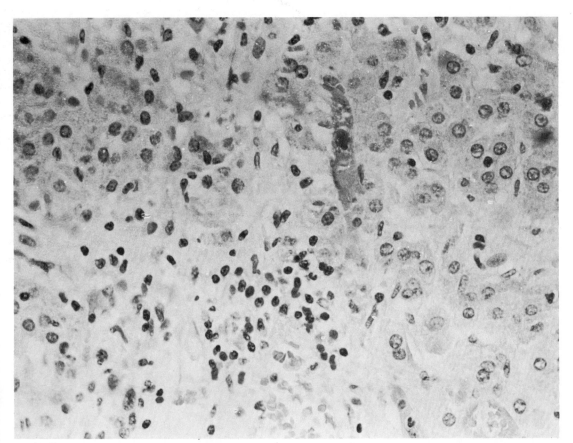

**Figure 2.** Higher-power view of CMV-infected cell adjacent to a lymphocytic infiltrate. Specimen from patient UPN 600.

patients with Fanconi's aplastic anemia who had both islet cell hyperplasia and benign liver cell tumors after 42 months of androgen therapy. In 1978, Foster et al.[217] reported familial liver adenomas in diabetes mellitus. Recently, Thung et al.[677] described diffuse nodular regenerative hyperplasia of the liver in a patient with diabetes. These cases suggest important relationships between pancreatic islet cell and hepatocytic neoplasia. There appears to be a hepatopancreatic syndrome comprising hyperplasia of both islet cells and hepatocytes which involves trophic effects of androgens, glucocorticoids, or polypeptide hormones such as insulin and glucagon. Alertness for more examples of such cases is needed. Pathologists assisting in the care of patients with hematologic diseases will have the most frequent opportunities for recognizing such cases, because without autopsy the pancreatic lesions will be missed.

### CONCLUSION

Table 1 suggests the current status of reported or proposed lesions and classifies them according to the likelihood with which they may be regarded as strongly associated with GVHD. The "definite" category is confined to noncontroversial lesions, or those which seem well supported statistically in more than one species or by more than one group of investigators. The other three categories are, by degrees, less well supported by the evidence.

### ADDENDUM

The small bile duct lesions in human liver should now be moved to the "definite" category (Table 1) as a result of the confirming study of Snover et al. (*Hepatology 4:* 127–130, 1984). Portal venous endothelialitis should be added to the "possible" list as a result of the same study.

**TABLE 1**
Current Status of Lesions Attributed to GVHD
(Degree of Certainty with Which
Lesion is Associated with GVHD)

*Definite:* agreed to and/or supported by statistics from at least two groups, or seen in humans and one other species.
1. Skin in acute and chronic GVHD
2. Gut in acute and "subacute" GVHD (from stomach to rectum)
3. Esophagus in acute GVHD
4. Hepatocyte in acute GVHD
5. Lip squamous epithelium
6. Cervical and vaginal squamous epithelium
7. Minor salivary gland ducts
8. Lacrimal gland ducts
9. Small bile ducts of liver in dogs and rats
10. Synovium (man and rat)
11. Serous surfaces:
     pericardium (man and rat), and
     peritoneum (man and rat)

*Probable:* not universally accepted, or not confirmed by a second group of investigators or in a second species.
1. Small bile ducts of liver in man (although confirmed in rat and horse, and agreed to by majority of published authors in human liver)
2. Conjunctiva
3. Skeletal muscle
4. Major salivary glands
5. Pancreatic islets in mice
6. Developing rat cerebellum
7. Esophageal fibrosis apart from infectious etiology

*Possible:* either not yet firmly buttressed by statistics, or controversial.
1. Human vessels
2. Pancreatic ducts
3. Limbus
4. Bronchial ciliary epithelium
5. Bronchial glands
6. Deep fibrosis of intestine
7. Esophageal submucosal glands
8. Larger order bile ducts in man and dog
9. Heart
10. Pleura

*Unlikely*
1. Cornea
2. Brain outside neonatal rats
3. Human pancreatic islets (although found in some rodents)
4. Human renal glomeruli (although found in rodents)

# Chapter 12

# Pathology of infections after bone marrow transplantation

**George E. Sale, M.D.**
**Robert C. Hackman, M.D.**

### Introduction

Infection and its clinical management after bone marrow transplantation have recently been reviewed at length.[440] This chapter will briefly review the clinical aspects in order to alert the pathologist to these infections. Infections tend to occur in three temporal groups: 1) the early granulocytopenic period (day 0–30) in which bacterial, fungal and herpes simplex virus infections predominate; 2) the recovery period (about day 30–100) when viral, protozoal, and idiopathic pneumonias predominate; and 3) the late period (after day 100) when varicella zoster, Gram-positive coccal, and Pneumocystis infections may occur, the latter two particularly in association with GVHD.

It is important to remain aware that microorganisms may behave in unexpected ways in these severely immunocompromised hosts. The incidence patterns are different from those in other patients. The predominant bacterial infections in our series have changed over several years from Gram-negative bacilli to Gram-positive organisms, such as *Staphylococcus epidermidis* and ordinary Corynebacteria. Any organism can be an invasive pathogen in these patients. Therefore, biopsy and autopsy cultures and special stains must be done thoroughly and any positive culture may be significant. Extensive study of the value of isolation, prophylactic antibiotics, and granulocyte transfusions have been carried out over the past several years. Buckner et al.[86] and Clift et al.[110–112] showed that laminar airflow room isolation and prophylactic granulocyte transfusions were strongly associated with a decrease in local and blood infections during the first 3 weeks after transplantation. Winston et al.[754,755] reported an increase in cytomegalovirus (CMV) infections associated with granulocyte transfusions, suggesting that the blood products were the source. Hersman et al.[289a] have now shown that this is likely to be due to the transfusion of granulocytes from CMV-seropositive donors into seronegative recipients. The latter study showed no significant increase in CMV infection rates in seropositive recipients of granulocytes whether the granulocyte donor was seropositive or seronegative.

### BACTERIAL INFECTIONS

Analyses of the first 52 Seattle marrow transplant patients by Clift et al.[110] and of 60 UCLA patients by Winston et al.[751–753] provide a detailed review of the early experience with infectious complications during the first 3 months after marrow transplantation for aplastic anemia or leukemia. In the former study, the frequency of septicemia was high between days 0–30 but then fell markedly in leukemic patients. Although half the aplasia patients developed septicemia after day 30, in most of these cases, either GVHD or rejection with neutropenia was present. The majority of the bacteremic episodes were due to *E. coli*, Pseudomonas, or Candida.

The study by Winston et al.[752] showed a similar distribution of early infections. Post-transplant bacterial and fungal infections showed a median onset before day 30. Fifty-three percent of the positive blood cultures showed Gram-negative bacteria (most commonly Pseudomonas, Klebsiella, and *E. coli*) and 33% were fungal (chiefly Candida, with two Aspergillus and one Trichophyton). Of the fungal infections, 14 were in the blood, eight in the lung, and one each in esophagus and peritoneum. Infections relatively uncommon in the United States also may occur. Active tuberculosis can occur as a reactivation or unsuspected active infection, as two of our patients demonstrated (Fig. 1). Atypical mycobacteria have infected a few patients, with fatal consequences in one. Nocardia infections may also occur (Fig. 2), although we have not yet seen Legionella.

A study of our late infections (in patients surviving at least 6 months) was reported by Atkinson.[19] Eighty-nine patients were analyzed, of whom 76 had received allogeneic, and 13 syngeneic grafts for aplastic anemia or leukemia. Significant late infections, defined as three or more episodes, occurred in 28% of the patients; 9% died from infection. Bacteria accounted for the majority of the infections occurring in the blood, respiratory tract, or skin, and one-third of the identified organisms were Gram-positive cocci. Bacterial infections were significantly associated with chronic GVHD. Varicella zoster virus (VZV) infections occurred in 22% of all patients but were not associated with chronic GVHD, although they were associated with negative skin tests to dinitrochlorobenzene. Fungal infections and interstitial pneumonia were uncommon late after transplantation.

### GRANULOCYTIC FUNCTION AFTER MARROW TRANSPLANTATION

The broad impairment of immune function, which occurs after marrow transplantation, and which may be due partially to delayed maturation of repopulating lymphoid cell types, is paral-leled by defects in granulocyte function. Sosa et al. studied 87 allogeneic marrow transplant recipients and 25 normal individuals.[605] They found depressed granulocyte chemotaxis in all marrow allograft recipients for the first 4 months after grafting, but normal chemotaxis in long-term survivors (days 175–2202 post transplant). However, patients with acute or chronic GVHD or infection had lower chemotactic responses than those without these entities. Impaired chemotaxis may, therefore, be regarded as another form of immunodeficiency associated with GVHD.

### FUNGAL INFECTIONS

Candida, Aspergillus, and zygomycete infections are well known to physicians treating leukemia patients with chemotherapy (Fig. 3). In the setting of marrow transplantation, the deep fungal infections show a similar species distribution, although rarer infections also occur. Histoplasmosis, blastomycosis, coccidioidomycosis, disseminated Torulopsis infection primary in the small bowel, brain infection with apiospermium, and rare zygomycetes have all occurred in marrow transplant recipients, in Seattle and elsewhere (Figs. 4–6).

Martin, Counts, and Thomas[411] analyzed 160 autopsy-proven cases of fungal infection in marrow recipients treated between March 1969 to January 1977. Excluding skin, gastrointestinal, or tracheobronchial infections, 55 fungal infections in 48 patients (30%) were identified histologically. Candida was the most frequent pathogen in this varied group of infections, of which 35 were disseminated and 20 local. At the time of death, marrow cellularity of less than 50% of normal for age was significantly associated with fungal infection ($p = 0.001$) and nearly half such patients were infected.

With early diagnosis, the treatment of fungal infections, especially with amphotericin B, may be successful. However, cure of deep fungal infections after invasion of vessels or viscera is still uncommon in immunocompromised patients. A young leukemic woman we transplanted in 1975 suffered a shunt infection with a zygomycete which invaded the radial artery (Fig. 3). This infection was successfully eradicated by combining intravenous amphotericin therapy with careful debridement. A more recent case was that of a teenaged male with aplastic anemia treated with

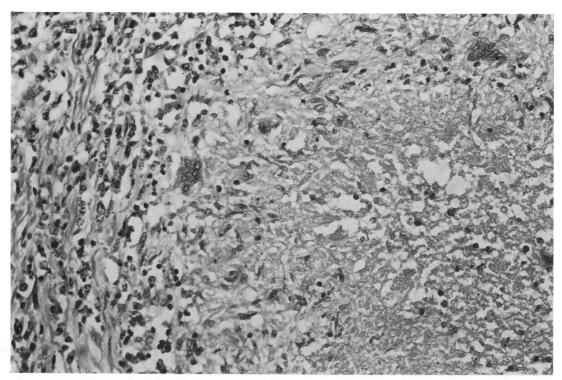

**Figure 1.**   One of two cases of tuberculosis we have seen after marrow transplantation. An 18-year-old male from Burma was transplanted for ALL in remission but died of CMV pneumonitis. Also discovered was focal, newly reactivated *Mycobacterium tuberculosis* infection, diagnosed at autopsy. Section is of small cavitating lesion in left upper lobe; hilar nodes were also involved.

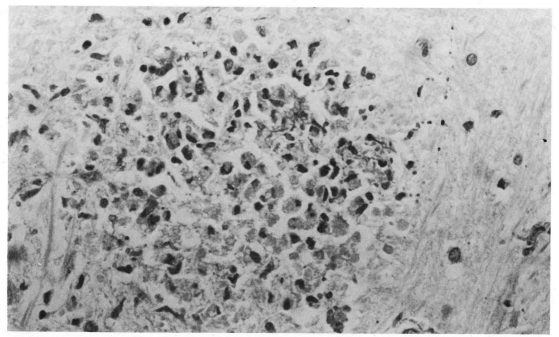

**Figure 2.**   Microscopic brain abscess stained with PAS reveals fibrillar organisms within nodular masses at 1 o'clock and 3 o'clock in this photograph of an autopsy. This 39-year-old male with AML died of disseminated infection with *Nocardia caviae* as well as CMV. Both organisms involved lung and liver, and the former involved brain. (See Fig. 18.)

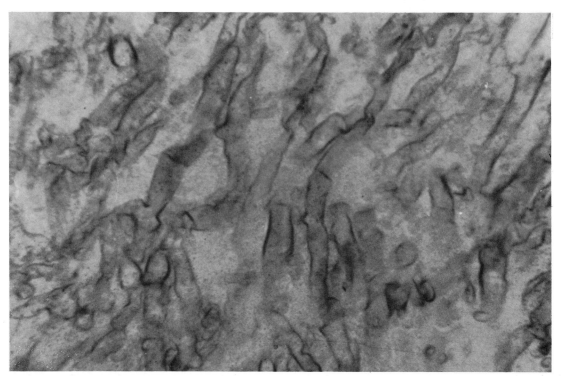

**Figure 3.** High-power photograph of the organisms (zygomycetes) found in the lumen of the infected radial artery near the Scribner shunt of patient described in text (fungal infections). This invasive infection disappeared in response to drugs and debridement.

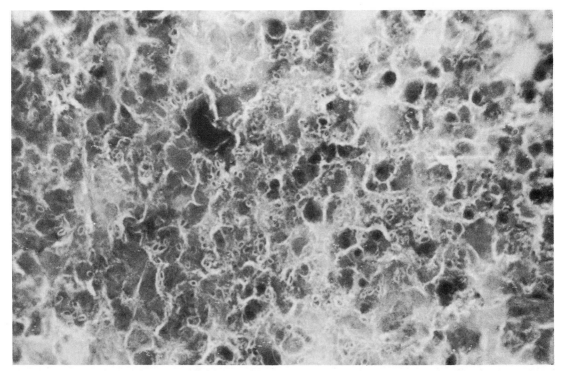

**Figure 4.** Active histoplasmosis as it appeared on a frozen section at open-lung biopsy. Stains and cultures confirmed *Histoplasma capsulatum* in this patient from the American midwest.

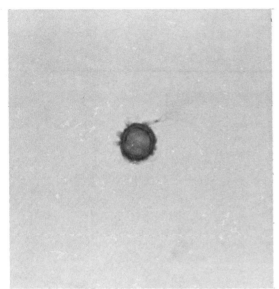

**Figure 5.** Culture of the same patient's lung biopsy confirmed characteristic morphology of *Histoplama capsulatum* as shown.

antithymocyte globulin (ATG), mismatched bone marrow, and androgens. Open-liver biopsy performed because of persistent fever and high alkaline phosphatase revealed miliary infection with *Candida albicans*. Despite a poor prognosis and continued dependence on platelet and red cell transfusions, this patient became afebrile while on amphotericin therapy and remains alive and afebrile over 12 months later. A laparotomy with repeat liver biopsy 6½ months after treatment revealed no evidence of residual infection. Newer agents for treatment of fungal infections, such as ketaconizole, are now available and are undergoing evaluation in patients with fungal infections, including marrow transplant recipients.[724]

A serious unsolved problem in the management of fungal infections is the difficulty of diagnosis. About half of the deep fungal infections we have diagnosed were not discovered until autopsy, as is often the case. Blood cultures commonly are not positive until very late in the course of infection, if at all. Serological or chemical methods for the detection of fungal antigen, particularly Candida, are available but carry a significant false-negative rate.[444] Fungi cause the most frequent granulomatous diseases in this population. As a general rule, histochemistry is twice as sensitive as culture for the diagnosis of lung granulomas,[704] and the rule may well extend to other organs in a transplanted population. Early and aggressive use of special stains on biopsies, therefore, provides the patient's best chance for a premortem fungal diagnosis and definitive treatment.

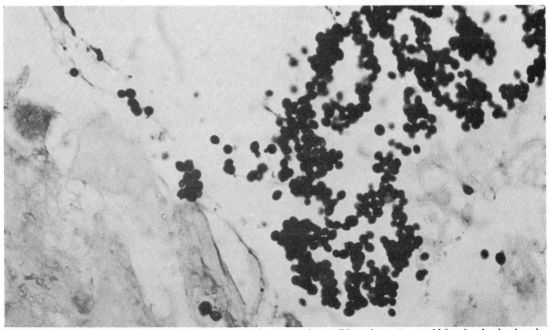

**Figure 6.** *Torulopsis glabrata* diagnosed in fibrinous exudate lining the small bowel in a 19-year-old female who developed a severe invasive infection of the entire small and large bowel due to this organism, and died with hemorrhage and fungemia. (Rapid methenamine silver stain.)[405]

## PARASITIC INFECTIONS

*Pneumocystis carinii* has been an important cause of pneumonia occurring in immunosuppressed patients. Originally called "plasma-cell" pneumonia, this entity was recently reviewed at length by Dutz.[165] The classical description is that of a diffuse process with interstitial and alveolar exudates, the latter particularly heavily laden with cysts. More recently, it has been realized that both the radiographic and the histologic patterns can be quite variable. In our patient population, these organisms are found in the interstitium as frequently as in alveoli, and the concentration of organisms per volume tissue is much lower than usually described. We developed a rapid modification of the methenamine silver technique because of the need for immediate study of smears and frozen sections at open-lung or transbronchial biopsy.[405] Prophylactic trimethoprim sulfa, first reported by Hughes and colleagues,[300] has resulted in the near elimination of this problem in patients able to take the medicine orally.[434,439]

Because of the rapid progression that can occur in patients suffering from this pneumonitis, rapid biopsy diagnosis is very important. We routinely include methenamine silver stains in our studies (Fig. 7). In our hands, the Giemsa method for the trophozoite forms has shown a very low sensitivity (about 5%) when compared directly to the silver method in multiple serial smears of the same infected rat or human lung specimen. Combined infection with CMV and Pneumocystis occurs in some cases of interstitial pneumonia, and an infrequent case of Pneumocystis is still diagnosed at autopsy, emphasizing the continuing importance of the disease in the differential diagnosis (Fig. 8). Fatal Pneumocystis pneumonia can appear suddenly in long-term survivors with chronic GVHD, particularly if they have had prior Pneumocystis infections. For this and other reasons, prophylactic trimethoprim sulfa is frequently continued in patients with chronic GVHD.

Toxoplasmosis is an unusual disseminated infection which occurs more frequently in immunosuppressed patients. We have found eight cases in the course of some 400 autopsies, of which only two were diagnosed premortem. The importance of this diagnosis is underscored when one discovers at autopsy a case for which strong premortem evidence had been present:

> A 19-year-old male underwent lymph node biopsy in 1973 for adenopathy. A diagnosis of toxoplasma lymphadenitis was made on the basis of the histology and a toxoplasma titer of 1/1024 by indirect fluorescence. No specific treatment was given. In May 1976, he underwent another lymph node biopsy for a 2-month febrile illness culminating in supraclavicular lymphadenopathy and anemia. The diagnosis was convoluted T-cell lymphoma in the leukemic phase. From May through July, the patient underwent chemotherapy accompanied by pyrimethamine and sulfadiazine therapy for toxoplasmosis. A remission, followed by a matched-sibling marrow allograft in August, ensued. Preconditioning was accomplished through use of dimethylbusulfan, cyclophosphamide (CY), and TBI. Unexplained headaches occurred in September and lasted several weeks. He developed fatal idiopathic interstitial pneumonia after an episode of epigastric pain and ileus, and died 120 days postgrafting. Autopsy disclosed idiopathic pneumonia and a gastric ulcer eroding into the pancreas. The brain and heart, however, showed active toxoplasma encephalitis and myocarditis (Figs. 9–12).

Vigilance for other parasitic infections continues to be necessary in a population drawn, as is ours, from the whole world. Ancylostoma and Strongyloides have both been found in our patients. Rarely, skin biopsy diagnoses of *Demodex follicularis* infestation have been made in sites (such as the forearm) not usually associated with this parasite.

## VIRAL INFECTIONS

The herpes viruses (CMV, herpes zoster, and herpes simplex) cause the vast majority of the diagnosed viral infections after marrow transplantation. Immune dysfunction caused by marrow and lymphoid irradiation, cytotoxic and immunosuppressive drugs, as well as by GVHD in many patients, is the chief predisposing factor to these infections. Between 1969 and 1979, the annual incidence of interstitial pneumonia in our total patient population varied from 10 to 58%, with a mean of 42%. CMV was the most prominent in this series.

### Cytomegalovirus (CMV) (Figures 13–19)

On the average, CMV pneumonia has constituted 40% of all pneumonias and 90% of these

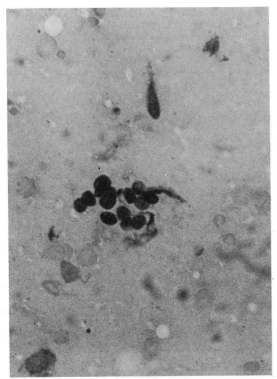

**Figure 7.** Rapid methenamine silver stain of lung smear from 9-year-old boy with ALL and a rapidly progressive pneumonia. He died of *Pneumocystis carinii* infection, diagnosed by identifying silver-stained clusters of cysts. (×40, air objective.)

cases have been fatal. The existence of a significant primary "interstitial" pneumonia caused by CMV and associated with early miliary lesions and focal necrosis now seems to be accepted. Miliary forms seem to progress, in animal models, to diffuse forms.[132] One recent study suggested that miliary and diffuse forms in man are separable clinicopathologic entities. Because blood and splenic infections were associated with rapidly progressive cases associated with miliary lesions in the lung in five patients, the authors propose miliary CMV as a separate entity with a worse prognosis.[52] However, in practice there are many exceptions to this dichotomy. In our series, miliary cases recover more often than diffuse cases do. The small percentage of biopsy-proven cases of CMV which have recovered have had a miliary pattern at biopsy with large areas of normal lung tissue between miliary foci (six cases). Furthermore, we frequently see miliary patterns at early biopsy in patients who progress over periods of weeks to display diffuse pulmonary damage. Some miliary cases do progress rapidly, as in the above-mentioned series. Our impression has been that the rate of progression varies greatly and is not predictable from the initial tissue pattern. Perhaps identification of different strains of CMV by a search for subtype-

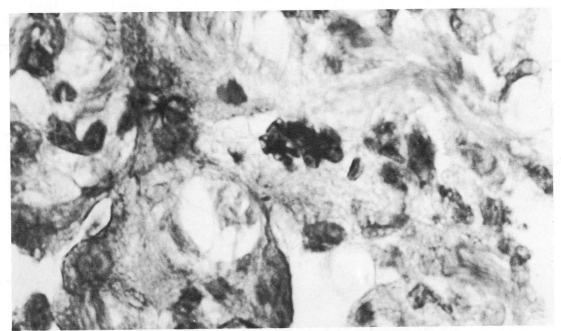

**Figure 8.** (UPN 396) Similar cluster (center) of paraffin section stained with rapid methenamine silver, H&E counterstain. This was a 38-year-old male who died of combined CMV-pneumocystis infection after allograft for AML. (See Fig. 15.)

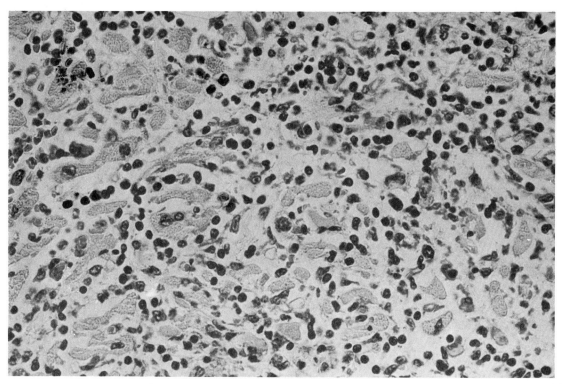

**Figure 9.**    Toxoplasma myocarditis in patient described in the text exhibits toxoplasma cyst (center) and extensive inflammation and destruction of adjacent myocardium. Free trophozoites were demonstrable in heart and brain by tissue Giemsa stain.

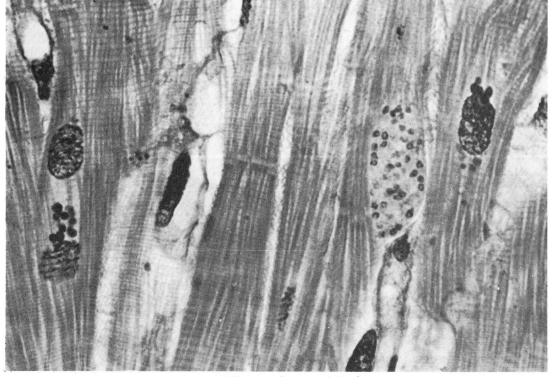

**Figure 10.**    Toxoplasmosis in heart of another patient. (×630 methacrylate, H&E.)

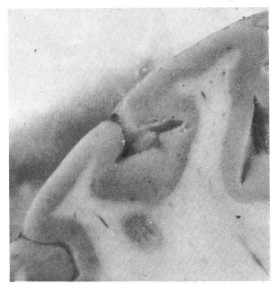

**Figure 11.** An 0.8-cm diameter focus of soft necrosis in cerebral white matter of patient with toxoplasmosis described in text.

disease. Brain infection is rare, and sufficient renal tubular involvement to produce many inclusions is unusual despite frequently positive urine cultures. Adrenal infection is common, and hepatic, splenic, and lymph node involvement are not unusual. Study of the latency of CMV infection by DNA hybridization techniques is one of the new methods which can be applied directly to biopsy and autopsy tissue. Briefly, RNA encoded for by segments of viral DNA can be detected by autoradiographic or immunoperoxidase methods in frozen sections or smears of infected tissue.[467] Results suggest that latent CMV infection is highly prevalent in general adult populations and that much remains to be learned about activation mechanisms.

specific antibodies would clarify the hypothesis postulating separable entities due to organisms of different virulence.

Fatal disseminated cases in adults after marrow transplant show a different distribution of viral lesions from that in neonates with congenital

We have recently shown that Wright-Giemsa, toluidine-blue, or Papanicolaou stained smears of open-lung biopsy specimens can provide immediate diagnosis of CMV pneumonia in nearly half the cases. Furthermore, the smear technique is thrice as sensitive as frozen section, which in itself can detect 13–15% of cases proven positive by culture or permanent section days to weeks later.[551,585a] Such methods might be rendered even more sensitive and specific by using pools of monoclonal antibodies to CMV antigens.[251,252]

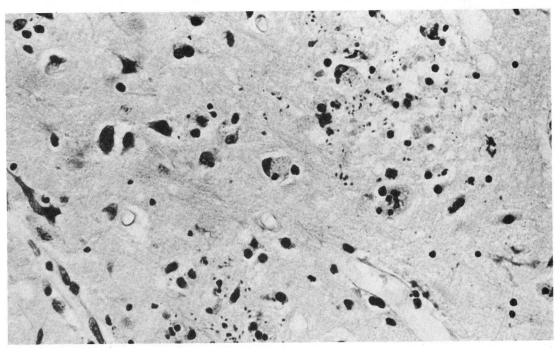

**Figure 12.** Focus of active toxoplasma encephalitis in brain of another patient showing multiple comma-shaped organisms of *Toxoplasma gondii.* (×250 Giemsa.)

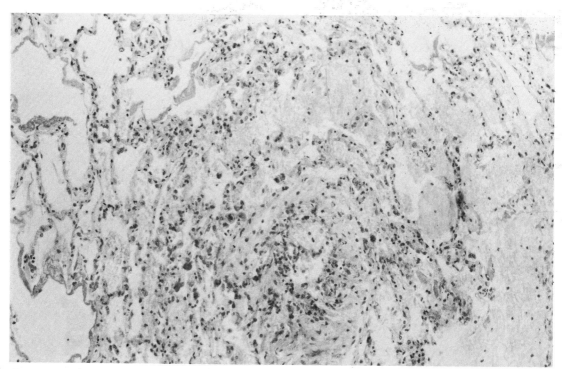

**Figure 13.** Miliary CMV pneumonia at low power. Concentric circles from the inside out exhibit: a) inflammatory infiltrate and hemorrhage; b) multiple CMV inclusions; c) zone of alveolar damage and pulmonary edema with alveolar proteinaceous fluid and small hyaline membranes; and d) region of intervening, nearly normal lung. The patient's radiograph suggested a miliary to interstitial pattern.

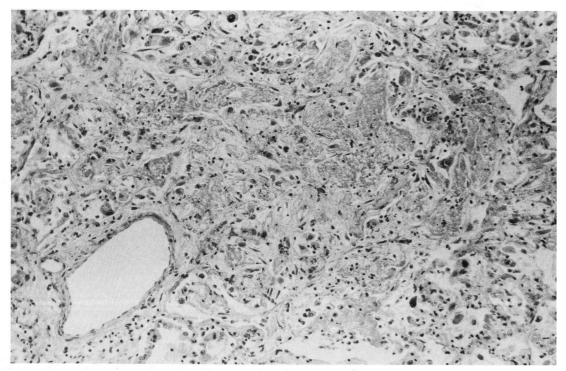

**Figure 14.** Similar region near a pulmonary venule (lower left) shows again dense perivascular damage to alveoli with proteinaceous fluid and with multiple CMV inclusion bodies concentrically arranged.

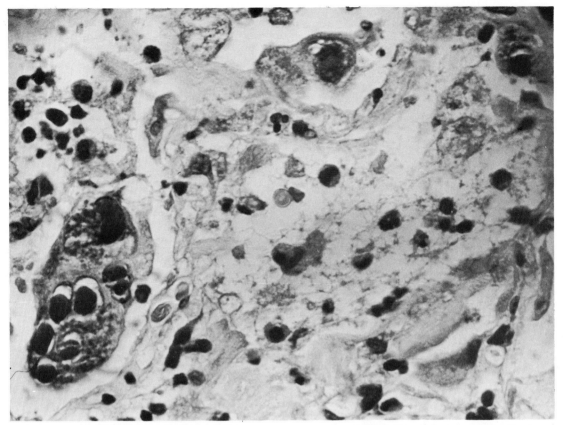

**Figure 15.** Example of spectacular nature of CMV inclusions in some cases. Multiple CMV inclusions in giant cell at lower left. More typical inclusions at upper middle and upper right. Same open-lung biopsy as Fig. 8 in fatal combined CMV-*Pneumocystis* infection.

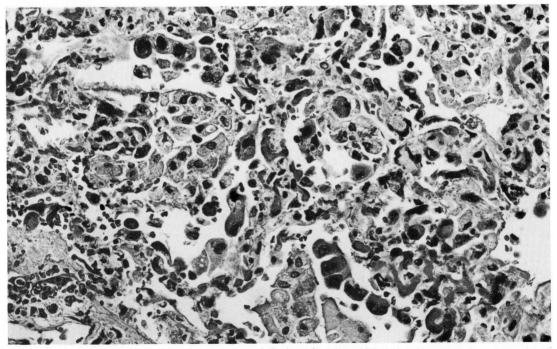

**Figure 16.** (UPN 1459) Diffuse CMV pneumonitis with high viral load and extreme diffuse alveolar damage in a 29-year-old woman with AML. Carnoy's fixation yields darker and crisper-appearing nuclear inclusions than does formalin fixation.

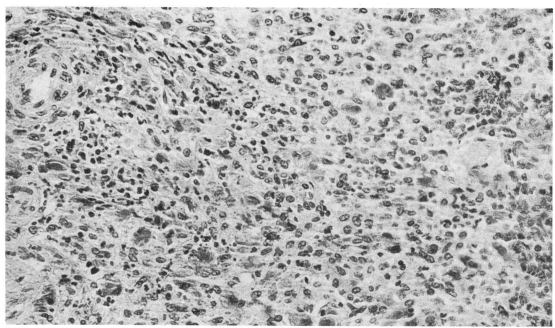

**Figure 17.**   Disseminated CMV infection involving the spleen in 18-year-old female with aplastic anemia. Large regions of necrosis near splenic arterioles show multiple cytopathic effects including CMV inclusion bodies. Hemorrhage, edema, and acellular PAS-positive interstitial material were readily demonstrable. Electron microscopy of the same block revealed multiple intranuclear and cytoplasmic herpes-type virus particles.

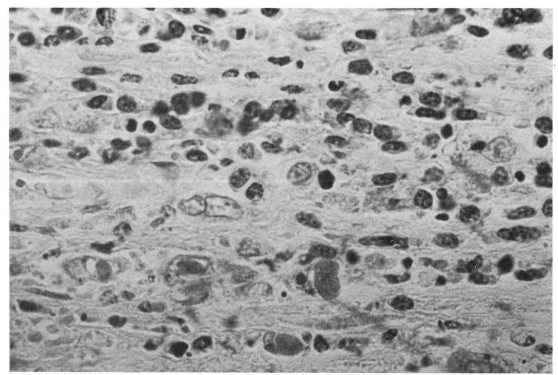

**Figure 18.**   High-power view of specimen in Fig. 3 of esophageal CMV involving lamina propria in patient with disseminated CMV and *Nocardia caviae* infections. Multiple cytopathic effects and several diagnostic inclusions in region of chronic inflammation and edema.

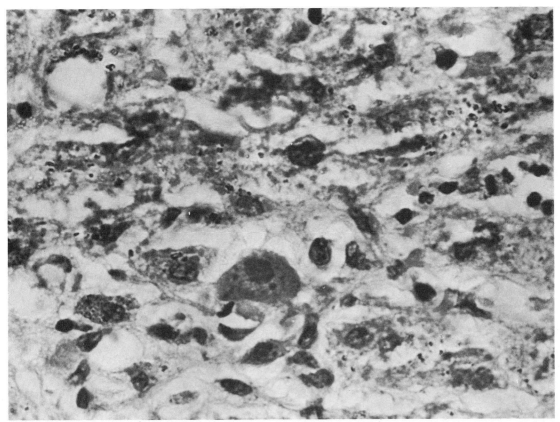

**Figure 19.** Hepatic involvement by disseminated CMV infection usually produced only scattered inclusion bodies in hepatocytes as seen in lower middle of this micrograph. Edema and necrosis are often nearby. Cell shows both nuclear and cytoplasmic inclusions. Particulate matter scattered about is due to increased iron stores.

In the future, these methods may serve to select patients rapidly for specific antiviral therapy of known effectiveness.

### Varicella zoster infections (VZV)

About half the patients in this setting develop VZV infections, most within the first year after engraftment, with a median onset of 5 months. Of 92 infected patients reported recently, 77 had herpes zoster and 15 had an infection resembling disseminated chickenpox. A 12% fatality rate of VZV in the first 4 months was seen, and was twice as high for the disseminated type as for the typical zoster case.[439] Disseminated VZV infections can be rapidly fatal and must be aggressively diagnosed to allow time for the initiation of therapy.

### Herpes simplex infections (HSV)

Most of these are oral infections and begin early post transplant. Sixteen reported patients with

prior oral or genital herpes developed pneumonia and were lung-culture positive: among serotyped cases, three were type II and had prior genital herpes, whereas two were type I and had previous oral involvement (Fig. 20). Clinically, oral cases had more focal pulmonary infiltrates and shorter courses than did genital cases. [518] The hypothesis is advanced that the oral cases more often spread locally, while genital cases may be blood-borne.

### Epstein-Barr virus (EBV)

Although EBV infection has been reported in one bone marrow recipient whose donor had evidenced a recent case of EBV-induced infectious mononucleosis,[652] the frequency of significant clinical events associated with EBV appears to be low in marrow transplant recipients. For example, Lange et al.[371] studied 50 or our marrow transplant recipients for serial EBV serology. They found the same exaggerated immune re-

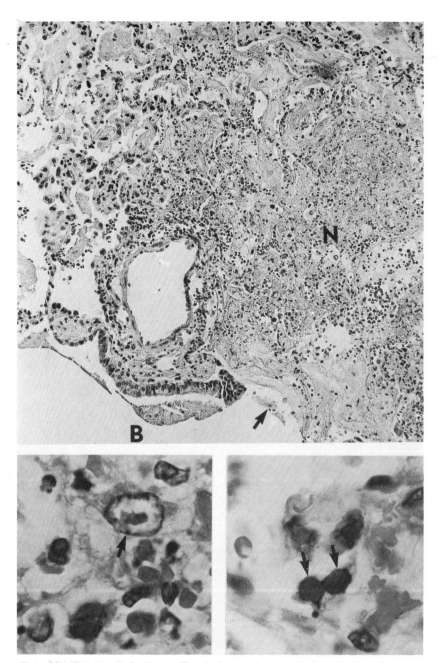

**Figure 20.**    Pneumonitis in 25-year-old male due to herpes simplex type I. At autopsy patient had positive pharyngeal culture and evidence of infection in adrenal gland as well as the illustrated pulmonary histology. (Top) An area of hemorrhage and necrosis (N) is contiguous with a bronchus (B) showing partial epithelial denudation marked by arrows. (Upper left) Alveoli contain a granular exudate and display septal widening and infiltration. (×320.) (Lower left) In the necrotic area, a cell (arrow) contains a characteristic eosinophilic intranuclear inclusion. (×320.) (Lower right) Other nearby nuclei (arrows) show chromatin margination and contain basophilic inclusion material which creates a ground-glass appearance. (×320.) (Reproduced with permission from Ramsey et al.[518] and the publisher of *Annals of Internal Medicine*.)

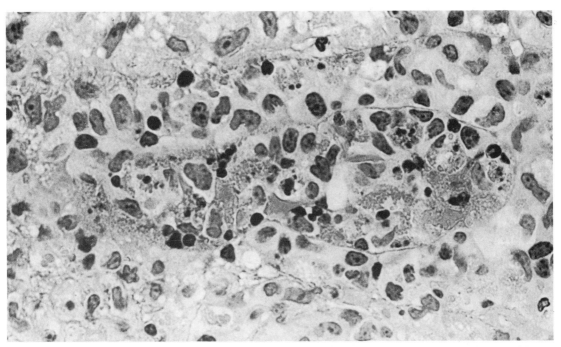

**Figure 21.** (UPN 1587) Adenovirus infection in 17-year-old male with aplastic anemia showing involvement of renal tubule. (Methacrylate, H&E.)

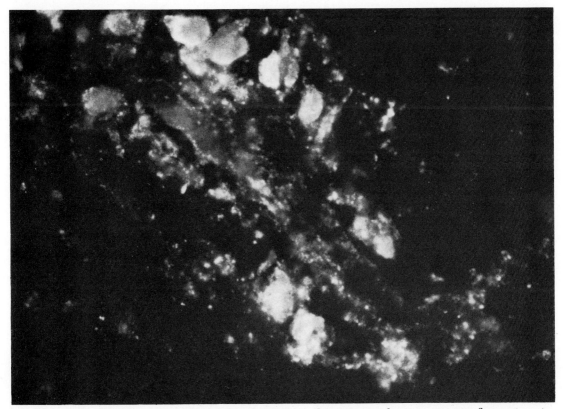

**Figure 22.** (UPN 1587) Adenovirus demonstrated by direct immunofluorescence on frozen section, using fluorescein-conjugated antibody to adenovirus. (×400.)

sponses to EBV in transplant patients as in other immunodeficient patients, but did not find clear evidence of infectious mononucleosis or other clinical syndromes associated with EBV. However, we have reported monoclonal B-cell immunoblastic sarcoma containing EBV genomic material.[273,569]

## Other viruses

Infectious gastroenteritis, associated with adenovirus, rotavirus, Coxsackie (as well as *Clostridium difficile*) was recently reported in 40% of 78 patients undergoing marrow transplantation in Baltimore.[764] This high percentage was detected by using sensitive immunoassay techniques on stool samples. These infections have not been so frequently reported in other centers using different methods, such as culture. About half these patients were thought to have GVHD. This issue should be thoroughly investigated in other centers, as some of these infections (such as *C. difficile*) are treatable and since much of the diarrhea in these patients is attributed to GVHD. Coxsackie infections also reported from Baltimore occurred in a single outbreak of seven cases over a 3-week period. Coxsackie myocarditis may occasionally masquerade as CY-induced cardiomyopathy in our unpublished experience. Adenovirus can sometimes infect the lung, liver, and kidney in this patient population as well (Figs. 21, 22).

## CONCLUSION

Rapid diagnosis of infections in marrow graft recipients may save their lives. The critical role of the histopathologist here is obvious. Nothing is faster than rapid smears, frozen sections, and direct histochemistry, and, in the case of fungi and parasites, nothing is more sensitive. Even minor, scientifically mundane, technical improvements can have a major impact on patient care if applied early in these settings. Newer rapid techniques are also becoming available, such as those using monoclonal antibodies. Similarly, in the fatal cases, autopsy is the only reliable source of data about infection by many of the organisms, especially fungi and parasites, plaguing this population.

## ADDENDUM

Several additional cases of EBV-associated lymphoproliferative disease in marrow transplant recipients have recently come to light. (Martin, Paul et al.: Fatal EBV associated proliferation of donor B cells following treatment of acute graft versus host disease with a murine monoclonal anti T cell antibody. *Blood* (in press). Also, latent CMV infection is widespread in human autopsy tissue in these patients. (Myerson, D. et al.: Widespread presence of histologically occult cytomegalovirus. *Hum Pathol* April, 1984.)

# Chapter 13

# Pathology of bone marrow with marrow transplantation

George E. Sale, M.D.

## BONE MARROW PRIOR TO TRANSPLANTATION

The inevitable broadening of the indications for marrow transplantation means that a number of different marrow diseases will pass across the attending pathologist's desk. These must be accurately evaluated in several stages of remission or relapse. All forms of myelogenous and acute lymphocytic leukemia, hairy cell leukemia, multiple myeloma, plasma cell leukemia, and most lymphomas, as well as various solid tumors have been treated with procedures involving marrow infusion. Severe but "nonmalignant" diseases, such as aplastic anemia, preleukemia, acute myelofibrosis, several hematologic and metabolic inborn errors, as well as severe combined immune deficiency (SCID) can be approached by marrow or immune cell therapy. To the anatomic and clinical laboratories, this translates into significant demands for special tests and unusually rapid responses for some "routine" tests, such as bone marrow histology, open-lung biopsies, and autopsies. The impact will be felt in all areas, including blood banking, cell surface marking, cytochemistry, and clinical chemistry.

The patient referred for marrow transplantation should be preceded or accompanied by all significant previous records. Tissue sampled for the original diagnosis must be reviewed carefully and described. When possible, representative slides of the diagnostic marrow or other tissue should be held (with permission) for a few weeks after grafting because reevaluation is required if recurrent disease is suspected. Nothing substitutes for the direct and simultaneous comparison of cytomorphology in a previous diagnostic specimen, for example, when, a few weeks after transplantation, a relapse is suspected in the marrow smear. Immediately on admission, a new marrow and blood examination is usually needed to confirm the previous diagnosis and to rule out a relapse since the last examination. Access to cytochemistry and cell surface marker laboratories is also essential for accurate diagnosis, which dictates the treatment protocol. The data are needed quickly, and marrow biopsies may have to be completed on weekends to afford timely decisions. The most critical data are the confirmation of referring diagnosis and the determination of remission status on arrival.

Two technical points regarding marrow evaluation in this setting require emphasis. First, the sample must be adequate, regardless of the technique used. The particle section technique, using anticoagulated fixative to prevent the aspirated material from clotting, is far more efficient than clot sectioning.[37] In most cases, particle sections and smears provide a more than adequate sample if the aspiration is vigorous. In some cases, the inability to aspirate prompts a biopsy. The Jamshidi needle provides good samples with the least equipment failure. Smears may be examined immediately by the clinical staff, but all parts of the specimen, when they are prepared, should be evaluated together by one morphologist so that a comprehensive synthesis of data is promptly available. Periodic acid–Schiff (PAS) staining is extremely effective and is a routine preparation. Methacrylate embedding, despite its reduced staining versatility, can be very useful, though not routinely used in all marrow cases. For the evaluation of aplastic anemia, methacrylate-embedded biopsies are obtained along with smears, and paraffin-embedded particle sections on all admissions. The second technical point concerns relapse evaluation in acute leukemia. A worldwide convention is to designate any marrow blast count between 5%–25% as partial remission. This has proven useful, but must not be applied rigidly when a patient has had very recent induction chemotherapy, producing a hypocellular, regenerating marrow. In this situation, nonmalignant blasts, in many cases undistinguishable morphologically from malignant ones, may be elevated. In the setting of conventional chemotherapy, overtreatment of the patient at this point can induce total aplasia and result in an infectious or hemorrhagic death. In the marrow transplant setting, remission status is an important determinant of the treatment protocol, but the decision is less immediately critical to survival than in the conventional setting since rescue is an aim of the transplant.

## HISTOLOGIC EVALUATION OF BONE MARROW AFTER TRANSPLANTATION

### Engraftment

Bone marrow from the donor is infused on what is conventionally designated as "day 0" of the transplantation course. Usually, from 10 to 30 billion nucleated cells can be obtained for the infusion. Serial marrow aspirates and biopsies plus data from prompt autopsies have shown that evidence of marrow engraftment can be found as early as day 7. This occurs in the form of colonies of cells differentiating into myeloid, erythroid, or megakaryocytic islands (Figs. 1–6). The kinetics of recovery in our first 42 allogeneic graft recipients were reviewed by Neiman.[464] The lowest point of the white blood cell count occurs about day 8. Mean granulocyte counts exceed 500/mm³ by day 17. By day 20, total white count is about 2000/mm³. On the average, recovery of platelets

and red cells is slower. Platelet transfusion support is usually necessary until about day 25. The recovery of cellularity to normal levels as estimated by marrow histology is quite variable: some patients show nearly normal cellularity by 3 weeks, whereas others show delays of 2–3 weeks before evidence of engraftment is obtained. The marrow reserve is impaired for some time, probably based on the sensitivity to marrow-challenging events. Some patients show prolonged or recurrent platelet transfusion dependence. Slow megakaryocyte engraftment in some of these is a longer-term problem. In others some evidence of antibodies to platelets, probably due to presensitization, is demonstrable by observing differential refractoriness to certain donors.

### Histology of rejection

Rejection is distinctly unusual in leukemia patients because their intensive preparative regimens are very immunosuppressive to the host. Rejection can, however, be a significant problem in aplastic anemia (AA), occurring in over one-third of patients who had received blood product transfusions prior to bone marrow transplantation. The mechanism of graft rejection is uncertain. In murine systems, a phenomenon known as natural resistance is characterized by an *a priori* failure of hematopoietic cell engraftment.[133] This is attributed to an MHC-linked genetic locus designated Hh. The phenomenon differs from acquired immunity and is relatively radioresistant. It has so far been observed only in hematopoietic grafts, not in solid organ grafts. Although there appears to be a minimum cell dose threshold in humans, primary failure of marrow graft to take is unusual.

Most graft failure is attributed to true rejection following take, an acquired immunity which is profoundly increased by presensitization of the recipient to histocompatibility antigens of the donor. Figure 7 diagrams the three possible fates of a bone marrow graft attempt. Studies in dogs had shown that presensitization of the recipient to blood products was a major determinant of graft rejection.[630,734] The frequency of rejection in untransfused human patients was much lower than that in transfused patients and the survival correspondingly much higher.[642] A predictive test for marrow rejection (the relative response index) was developed, based on the mixed leukocyte culture. This index compared the responsiveness

Specimens in Figures 1–5 illustrate the sequential picture of marrow engraftment in an autograft recipient, a 58-year-old white male (UPN 364) with CML in blast crisis.

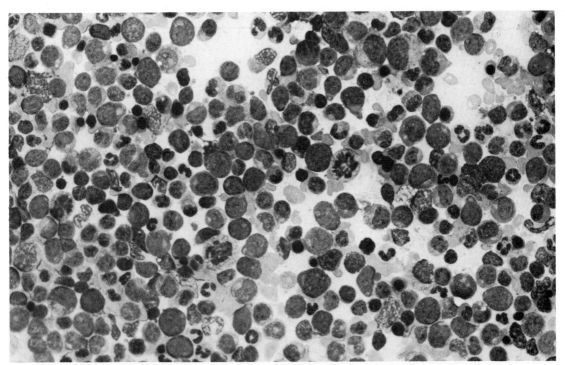

**Figure 1.** Hypercellular pretransplant marrow smear exhibits immature myeloid cells.

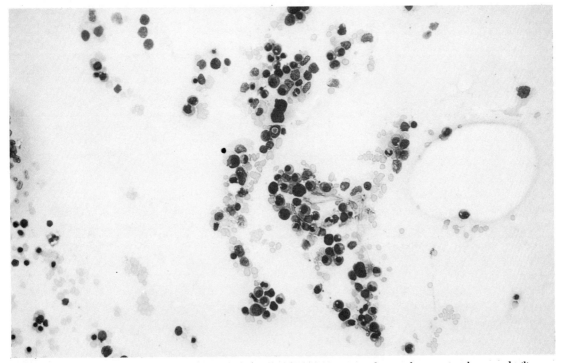

**Figure 2.** On day 14 after an autograft of his own marrow, stored while he was in chronic phase, patient has a good trilineage graft on this smear stained with Wright-Giemsa (W-G).

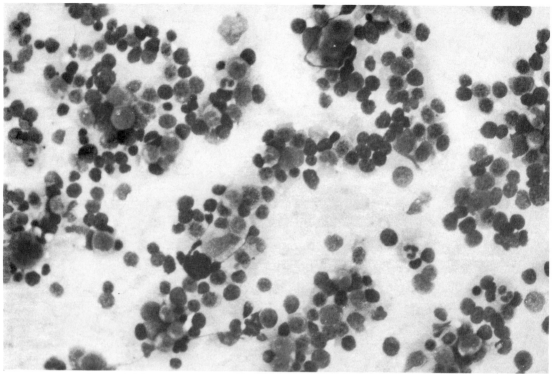

**Figure 3.** On day 21 the cellularity is higher and the erythroid series is megaloblastic. (W-G smear.)

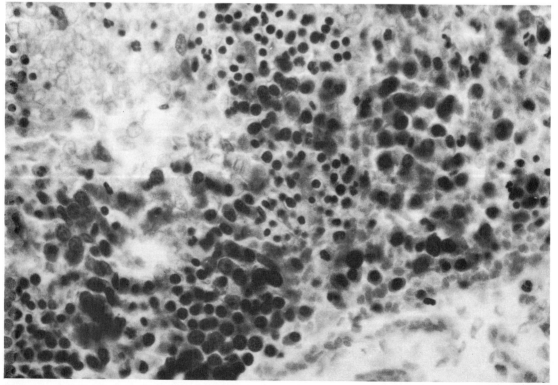

**Figure 4.** A PAS-stained paraffin section of patient's marrow on day 31 shows normal cellularity with continuing preponderance of erythroid cells, but fewer megaloblastic changes.

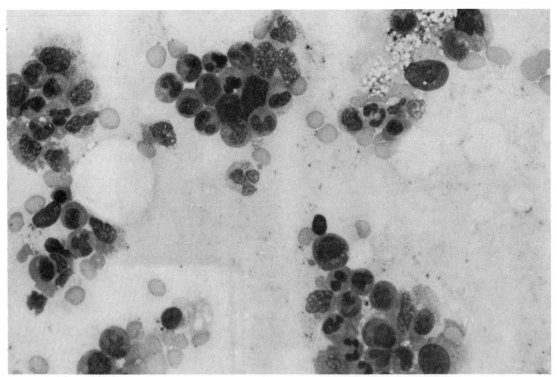

**Figure 5.** By day 42, marrow is normocellular to hypercellular with a full range of myeloid maturation. The myeloid–erythroid ratio is now elevated and the overall histology is identical to that which his marrow exhibited during the previous chronic phase when his marrow was stored. (W-G smear.)

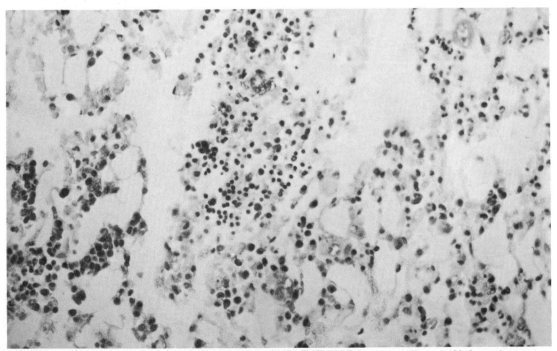

**Figure 6.** (UPN 387) Example of a brisk graft with cellularity more than half normal in paraffin-embedded particle section at day 25, of a 31-year-old woman with aplastic anemia. The tendency of cell lines to form colonies is illustrated by myeloid cells at lower left and erythroid group in center of photograph.

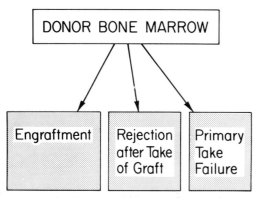

Figure 7. The three possible fates of a bone marrow transplant. Rejection and primary take failure are regarded as different events because they may have different mechanisms. Primary take failure in murine systems is considered a manifestation of natural immunity (natural resistance), as distinguished from the acquired immunity which characterizes true rejection.[133]

of patient cells to sibling donor cells to that of patient cells to unrelated cells, and expressed this dual comparison as a ratio. A ratio of greater than 1.6% was found to predict rejection with a *p* value of less than 0.01. Marrow cell dose as a positive factor in successful engraftment in the same study.[639] The test appears useful only in transfused patients.

Morphologically, marrow graft rejection is usually a nonspecific disappearance of hematopoietic cells, and any of the three primary lines may fail first (Figs. 8–10). An increase in mast cell counts in the marrow and a reversal of the myeloid:erythroid (M:E) ratio were both reported to be possibly predictive for rejection,[459a] but we were unable to confirm either relationship in our study of 73 patients who underwent transplantation for AA.[549] The usual general and nonspecific signs of marrow damage are frequent; e.g., fat necrosis, nonspecific granulomas, congestion, and hemorrhage, with new development of nonuniform cellularity and patchiness of marrow distribution. Pancytopenia frequently develops. Study of the marrow or peripheral blood may show evidence of early mixed chimerism in that host cells will be detectable and may increase with time. Rarely, autogenous regeneration of the host marrow may recur unexpectedly with complete recovery.[670]

Infrequent cases of rejection have shown a marked, unexplained increase in reactive marrow and peripheral blood lymphocytes or plasmacytosis of marrow prior to rejection which resembles brisk rejection like that reported in renal and skin grafts (Figs. 11–13). Autopsy lymph

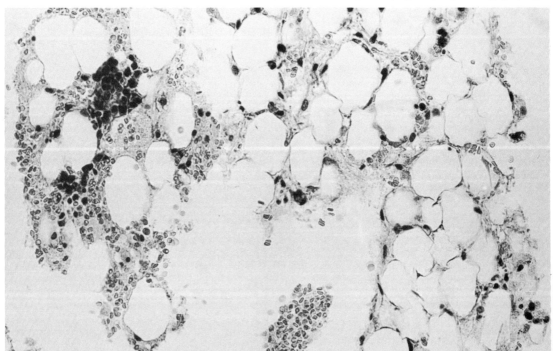

Figure 8. Day 6 marrow shows one of several foci of engraftment by colonies of hematopoietic cells—in this case, myeloid. The graft was rejected, however. (Marrow specimen from a 23-year-old female (UPN 779) transplanted for aplastic anemia.)

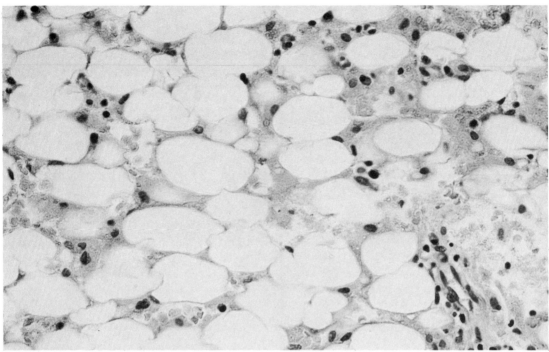

**Figure 9.** By day 14, the marrow is devoid of hematopoiesis, exhibiting only interstitial damage and sparse mononuclear cells. This is the typical histologic pattern for the great majority of marrow rejections, although later rejections are common. (Marrow specimen from a 23-year-old female (UPN 779) transplanted for aplastic anemia.)

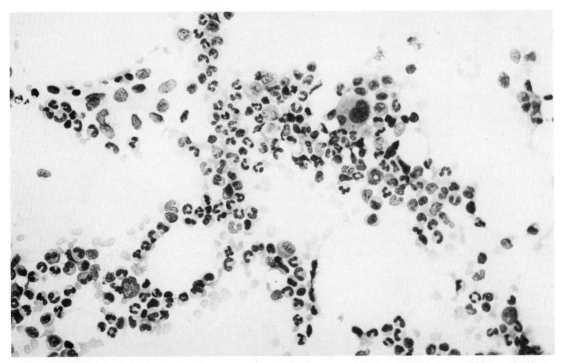

**Figure 10.** (UPN 610) Pure red cell aplasia is an unusual first sign of rejection, here occurring in a 6-year-old boy with aplastic anemia on day 69 after a previously good trilineage graft. First marrow histologic evidence of graft had been on day 7. A second graft showed an early marrow take, but septicemia intervened and patient died of infection 4 months after first graft and about 1½ months after this examination. (W-G smear.)

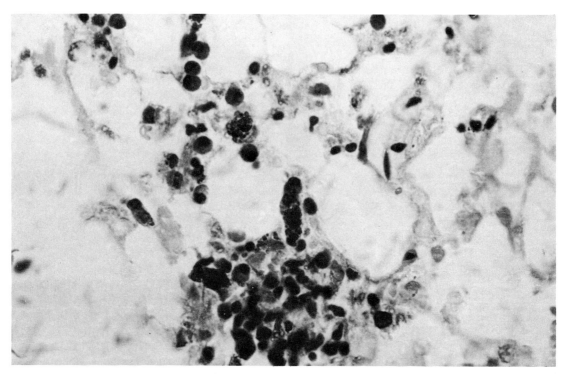

**Figure 11.** This marrow shows an unusual pattern of rejection which occurred twice in successive graft attempts. Paraffin marrow particle section shows severe damage with increased iron and a pronounced plasmacytosis. (Marrow specimen from a 3-year-old boy (UPN 614) with idiopathic aplastic anemia.)

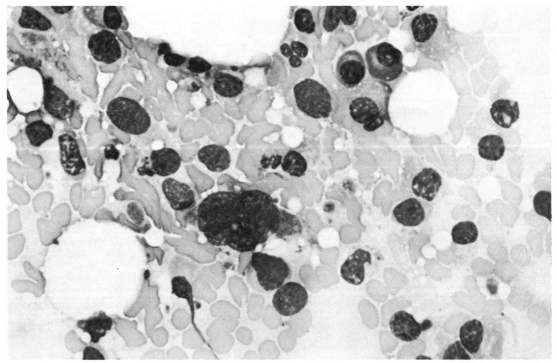

**Figure 12.** A Wright-Giemsa smear of the same marrow demonstrates the plasmacytosis (pair of cells at upper right). (Marrow specimen from a 3-year-old boy (UPN 614) with idiopathic plastic anemia.)

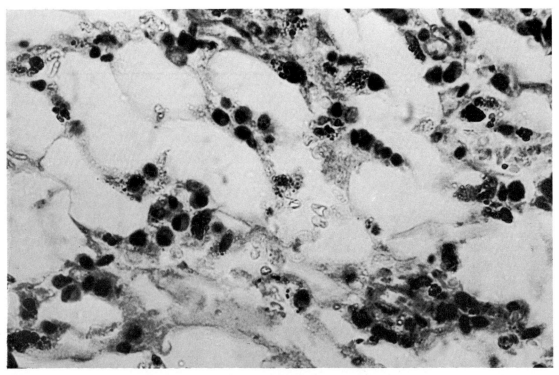

**Figure 13.** Particle section of the second rejection had an identical pattern. Many plasma cells are interspersed with iron-laden histiocytes producing the pattern of particulate, refractile cell-bound materials. (Marrow specimen from a 3-year-old boy (UPN 614) with idiopathic plastic anemia.)

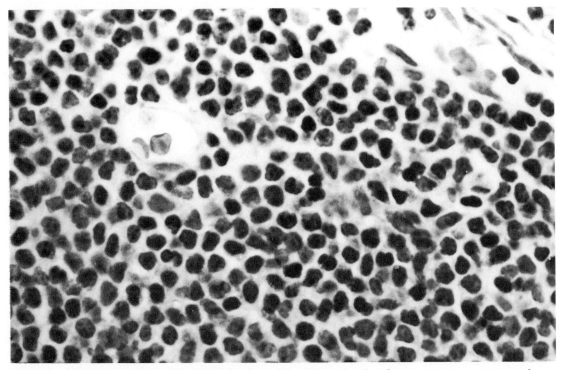

**Figure 14.** Diffuse intermediately differentiated lymphocytic lymphoma in lymph node section prior to marrow transplantation. (Specimen from a 62-year-old male, UPN 1422).

nodes of both primary marrow failure and true rejection patients may show the same degree of diffuse plasmacytoid hyperplasia, which is characteristic of nonrejecting allograft recipients with or without GVHD (Chapter 10).

### Recurrent tumor (Figures 14–18)

Refractoriness of some tumors even to radical therapy occurs, particularly in acute lymphocytic leukemia (ALL). Our experience with 136 patients transplanted for end-stage acute leukemia reviewed by Harrison[281] revealed that 35% of 72 patients with acute *non*lymphocytic leukemia (ANL) and 44% of 64 patients with ALL suffered relapse. Several pretransplant factors were associated with relapse. A high total white cell count at admission was significant for the whole group ($p = 0.02$). If the white count was over 20,000/mm$^3$, the $p$ value was less than 0.003. In ANL patients, an enlarged spleen showed a $p$ of less than 0.006, whereas in the ALL group, active central nervous system leukemia showed a $p$ of less than 0.01. The persistence of blast cells in the marrow during the first 3 weeks after transplantation was a predictor of relapse. For blast persistence, the $p$ value was less than 0.001.

Cytogenetic analyses have been important in such studies. The above study showed that if the tumor cells obtained before transplantation had demonstrable cytogenetic abnormalities, relapse was more likely with a $p$ of less than 0.04. Cytogenetic data were also responsible, through Y-body analysis in opposite-sex-donor–host combinations, for the first report of donor-cell leukemia recurrence in human marrow graft recipients. This was demonstrated in two of six patients treated for leukemia with 1000 rad total body irradiation only, followed by allografting.[464] The incidence of donor recurrences is about 5%[77] Occasional recurrences will present with unusual manifestations and "pseudorecurrences" also appear in cases with unexplained but apparently benign lymphocytosis. Patients with viral infection or benign infectious mononucleosis exemplify the latter situation. Two cases illustrate this:

1). A young male with cytogenetically and morphologically proven host-type recurrence of ALL in the bone marrow was returned home to be considered for conventional therapy but underwent an apparently spontaneous remission. He remains well over 2 years later with mixed chimerism and the explanation remains uncertain. (Singer et al.: *Blood 62: 869, 1984.*)

2). An adult female with acute myelogenous leukemia (AML) developed a benign histiocytic infiltrate of the marrow on day 60, accompanied by an "autoimmune" syndrome characterized by a Coomb's-positive hemolytic anemia, thrombocytopenia, fever, and constitutional symptoms. The episode resolved clinically and histologically, but 5 weeks later a clear relapse of AML was diagnosed in the marrow and peripheral blood (Figs. 19–21). Such examples may represent clinical evidence of a graft-vs.-leukemia effect, but only speculation supports such an interpretation and individual cases.

The detection sensitivity in leukemia cases for the recurrence of fewer than 10$^9$ tumor cells (the number required to produce marrow blast counts of over 5%) remains unsatisfactory. Occasional cases provide the opportunity to look for known markers (cytogenetic, immunological, or morphological), but what is needed is a highly sensitive, quantitative marker assay for the patient's tumor. Cell sorting technology, oncogene detection, and sensitive quantitative immunochemical or radioimmune assays promise to contribute significantly to this field.

### Secondary marrow damage

Several drugs given marrow graft recipients are potentially or consistently toxic to marrow. The low-dose methotrexate frequently given for prophylaxis of GVHD must be monitored constantly and adjusted frequently. Antibiotic drugs have variably well-evidenced effects on the marrow. Of these, the best known is chloramphenicol, but trimethoprim sulfa and other agents have been implicated in direct, idiosyncratic, or allergic effects. Marrow failure after grafting is a situation, therefore, whose etiology can be difficult to pinpoint. Antiviral agents, such as interferon, adenine arabinoside (Ara-A) or acyclovir, must also be administered judiciously to these patients (Fig. 22).

Viral infections may cause severe marrow failure as evidenced by aplasia after viral hepatitis. Cytomegalovirus (CMV) infection after marrow transplantation seems frequently to be myelosuppressive in and of itself.[440] We have seen

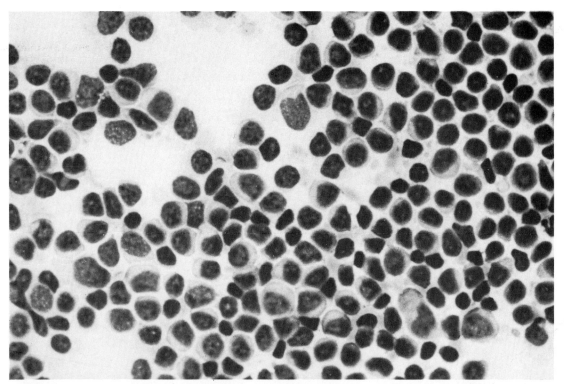

**Figure 15.**    Wright-Giemsa smear of lymph node showing tumor cells. (Specimen from a 62-year-old male, UPN 1422.)

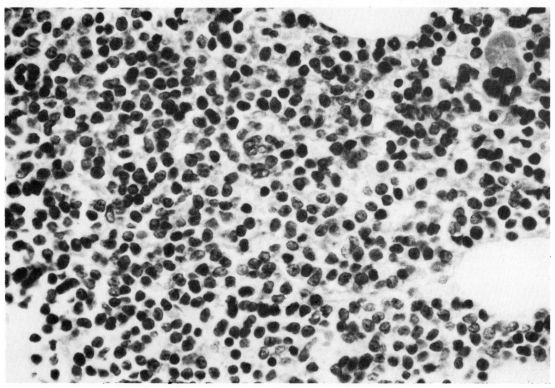

**Figure 16.**    Bone marrow particle section at admission shows diffuse marrow involvement. (Specimen from a 62-year-old male, UPN 1422.)

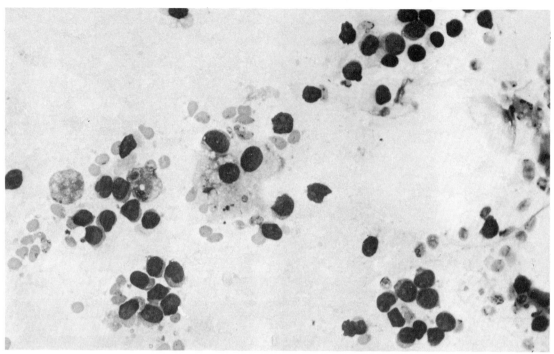

**Figure 17.**    Day 7 marrow reveals lymphoma cells. Except for macrophages, these persistent cells are the only viable nucleated elements remaining. This patient's marrow tumor very gradually disappeared over several weeks but he relapsed a few months later. Residual marrow tumor in acute leukemia after day zero carries a high probability of recurrence, as shown by Harrison et al.[281] (Specimen from a 62-year-old male, UPN 1422.)

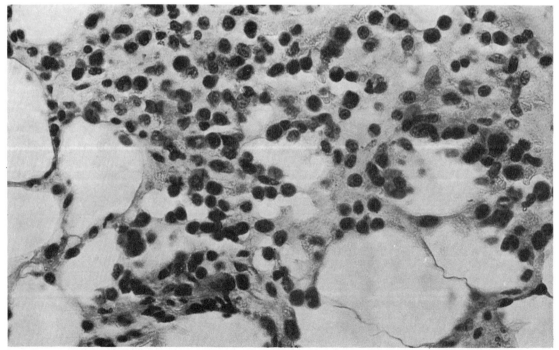

**Figure 18.**    (UPN 378) Residual tumor on day 21 in 20-year-old woman transplanted for plasma cell leukemia. Although she showed minimal evidence of engraftment, the tumor cells seemed totally refractory to superlethal irradiation and chemotherapy, and she only survived for a few weeks.

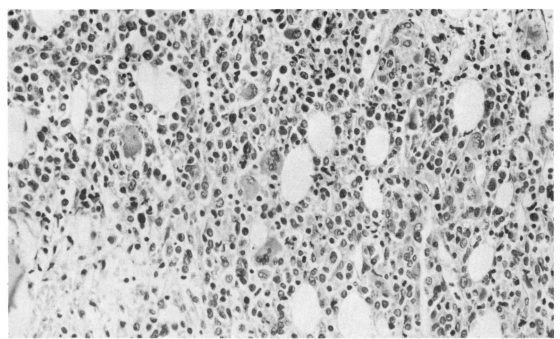

**Figure 19.** Unexplained histocytic reaction in bone marrow accompanied clinically by Coomb's-positive hemolytic anemia and thrombocytopenia about day 50. There is a diffuse increase in histiocytes with abundant cytoplasm. Several weeks later this patient developed frank relapse of her AML, but not before the marrow became more nearly normal (Fig. 20). (Specimen from a 40-year-old female (UPN 1350) with AML.)

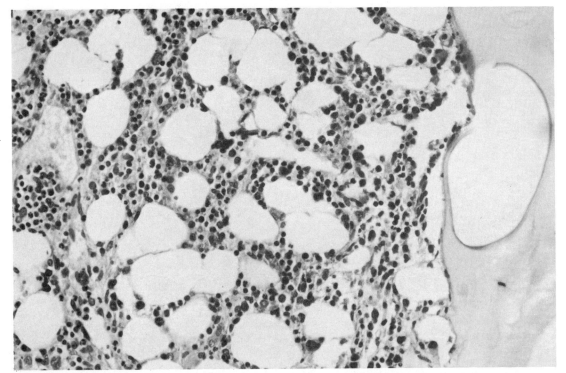

**Figure 20.** Two weeks after the previous marrow examination, the cellular composition is nearly normal with fewer histiocytes and normal myeloid and erythroid precursors, yet 5 weeks later the patient relapsed (Fig. 21). (Specimen from a 40-year-old female (UPN 1350) with AML.)

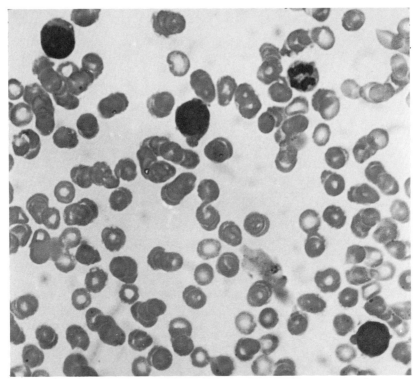

**Figure 21.** Five weeks later, peripheral blood smear exhibits myeloblasts. Was this a graft-vs.-leukemia reaction? (Specimen from a 40-year-old female (UPN 1350) with AML.)

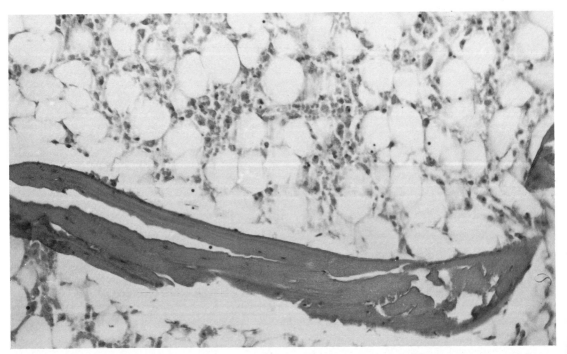

**Figure 22.** (UPN 519) PAS-stained autopsy marrow section of leukemia patient with fatal CMV pneumonia who received Ara-A in an unsuccessful treatment attempt. Peripheral white blood count fell profoundly when the daily dose was increased from 5 to 10, then to 15 mg/kg. CMV itself is also marrow toxic and probably contributed to the illustrated total aplasia. Death was from irreversible pulmonary insufficiency.

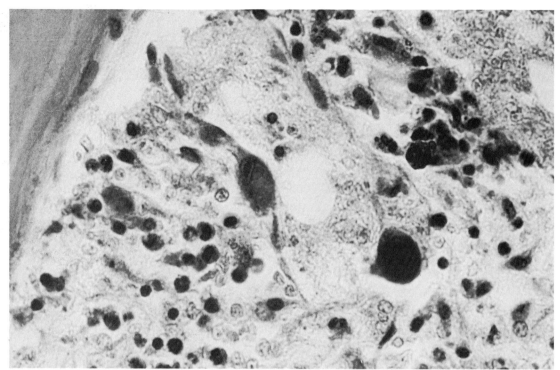

**Figure 23.** (UPN 518) Bone marrow infection with CMV was first clue to the diagnosis in a 25-year-old woman who later died of CMV pneumonia. Note that of the two cells with cytomegaly, the one at upper left has characteristic peri-inclusion halo.

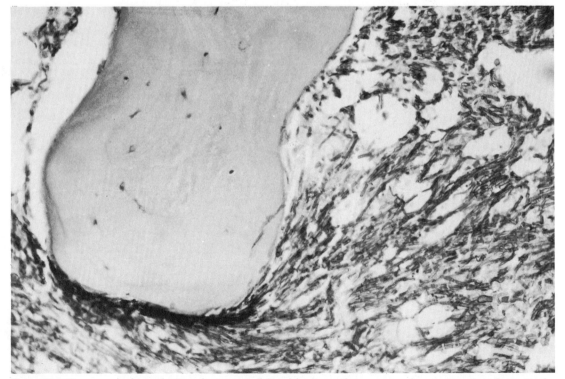

**Figure 24.** Bone marrow biopsy section shows mass of fungal hyphae with true septa, characteristic of another patient's disseminated infection with Aspergillus. It is unusual to diagnose this on a marrow biopsy. (Rapid methenamine silver stain.[405])

direct marrow infection at biopsy (Fig. 23). Other systemic infections such as disseminated fungi can also involve the marrow (Fig. 24).

## Marrow elements as targets of the graft-host reaction (GVHR)

Although still controversial, it is fair to suggest that the bone marrow is not a target of the true GVHR in patients prepared by ablation of their host marrow. The marrow they have after grafting is of donor origin and, if even the target of immune attack, is best classified as the victim of an autoimmune reaction. However, in cases in which the recipient's marrow is not ablated, such as transplantation for SCID in children, or in accidental engraftment and GVHD due to transfusion of viable lymphocytes to leukemic patients while immunosuppressed, the marrow is a direct target, and marrow damage and hypoplasia can result. The latter situation is usually severe— first, because the patient's marrow may be suppressed by prior chemotherapy, and second, because the grafted cells are likely to be HLA-mismatched to the patient. Our recently reported case of this situation underscores the severity of such GVHR,[739] and the incidence and prevalence may be underestimated as yet. The recommendation that blood products given such patients be irradiated has far-reaching implications in blood banking.

## Marrow sampling at autopsy

When remission or graft status are important questions, there is need for very prompt autopsy due to rapid autolysis that occurs in the marrow (as well as gut). We sample rib, vertebrae, iliac crest, and sternum in all autopsies. Excellent smears of autopsy marrow can be obtained by gently pressing fresh marrow particles between two glass slides.[333] When the time of death renders a prompt, complete autopsy difficult, immediate sampling of the most critical tissues is a useful substitute. Lung, liver, and kidney, as well as marrow, can be obtained with large-bore needle biopsy tools, then fixed, and studied at a more convenient time. If gut histology is critical, samples of large and small bowel can be obtained through a small midline incision for immediate fixation, although rapid fixation of the removed whole gut is optimal. Viable marrow stem cells and immune spleen cells can be cultured after postmortem intervals as long as 12 hours, and fibroblasts after even longer intervals, so that even tissue culture studies may be done in selected cases.

# References

1. Abe, H., Beninger, P.R., Ikejiri, N., Setoyama, H., Sata, M., and Tanikawa, K.: Light microscopic findings of liver biopsy specimens from patients with hepatitis type A and comparison with type B. *Gastroenterology* 82: 938–947, 1982.

2. Ackerman, A.B.: Superficial perivascular dermatitis. In *Histologic Diagnosis of Inflammatory Skin Diseases*, Lee & Febiger, Philadelphia, 1978, pp. 169–279.

3. Ackerman, L.V., and Rosai, J.: Breast. In *Surgical Pathology* (5th ed.)., C.V. Mosby, St. Louis, 1974, Figs. 893, 896, and 901 on pp. 904–910.

4. Aisenberg, A.C., Wilkes, B., and Waksman, B.H.: The production of runt disease in rats thymectomized at birth. *J Exp Med 116: 759–772, 1962.*

5. Allen, J.I., Silvis, S.E., Sumner, H.W., and McLain, C.J.: Cytomegalic inclusion disease diagnosed endoscopically. *Dig Dis Sci 26: 133–135, 1981.*

6. Allen, J.R., Carstens, L.A., and Katagiri, G.J.: Hepatic veins of monkeys with veno-occlusive disease. Sequential ultrastructural changes. *Arch Pathol 87: 279–289, 1969.*

7. Ament, M.E., Ochs, H.D., and Davis, S.D.: Structure and function of the gastrointestinal tract in primary immunodeficiency syndromes: A study of 39 patients. *Medicine 52: 227–248, 1973.*

8. Appelbaum, F.R., Herzig, G.P., Zeigler, J.L., Graw, R.G., Levine, A.S., and Deisseroth, A.B.: Successful engraftment of cryopreserved autologous bone marrow in patients with malignant lymphoma. *Blood 52: 85–95, 1978.*

9. Appelbaum, F.R., Fefer, A., Cheever, M.A., Saunders, J.E., Singer, J.W., Adamson, J.W., Mickelson, E.M., Hansen, J.A., Greenberg, P.D., and Thomas, E.D.: Treatment of aplastic anemia by bone marrow transplantation in identical twins. *Blood 55: 1033–1039, 1980.*

10. Appelbaum, F.R., and Fefer, A.: The pathogenesis of aplastic anemia. *Semin Hematol 18: 241–257, 1981.*

11. Appelbaum, F.R., Meyers, J.D., Fefer, A., Flournoy, N., Cheever, M.A., Greenberg, P.D., Hackman, R., and Thomas, E.D.: Nonbacterial nonfungal pneumonia following marrow transplantation in 100 identical twins. *Transplantation 33: 265–268, 1982.*

12. Appelbaum, F.R., and Shulman, H.M.: Fatal hepatotoxicity associated with AMSA therapy. *Cancer Treat Rep 66: 1863–1865, 1982.*

13. Arakawa, K., Jézéquel, A.M., Macvie, S.I., Johnston, R., Perz, Z.M., and Steiner, J.W.: The liver in murine transplantation (runt) disease. Observations of the acute lesions by light and electron microscopy. *Am J Pathol 49: 257–299, 1966.*

14. Armitage, J.O., Burns, C.P., and Kent, T.H.: Liver disease complicating the management of acute leukemia during remission. *Cancer 41: 737–742, 1978.*

15. Armstrong, D.: Interstitial pneumonia in the immunosuppressed patient. *Transplant Proc 8: 657–661, 1976.*

16. Armstrong, M.Y.K., Gleichmann, E., Gleichmann, H., Beldotti, L., André-Schwartz, J., and Schwartz, R.S.: Chronic allogeneic disease. II. Development of lymphomas. *J Exp Med 132: 417–439, 1970.*

17. Asbury, R.F., Rosenthal, S.N., Descalzi, M.E., Ratcliffe, R.L., and Arseneau, J.C.: Hepatic veno-occlusive disease due to DTIC. *Cancer 45: 2670–2674, 1980.*

18. Askin, F.B., and Katzenstein, A.L.: *Pneumocystis* infection masquerading as diffuse alveolar damage: A potential source of diagnostic error. *Chest 79: 420–422, 1981.*

19. Atkinson, K., Storb, R., Prentice, R.L., Weiden, P.L., Witherspoon, R.P., Sullivan, K., Noel, D., and Thomas, E.D.: Analysis of late infections in 89 long-term survivors of bone marrow transplantation. *Blood 53: 720–731, 1979.*

20. Atkinson, K., Meyers, J.D., Storb, R., Prentice, R.L., and Thomas, E.D.: Varicellazoster virus infection after marrow transplantation for aplastic anemia or leukemia. *Transplantation 29: 47–50, 1980.*

21. Atkinson, K., Farewell, V., Storb, R., Tsoi, M.S., Sullivan, K.M., Witherspoon, R.P., Fefer, A., Clift, F., Goodell, B., and Thomas, E.D.: Analysis of late infections after human bone marrow transplantation. Role of genotypic nonidentity between marrow donor and recipient and of nonspecific suppressor cells in patients with chronic graft-vs.-host disease. *Blood 60: 714–720, 1982.*

22. Atkinson, K., Hansen, J., Storb, R., Goehle, S., Goldstein, G., and Thomas, E.D.: T-cell subpopulations identified by monoclonal antibodies after human marrow transplantation. I. Helper-inducer and cytotoxic-suppressor subsets. *Blood 59: 1292–1298, 1982.*

23. Atkinson, K., Shulman, H.M., Deeg, H.J., Weiden, P.L., Graham, T.C., Thomas, E.D., and Storb, R.: Acute and chronic graft-vs.-host disease in dogs given hematopoietic grafts from DLA-nonidentical littermates: Two distinct syndromes. *Am J Pathol 108: 196–205, 1982.*

24. Atkinson, K., Storb, R., Ochs, H.D., Goehle, S., Sullivan, K.M., Witherspoon, R.P., Lum, L.G., Tsoi, M.S., Sanders, J.E., Parr, M., Stewart, P., and Thomas, E.D.: Thymus transplantation after allogeneic bone marrow graft to prevent chronic graft-vs.-host disease in humans. *Transplantation 33: 168–173, 1982.*

25. Atkinson, K., Incefy, G.S., Storb, R., Sullivan, K.M., Iwata, T., Dardenne, M., Ochs, H.D., Good, R.A., and Thomas, E.D.: Low serum thymic hormone levels in patients with chronic graft-vs.-host disease. *Blood 59: 1073–1077, 1982.*

26. Ayulo, M., Aisner, S.C., Margolis, K., and Moravec, C.: Cytomegalovirus-associated gastritis in a compromised host. *JAMA 243: 1364, 1980.*

27. Baert, A.L., Fevery, J., Marchal, G., Goddeeris, P., Wilms, G., Ponette, E., and De Groote, J.: Early diagnosis of Budd-Chiari syndrome by computed tomography and ultrasonography: Report of five cases. *Gastroenterology 84: 587–595, 1983.*

28. Baggenstoss, A.H., Foulk, W.T., Butt, H.R., and Bahn, R.C.: The pathology of primary biliary cirrhosis with emphasis on histogenesis. *Am J Clin Pathol 42: 259–276, 1964.*

29. Baggenstoss, A.H.: Morphologic and etiologic diagnoses from hepatic biopsies without clinical data. *Medicine 45: 435–443, 1966.*

30. Bain, G.O.: Distribution, dose dependency, and effect of donor presensitization on liver infiltration in the graft-vs.-host reaction. *Transplantation 9: 383–394, 1970.*

31. Baker, J.R., Fleischman, R.W., Thompson, G.R., Schaeppi, U., Ilievski, V., Cooney, D.A., and Davis, R.D.: Pathological effects of bleomycin on the skin of dogs and monkeys. *Toxicol Appl Pharmacol 25: 190–200, 1973.*

32. Balner, H., DeVries, M.J., and van Bekkum, D.W.: Secondary disease in rat radiation chimeras. *J Natl Cancer Inst 32: 419–459, 1964.*

33. Barnes, D.W.H., and Loutit, J.F.: Radiation recovery factor: Preservation by Polge-Smith-Parkes technique. *J Natl Cancer Inst 15: 901–905, 1955.*

34. Barnes, D.W.H., Loutit, J.F., and Michlem, H.S.: "Secondary disease" of radiation chimeras: A syndrome due to lymphoid aplasia. *Ann NY Acad Sci 99: 374–385, 1962.*

35. Barnes, D.W.H., and Loutit, J.F.: Acute graft-vs.-host disease in recipients of bone-marrow transplants from identical twin donors. *Lancet 2: 905–906, 1979.*

36. Barton, J.C., and Conrad, M.E.: Beneficial effects of hepatitis in patients with acute myelogenous leukemia. *Ann Intern Med 90: 188–190, 1979.*

37. Batjer, J.D.: Preparation of optimal bone marrow samples. *Lab Med 10: 101–106, 1979.*

38. Belldegrun, A., Berlatzky, Y., and Cohen, I.R.: Immunospecific depletion of effector lymphocytes and graft-vs.-host reactive lymphocytes using a recruitment model of cell-mediated immunity. In Gale and Fox, *op cit,* pp. 247–256.

39. Benjamin, D.R.: Hepatobiliary dysfunction in infants and children associated with long-term total parenteral nutrition. A clinico-pathologic study. *Am J Clin Pathol 76: 276–283, 1981.*

40. Bennett, M.: Alloantigen sensitive units (AASU) of mouse lymphoid tissues. *Fed Proc 28: 553, 1969.*

41. Berk, P.D., Popper, H., Krueger, G.R.F., Decter, J., Herzig, G., and Graw, R.G., Jr.: Venocclusive disease of the liver after allogeneic bone marrow transplantation: Possible association with graft-vs.-host disease. *Ann Intern Med 90: 158–164, 1979.*

42. Berke, G., Ax, W., Ginsburg, H., and Feldman, M.: Graft reaction in tissue culture. II. Quantification of the lytic action on mouse fibroblasts by rat lymphocytes sensitized on mouse embryo fibroblast monolayers. *Immunology 16: 643–657, 1969.*

43. Berkowitz, I.D., Robboy, S.J., Karchmer, A.W., and Kunz, L.J.: *Torulopsis glabrata* fungemia—A clinical pathological study. *Medicine 58: 430–440, 1979.*

44. Berman, M., Alter, H.J., Ishak, K.G., Purcell, R.H., and Jones, E.A.: The chronic sequelae of non-A, non-B hepatitis. *Ann Intern Med 91: 1–6, 1979.*

45. Berman, M.D., Rabin, L., O'Donnell, J., Gratwohl, A.A., Graw, R.G., Deisseroth, A.B., and Jones, E.A.: The liver in long-term survivors of marrow transplant—chronic graft-vs.-host disease. *J Clin Gastroenterol 2: 53–63, 1980.*

46. Bernuau, D., Gisselbrecht, C., Devergie, A., Feldmann, G., Gluckman, E., Marty, M., and Boiron, M.: Histological and ultrastructural appearance of the liver during graft-vs.-host disease complicating bone marrow transplantation. *Transplantation 29: 236–244, 1980.*

47. Bernuau, D., Feldman, G., Degott, C., and Gisselbrecht, C.: Ultrastructural lesion of bile ducts in primary biliary cirrhosis. A comparison with the lesions observed in graft-vs.-host disease. *Hum Pathol 12: 782–793, 1981.*

48. Berthrong, M., and Fajardo, L.F.: Radiation injury in surgical pathology. Part II. Alimentary tract. *Am J Surg Pathol 5: 153–178, 1981.*

49. Beschorner, W.E., Hutchins, G.M., Elfenbein, G.J., and Santos, G.W.: The thymus in patients with allogeneic bone marrow transplants. *Am J Pathol 92: 173–181, 1978.*

50. Beschorner, W.E., Saral, R., Hutchins, G.M., Tutschka, P.J., and Santos, G.W.: Lymphocytic bronchitis associated with graft-vs.-host disease in recipients of bone-marrow transplants. *N Engl J Med 299: 1030–1036, 1978.*

51. Beschorner, W.E., Pino, J., Boitnott, J.K., Tutschka, P.J., and Santos, G.W.: Pathology of the liver with bone marrow transplantation. Effects of busulfan, carmustine, acute graft-vs.-host disease, and cytomegalovirus infection. *Am J Pathol 99: 369–385, 1980.*

52. Beschorner, W.E., Hutchins, G.M., Burns, W.H., Saral, R., Tutschka, P.J., and Santos, G.W.: Cytomegalovirus pneumonia in bone marrow transplant recipients: miliary and diffuse patterns. *Am Rev Respir Dis 122: 107–114, 1980.*

53. Beschorner, W.E., Yardley, J.H., Tutschka, P., and Santos, G.: Deficiency of intestinal immunity with graft-vs.-host disease in humans. *J Infect Dis 144: 38–46, 1981.*

54. Beschorner, W.E., Tutschka, P.J., and Santos, G.W.: Sequential morphology of graft-vs.-host disease in the rat radiation chimera. *Clin Immunol Immunopathol 22: 203–224, 1982.*

55. Beschorner, W.E., Tutschka, P.J., and Santos, G.W.: Chronic graft-vs.host disease in rat radiation chimera. I. Clinical features, hematology, histology, and immunopathology in long-term chimeras. *Transplantation 33: 393–399, 1982.*

56. Beschorner, W.E., Tutschka P.J. and Santos, G.W.: Characterization of T-lymphocyte subsets in target tissues with acute and chronic graft-vs.-host disease (GVHD) (Abstract). *Fed Proc 41: 620, #2048, 1982.*

57. Bhan, A.K., Harris, T.J., Murphy, G.F., and Mihm, M.C., Jr.: T-cell subsets and Langerhans' cells in lichen

planus: *in situ* characterization using monoclonal antibodies. *Br J Dermatol 105: 617–622, 1981.*

58. Biberfield, P., and Johansson, A.: Contact areas of cytotoxic lymphocytes and target cells. An electron microscopic study. *Exp Cell Res 94: 79–87, 1975.*

59. Billingham, R.E.: The biology of graft-versus-host reactions. *Harvey Lecture 62: 21–78, 1966–1967.*

60. Bjerke, J.R., and Krogh, H.K.: Identification of mononuclear cells *in situ* in skin lesions of lichen planus. *Br J Dermatol 98: 605–610, 1978.*

61. Bleyer, W.A.: The clinical pharmacology of methotrexate: New applications of an old drug. *Cancer 41: 36–51, 1978.*

62. Bleyer, W.A.: Neurologic sequelae of methotrexate and ionizing radiation: A new classification. *Cancer Treat Rep 65 (Suppl 1): 89–98, 1981.*

63. Bloch, K.J., Buchanan, W.W., Wohl, M.J., and Bunim, J.J.: Sjogren's syndrome. A clinical, pathological, and serological study of 62 cases. *Medicine 44: 187–231, 1965.*

64. Blum, R.H., Carter, S.K., and Agre, K.: A clinical review of bleomycin—A new antineoplastic agent. *Cancer 31: 903–914, 1973.*

65. Blume, K.G., Beutler, E., Bross, K.J., Chillar, R.K., Ellington, O.B., Fahey, J.L., Farbstein, M.J., Forman, S.J., Schmidt, G.M., Scott, E.P., Spruce, W.E., Turner, M.A., and Wolf, J.L.: Bone-marrow ablation and allogeneic marrow transplantation in acute leukemia. *N Engl J Med 302: 1041–1046, 1980.*

66. Blume, K.G., Spruce, W.E., Forman, S.J., Wolf, J.L., Farbstein, M.J., Scott, E.P., and Fahey, J.L.: Bone-marrow transplantation for acute leukemia (Letter). *N Engl J Med 305: 101–103, 1981.*

67. Blumenkrantz, N., and Asboe-Hansen, G.: Subhydroxylated collagen in scleroderma. *Acta Derm Venereol (Stockh) 58: 359–361, 1978.*

68. Bondestam, S., Jansson, S.E., Kivisaari, L., Elonen, E., Ruutu, T., and Antinnen, I.: Liver and spleen candidiasis: Imaging and verification by fine-needle aspiration biopsy. *Br Med J (Clin Res) 282: 1514–1515, 1981.*

69. Bonkowsky, H.L., Lee, R.V., and Klatskin, G.: Acute granulomatous hepatitis. Occurrence in cytomegalovirus mononucleosis. *JAMA 233: 1284–1288, 1975.*

70. Boranić, M.: Time pattern of antileukemic effect of graft-versus-host reaction in mice. *Transplant Proc 3: 394–396, 1971.*

71. Boranić M.: Transient graft-versus-host reaction in the treatment of leukemia in mice. *J Natl Cancer Inst 41: 421–437, 1968.*

72. Borel, J.F., Feurer, C., Magnée, C., and Stahelin, H.: Effects of the new antilymphocytic peptide cyclosporin A in animals. *Immunology 32: 1017–1025, 1977.*

73. Bortin, M.M., and Rimm, A.A.: Severe combined immunodeficiency disease. Characterization of the disease and results of transplantation. *JAMA 238: 591–600, 1977.*

74. Bortin, M.M., Kay, H.E.M., Gale, R.P., and Rimm, A.A.: Factors associated with interstitial pneumonitis after bone-marrow transplantation for acute leukemia. *Lancet 1: 437–439, 1982.*

75. Borzy, M.S., Hong, R., Horowitz, S.D., Gilbert, E., Kaufman, D., DeMendonca, W., Oxelius, V.A., Dic-

tor, M., and Pachman, L.: Fatal lymphoma after transplantation of cultured thymus in children with combined immunodeficiency disease. *N Engl J Med 301: 565–568, 1979.*

76. Botstein, G.R., Sherer, G.K., and LeRoy, E.C.: Fibroblast selection in scleroderma: An alternative model of fibrosis. *Arthritis Rheum 25: 189–195, 1982.*

77. Boyd, C.N., Rambert, R.C., and Thomas, E.D.: The incidence of recurrence of leukemia in donor cells after allogeneic bone marrow transplantation. *Leuk Res 6: 833–837, 1982.*

78. Bozdech, M.J., Sondel, P.M., Hong, R., Prendergast, E.J., Exten, R.E., Flynn, B.A., and Muellenbach, R.: Acute graft-versus-host disease (GVHD) following a syngeneic bone marrow transplant: an "autoimmune disorder" associated with non-specific T-cell suppression (Abstract). *Blood 58 (Suppl 1): 171a, 1981.*

79. Braine, H.G., Sensenbrenner, L.L., and Bone Marrow Transplant Team: RBC incompatible bone-marrow transplants. *Exp Hematol 6 (Suppl 3): 9, 1978.*

80. Brandborg, L.L.: Parasitic diseases. In *Gastrointestinal Disease: Pathophysiology, Diagnosis, Management,* Vol. 2, (2nd ed.), M.H. Sleisenger and J.S. Fordtran, Eds., W.B. Saunders, Philadelphia, 1978, pp 1154–1181.

81. Breshot, C., Hadchouel, M., Scotto, J., Fonck, M., Potet, F., Vyas, G.N., and Tiollais, P.: State of hepatitis B virus DNA in hepatocytes of patients with hepatitis B surface antigen-positive and -negative liver diseases. *Proc Natl Acad Sci 78: 3906–3710, 1981.*

82. Buckingham, R.B., Prince, R.K., Rodnan, G.P., and Taylor, F.: Increased collagen accumulation in dermal fibroblast cultures from patients with progressive systemic sclerosis (scleroderma). *J Lab Clin Med 92: 5–21, 1978.*

83. Buckingham, R.B., Prince, R.K., Rodnan, G.P., and Barnes, E.L.: Collagen accumulation by dermal fibroblast cultures of patients with linear localized scleroderma. *J Rheumatol 7: 130–142, 1980.*

84. Buckner, C.D., Clift, R.A., Fefer, A., Neiman, P.E., Storb, R., and Thomas, E.D.: Treatment of blastic transformation of chronic granulocytic leukemia by high-dose cyclophosphamide, total body irradiation, and infusion of cryopreserved autologous marrow. *Exp Hematol 2: 138–146, 1974.*

85. Buckner, C.D., Clift, R.A., Sanders, J.E., Meyers, J.D., Counts, G.W., Farewell, V.T., Thomas, E.D., and the Seattle Marrow Transplant Team: Protective environment for marrow transplant recipients: A prospective study. *Ann Intern Med 89: 893–901, 1978.*

86. Buckner, C.D., Clift, R.A., Sanders, J.E., Williams, B., Gray, M., Storb, R., and Thomas, E.D.: ABO-incompatible marrow transplants. *Transplantation 26: 233–238, 1978.*

87. Buckner, C.D., Stewart, P.S., Bensinger, W., Clift, R., Appelbaum, F., Martin, P., Sanders, J., Fefer, A., Lum, L., Storb, R., Hill, R., and Thomas, E.D.: Critical issues in autologous marrow transplantation for hematologic malignancies. In *Recent Advances in Bone Marrow Transplantation*, R.P. Gale, Ed., Alan R. Liss, New York, 1983.

88. Burnet, F.M., and Boyer, G.S.: The chorioallantoic lesion in the Simonsen phenomenon. *J Pathol Bacteriol 81: 141–150, 1961.*

89. Burnet, F.M.: *Immunological Surveillance.* Pergamon Press, Oxford, 1970.

90. Calne, R.Y., Rolles, K., White, D.J.G., Thiru, S., Evans, D.B., McMaster, P., Dunn, D.C., Craddock, G.N., Henderson, R.G., Aziz, S., and Lewis, P.: Cyclosporin A initially as the only immunosuppressant in 34 recipients of cadaveric organs: Thirty-two kidneys, two pancreases, and two livers. *Lancet 2: 1033–1036, 1979.*

91. Camitta, B.M., and Thomas, E.D.: Severe aplastic anaemia: A prospective study of the effect of androgens or transplantation on haematological recovery and survival. *Clin Haematol 7: 587–595, 1978.*

92. Campbell, P.M., and LeRoy, E.C.: Pathogenesis of systemic sclerosis: A vascular hypothesis. *Semin Arthritis Rheum 4: 351–368, 1975.*

93. Campbell, D.A., Piercey, J.R.A., Schnitka, T.K., Goldsand, G., Devine, R.D.O., and Weinstein, W.M.: Cytomegalovirus-associated gastric ulcer. *Gastroenterology 72: 533–535, 1977.*

94. Carrington, C.B., and Gaensler, E.A.: Clinical-pathologic approach to diffuse infiltrative lung disease. In *The Lung: Structure, Function and Disease,* IAP Monographs in Pathology, No. 19, W.M. Thurlbeck and M.R. Abell, Eds., Williams and Wilkins, Baltimore, 1978, pp. 58–87.

95. Casarett, G.W.: *Radiation Histopathology.* CRC Press, Boca Raton, Florida, 1980, Vols. I and II.

96. Case, J.T., and Warthin, A.S.: The occurrence of hepatic lesions in patients treated by intensive deep roentgen irradiation. *Am J Roentgenol Radiat Ther 12: 27–46, 1924.*

97. Cathcart, M.K., and Krakauer, R.S.: Immunologic enhancement of collagen accumulation in progressive systemic sclerosis (PSS). *Clin Immunol Immunopathol 21: 128–133, 1981.*

98. Catty, D., and Ross, I.N.: Immunological aspects of infection with gastrointestinal parasites (protozoa and nematodes). In *Immunology of the Gastrointestinal Tract,* P. Asquith, Ed., Churchill Livingstone, Edinburgh, 1979, pp. 246–267.

99. Cech, P., Stalder, H., Widmann, J.J., Rohner, A., and Miescher, P.A.: Leukocyte myeloperoxidase deficiency and diabetes mellitus associated with *Candida albicans* liver abscess. *Am J Med 66: 149–153, 1979.*

100. Cerottini, J.C., Nordin, A.A., and Brunner, K.T.: Cellular and humoral response to transplantation antigens. I. Development of alloantibody-forming cells and cytotoxic lymphocytes in the graft-versus-host reaction. *J Exp Med 134: 553–564, 1971.*

101. Chen, P.S., and Alipoulious, M.A.: Acute acalculous cholecystitis. Ultrasonic appearance. *Arch Surg 113: 1461–1462, 1978.*

102. Cherry, C.P., and Glucksmann, A.: Injury and repair following irradiation of salivary glands in male rats. *Br J Radiol 32: 596–608, 1959.*

103. Cho, S.R., Tisnado, J., Liu, C.I., Beachley, M.C., Shaw, C.I., Kipreos, B.E., and Schneider, V.: Bleeding cytomegalovirus ulcers of the colon: Barium enema and angiography. *AJR 136: 1213–1215, 1981.*

104. Chomette, G., Mathé, G., Auriol, M., Brocheriou, C., and Pinaudeau, Y.: Le syndrome secondaire chez l'homme. Études anatomique de six cas de leucémie traités par graffe allogénique de moelle osseuse après

irradiation totale. *Virchows Arch (Pathol Anat) 349; 98–114, 1970.*

105. Chomette, G., Auriol, M., Van Cat, N., Szpirglas, H., Tranbaloc, P., and Vaillant, J.M.: Biopsie des glandes salivaires labials dans le syndrome de Gougerot-Sjögren. Étude clinico-pathologique, histoenzymologique, et ultrastructurale. *Virchows Arch (Pathol Anat) 392: 339–354, 1981.*

106. Chung, C.K., Stryker, J.A., Cruse, R., Vanucci, R., and Towfighi, J.: Glioblastoma multiforme following prophylactic cranial irradiation and intrathecal methotrexate in a child with acute lymphocytic leukemia. *Cancer 47: 2563–2566, 1981.*

107. Chused, T.M., Hardin, J.A., Frank, M.M., and Green, I.: Identification of cells infiltrating the minor salivary glands in patients with Sjögren's syndrome. *J Immunol 112: 641–648, 1974.*

108. Clarke, J., Craig, R.M., Saffro, R., Murphy, P., and Yokoo, H.: Cytomegalovirus granulomatous hepatitis. *Am J Med 66: 264–269, 1979.*

109. Clarysse, A.M., Cathay, W.J., Cartwright, G.E., and Wintrobe, M.M.: Pulmonary disease complicating intermittent therapy with methotrexate. *JAMA 209: 1861–1868, 1969.*

110. Clift, R.A., Buckner, C.D., Fefer, A., Lerner, K.G., Neiman, P.E., Storb, R., Murphy, M., and Thomas, E.D.: Infectious complications of marrow transplantation. *Transplant Proc 6: 389–393, 1974.*

111. Clift, R.A., Buckner, C.D., Williams, B., and Thomas, E.D.: Granulocyte transfusions in marrow transplant recipients. In *Leukocytes: Separation, Collection, and Transfusions,* J.M. Goldman, and R.M. Lowenthal, Eds. Academic Press, New York, 1975, pp. 340–348.

112. Clift, R.A., Sanders, J.E., Thomas, E.D., Williams, B., and Buckner, C.D.: Granulocyte transfusions for the prevention of infection in patients receiving bone-marrow transplants. *N Engl J Med 298: 1052–1057, 1978.*

113. Clift, R.A., Hansen, J.A., Thomas, E.D., Buckner, C.D., Sanders, J.E., Mickelson, E.M., Storb, R., Johnson, F.L., Singer, J.W., and Goodell, B.W.: Marrow transplantation from donors other than HLA-identical siblings. *Transplantation 28: 235–242, 1979.*

114. Clift, R.A., Hansen, J.A., and Thomas, E.D.: The role of HLA in marrow transplantation. *Transplant Proc 13: 234–236, 1981.*

115. Clift, R., Buckner, C.D., Thomas, E.D., Doney, K., Fefer, A., Neiman, P.E., Singer, J., Sanders, J., Stewart, P., Sullivan, K.M., Deeg, J., and Storb, R.: The treatment of chronic granulocytic leukemia in chronic phase by allogeneic bone marrow transplantation. *Lancet 2: 621–624, 1982.*

115a. Coccia, P.F., Krivit, W., Cervenka, J., Clawson, C., Kersey, J.H., Kim, T.H., Nesbit, M.E., Ramsay, N.K.C., Warkentin, P.I., Teitelbaum, S.L., Kahn, A.J., and Brown, D.M.: Successful bone-marrow transplantation for infantile malignant osteopetrosis. *N Engl J Med 302: 701–708, 1980.*

116. Cohen, C., and Olsen, M.M.: Pediatric total parenteral nutrition. Liver histopathology. *Arch Pathol Lab Med 105: 152–156, 1981.*

117. Cohen, I.S., Mosher, M.B., O'Keefe, E.J., Klaus, S.N., and DeConti, R.C.: Cutaneous toxicity of bleomycin therapy. *Arch Dermatol 107: 553–555, 1973.*

118. Congdon, C.C., Uphoff, D., and Lorenz, E.: Modification of acute irradiation injury in mice and guinea pigs by injection of bone marrow: A histopathologic study. *J Natl Cancer Inst 13: 73–107, 1952.*

119. Congdon, C.C., and Urso, I.S.: Homologous bone marrow in the treatment of radiation injury in mice. *Am J Pathol 33: 749–767, 1957.*

120. Congdon, C.C., Makinodan, T., Gengozien, N., Shekarchi, I.C., and Urso, I.S.: Lymphatic tissue changes in lethally irradiated mice given spleen cells intravenously. *J Natl Cancer Inst 21: 193–211, 1958.*

121. Congdon, C.C.: The destructive effect of radiation on lymphatic tissue. *Cancer Res 26: 1211–1220, 1966.*

122. Connell, M.S., and Wilson, R.: The treatment of x-irradiated germfree CFW and C3H mice with isologous and homologous bone marrow. *Life Sci 4: 721–729, 1965.*

123. Connor, R.E., Ramsay, N.K.C., McGlave, P., Snover, D.C., Kersey, J.H., and Burke, B.A.: Pulmonary pathology in bone marrow transplant recipients (Abstract). *Lab Invest 46: 3P, 1982.*

124. Conrad, M.E., and Barton, J.C.: Hepatitis and leukemia (Letter). *Ann Intern Med 93: 780, 1980.*

125. Coppelson, L.W., and Michie, D.: A quantitative study of the chorioallantoic membrane reaction in the chick embryo. *Proc R Soc Lond (Biol) 163: 555–563, 1965.*

126. Cornelius, E.A., Yunis, E.J., Martinez, C., and Good, R.A.: Pathologic feature of parabiosis intoxication. *Lab Invest 19: 324–332, 1968.*

127. Cornelius, E.A.: Protein-losing enteropathy in the graft-versus-host reaction. *Transplantation 9: 247–252, 1970.*

128. Cornelius, E.A.: Rapid viral induction of murine lymphomas in the graft-versus-host reaction. *J Exp Med 136: 1533–1544, 1972.*

129. Corson, S.L., Sullivan, K., Batzer, F., August, C., Storb, R., and Thomas, E.D.: Gynecologic manifestations of chronic graft-versus-host disease. *Obstet Gynecol 60: 488–492, 1982.*

130. Cottier, H., Turk, J., and Sobin, L.: A proposal for a standardized system of reporting human lymph node morphology in relation to immunological function. *Bull WHO 47: 375–417, 1972.*

131. Crystal, R.G., Gadek, J.E., Ferrans, V.J., Fulmar, J.D., Line, B.R., and Hunninghake, G.W.: Interstitial lung disease. Current concepts of pathogenesis, staging, and therapy. *Am J Med 70: 542–568, 1981.*

132. Craighead, J.E.: Cytomegalovirus pulmonary disease. In *Pathobiology Annual*, Vol. 5, H.L. Ioachim, Ed., Appleton-Century-Crofts, New York, 1975, pp. 197–220.

133. Cudkowicz, G., Landy, M., and Shearer, G.M., Eds.: *Natural Resistance Systems Against Foreign Cells, Tumors, and Microbes*. (Perspectives in Immunology Series, Vol. 7). Academic Press, New York, 1978.

134. Cummings, N.A., Schall, G.L., Asofsky, R., Anderson, L.G., and Talal, N.: Sjörgren's syndrome. Newer aspects of research, diagnosis, and theory. *Ann Intern Med 75: 937–950, 1971.*

135. Dahl, M.G.C., Gregory, M.M., and Scheuer, P.J.: Liver damage due to methotrexate in patients with psoriasis. *Br Med J 1: 625–630, 1971.*

136. Dahl, M.G.C., Gregory, M.M., and Scheuer, P.J.: Methotrexate hepatotoxicity in psoriasis: comparison of different dose regimens. *Br Med J 1: 654–656, 1972.*

137. Dahms, B.B., and Halpin, T.C., Jr.: Serial liver biopsies in parenteral nutrition-associated cholestasis of early infancy. *Gastroenterology 81: 136–144, 1981.*

138. Danchakoff, V.: Equivalence of different hematopoietic analogs (by method of stimulation of their stem cells). *Am J Anat 20: 255, 1916.*

139. Deeg, H.J., Storb, R., Thomas, E.D., Appelbaum, F., Buckner, C.D., Clift, R.A., Doney, K., Johnson, L. Sanders, J.E., Stewart, P., Sullivan, K.M., and Witherspoon, P.: Fanconi's anemia treated by allogeneic marrow transplantation. *Blood 61: 954–959, 1983.*

140. D'Angio, G.J., Farber, S., and Maddock, C.L.: Potentiation of x-ray effects by actinomycin D. *Radiology 73: 175–177, 1959.*

141. Dann, J.A., Wachtel, S.S., and Rubin, A.L.: Possible involvement of the central nervous system in graft rejection. *Transplantation 27: 223–226, 1979.*

142. de Bruin, H.G., Astaldi, A., Leupers, T., van de Griend, R.J., Dooren, L.J., Schellekens, P.T.A., Tanke, H.J., Roos, M., and Vossen, J.M.: T-lymphocyte characteristics in bone marrow-transplanted patients. II. Analysis with monoclonal antibodies. *J Immunol 127: 244–251, 1981.*

143. De Dobbeleer, G.D., Ledoux-Corbusier, M.H., and Achten, G.A.: Graft versus host reaction. An ultrastructural study. *Arch Dermatol III: 1597–1602, 1975.*

144. Deeg, H.J., Storb, R., Prentice, R., Fritz, T.E., Weiden, P.L., Sale, G.E., Graham, T.C., and Thomas, E.D.: Increased cancer risk in canine radiation chimeras. *Blood 55: 233–239, 1980.*

145. Deeg, H.J., Storb, R., Weiden, P.L., Graham, T., Atkinson, K., and Thomas, E.D.: Cyclosporin-A: Effect on marrow engraftment and graft-versus-host disease in dogs. *Transplant Proc 13: 402–409, 1981.*

146. Deeg, H.J., Storb, R., Weiden, P.L., Raff, R.F., Sale, G.E., Atkinson, K., Graham, T.C., and Thomas, E.D.: Cyclosporin A and methotrexate in canine marrow transplantation: Engraftment, graft-versus-host disease, and induction of tolerance. *Transplantation 34: 30–35, 1982.*

146a. Deeg, H.J., Prentice, R., Fritz, T.E., Sale, G.E., Lombard, L.S., Thomas, E.D., and Storb, R.: Increased incidence of malignant tumors in dogs after total body irradiation and marrow transplantation. *Int J Radiat Oncol Biol Phys 9: 1505–1511, 1983.*

147. Degott, C., Rueff, B., Kreis, H., Duboust, A., Potet, F., and Benhamou, J.P.: Peliosis hepatis in recipients of renal transplants. *Gut 19: 748–753, 1978.*

148. Deisseroth, A., Abrans, R., Bode, U., Colbert, D., Fontana, J., Holihan, T., and Wright, D.: Current status of autologous bone marrow transplantation. In Gale and Fox, *op cit*, pp. 145–157.

149. Denko, J.D.: The histopathology of the irradiation syndrome after homologous injections in mice (Abstract). *Radiat Res 5: 607, 1956.*

150. deVries, M.J., and Vos, O.: Delayed mortality of radiation chimeras: A pathological and hematological study. *J Natl Cancer Inst 23: 1403–1439, 1959.*

151. deVries, M.J., Crouch, B.G., van Putten, L.M., and van Bekkum, D.W.: Pathologic changes in irradiated monkeys treated with bone marrow. *J Natl Cancer Inst 27, 67–97, 1961.*

152. deVries, M.J.: Pathology of secondary disease in primates. *Proceedings of the International Symposium on Bone Marrow Therapy and Chemical Protection in Irradiated Primates.* The Netherlands Krips, 1962, pp. 101–111.

153. Dicke, K.A., Vellekoop, L., Spitzer, G., Zander, A.R., Schell, F., and Verma, D.S.: Autologous bone marrow transplantation in neoplasia. In Gale and Fox, *op cit*, pp. 159–165.

154. Dienstag, J.L.: Immunologic abnormalities in chronic hepatitis. Postgraduate course in chronic hepatitis and primary biliary cirrhosis for the American Association for the Study of Liver Diseases Symposium, 1982.

155. Dobbins, W.O., 3rd: Colonic epithelial cells and polymorphonuclear leukocytes in ulcerative colitis: An electron-microscopic study. *Am J Dig Dis 20*: 236–252, 1975.

156. Doherty, P.C., and Zinkernagel, R.M.: A biological role for the major histocompatibility antigens. *Lancet 1*: 1406–1409, 1975.

157. Dokhelar, M.C., Wiels, J., Lipinski, M., Tetaud, C., Devergie, A., Gluckman, E., and Tursz, T.: Natural killer cell activity in human bone marrow recipients: Early reappearance of peripheral natural killer activity in graft-versus-host disease. *Transplantation 31*: 61–65, 1981.

158. Donaldson, S.S., Glick, J.M., and Wilber, J.R.: Adriamycin activating a recall phenomenon after radiation therapy (Letter). *Ann Intern Med 81*: 407–408, 1974.

159. Doney, K., Buckner, C.D., Sale, G.E., Ramberg, R., Boyd, C., and Thomas, E.D.: Treatment of chronic granulocytic leukemia by chemotherapy, total body irradiation, and allogeneic bone marrow transplantation. *Exp Hematol 6*: 738–747, 1978.

160. Doney, K.C., Weiden, P.L., Storb, R., and Thomas E.D.: Treatment of graft-versus-host disease in human allogeneic marrow graft recipients: A randomized trial comparing antithymocyte globulin and corticosteroids. *Am J Hematol 11*: 1–8, 1981.

161. Doney, K.C., Weiden, P.L., Storb, R., and Thomas, E.D.: Failure of early administration of antithymocyte globulin to lessen graft-versus-host disease in human allogeneic marrow transplant recipients. *Transplantation 31*: 141–143, 1981.

162. Donnellan, W.L.: Early histological changes in ulcerative colitis. A light and electron microscopic study. *Gastroenterology 50*: 519–540, 1966.

163. Douer, D., Champlin, R.E., and Winston, G.H.: High-dose combined-modality therapy and autologous bone marrow transplantation in resistant cancer. *Am J Med 71*: 973–976, 1981.

164. Drenguis, W.R., and Sale, G.E.: Lymph node repopulation after bone marrow transplantation (Abstract). *Clin Res 26*: 161A, 1978.

165. Dutz, W.: *Pneumocystis carinii* pneumonia. In *Pulmonary Pathology Decennial, 1966-75*, S.C. Sommers, Ed., Appleton-Century-Crofts, New York, 1975, pp. 217–258.

166. Dvorak, H.F., Mihm, M.C., Jr., Dvorak, A.M., Barnes, B.A., and Galli, S.J.: The microvasculature is the critical target of the immune response in vascularized skin allograft rejection. *J Invest Dermatol 74*: 280–284, 1980.

167. Edelson, R.L., Smith, R.W., Frank, M.M., and Green, J.: Identification of subpopulations of mononuclear cells in cutaneous infiltrates. I. Differentiation between B-cells, T-cells and histiocytes. *J Invest Dermatol 61*: 82–89, 1973.

168. Eidelman, S. and Lagunoff, D.: The morphology of the normal human rectal biopsy. *Hum Pathol 3*: 389–401, 1972.

169. Einhorn, L., Krause, M., Hornback, N., and Furnas, B.: Enhanced pulmonary toxicity with bleomycin and radiotherapy in oat cell lung cancer. *Cancer 37*: 2414–2416, 1976.

170. Einstein, A.B., Jr., Cheever, M.A., and Fefer, A.: Induction of increased graft-versus-host disease by mouse spleen cells sensitized *in vitro* to allogeneic tumor. *Transplantation 22*: 589–594, 1976.

171. Elfenbein, G.J., Anderson, P.N., Humphrey, R.L., Mullins, G.M., Sensenbrenner, L.L., Wands, J.R., and Santos, G.W.: Immune system reconstitution following allogeneic bone marrow transplantation in man: A multiparameter analysis. *Transplant Proc 8*: 641–646, 1976.

172. Elfenbein, G.J., Bellis, M.B., and Santos, G.W.: Peanut agglutinin receptor-bearing nonadherent mononuclear cells circulating in the blood after bone marrow transplantation in man. *Transplant Proc 13*: 273–277, 1981.

173. Elfenbein, G.J., and Santos, G.W.: Immunodeficiency after human allogeneic bone marrow transplantation: Lack of evidence for maintenance by nonspecific suppressor cells. In *Experimental Hematology Today*, S.J. Baum, G.D. Ledney, and A. Kahn, Eds., Karger, Basel, Switzerland, 1981, pp. 39–48.

174. Elfenbein, G.J., and Saral, R.: Infectious disease during immune recovery after bone marrow transplantation. In *Infection and the Compromised Host: Clinical Correlations and Therapeutic Approaches* (2nd ed.), J.C. Allen, Ed., Williams & Wilkins, Baltimore, 1981, pp. 157–196.

175. Elie, R., and Lapp, W.S.: Graft versus host-induced immunosuppression: Mechanism of depressed T-cell helper function *in vitro*. *Cell Immunol 34*: 38–48, 1977.

176. Elkins, W.L.: Invasion and destruction of homologous kidney by locally inoculated lymphoid cells. *J Exp Med 120*: 329–348, 1964.

177. Elkins, W.L., and Guttmann, R.D.: Pathogenesis of a local graft-versus-host reaction. Immunogenicity of circulating host leukocytes. *Science 159*: 1250–1251, 1968.

178. Elkins, W.L.: Cellular immunology and the pathogenesis of graft-versus-host reaction. *Prog Allergy 15*: 78–187, 1971.

179. Elkins, W.L.: Graft-versus-host disease as a consequence of bone marrow grafting. In Cudkowicz, Landy, and Shearer, *op cit*, pp. 73–90.

180. Elkins, W.L.: An immunogenetic approach to the graft-vs.-host reaction and secondary disease. In Gale and Fox, *op cit*, pp. 195–207.

181. Elson, C.O., Reilly, R.W., and Rosenberg, I.H.: Small intestinal injury in the graft-versus-host reaction: An innocent-bystander phenomenon. *Gastroenterology 72*: 886–889, 1977.

182. Engeset, A.: Irradiation of lymph nodes and vessels. Experiments in rats with reference to cancer therapy. *Acta Radiol (Diagn) (Stockh) Suppl 229: 1+, 1964.*

183. English, J.A., and Tullis, J.L.: Oral manifestations of ionizing radiation. I. Oral lesions and effect on developing teeth of swine exposed to 2000 K.V. total body x-ray irradiation. *J Dent Res 30: 33–52, 1951.*

184. English, J.A.: Morphologic effects of irradiation on the salivary glands of rats. *J Dent Res 34: 4–11, 1955.*

185. English, J.A., Wheatcroft, M.G., Lyon, H.W., and Miller, C.: Long-term observations of radiation changes in salivary glands and the general effects of 1000 R to 1750 R of x-ray radiation locally administered to heads of dogs. *Oral Surg: 87–99, 1955.*

186. Epstein, O., Thomas, H.C., and Sherlock, S.: Primary biliary cirrhosis in a dry gland syndrome with features of chronic graft-versus-host disease. *Lancet 1: 1166–1168, 1980.*

187. Epstein, R.B., Graham, T.C., Buckner, C.D., Bryant, J., and Thomas, E.D.: Allogeneic marrow engraftment by cross circulation in lethally irradiated dogs. *Blood 28: 692–707, 1966.*

188. Epstein, R.B., Bryant, J., and Thomas, E.D.: Cytogenetic demonstration of permanent tolerance in adult outbred dogs. *Transplantation 5: 267–272, 1967.*

189. Epstein, R.B., Storb, R., Radge, H., and Thomas, E.D.: Cytotoxic typing antisera for marrow grafting in littermate dogs. *Transplantation 6: 45–58, 1968.*

190. Epstein, R.B., Storb, R., Clift, R.A., and Thomas, E.D.: Transplantation of stored allogeneic bone marrow in dogs selected by histocompatibility typing. *Transplantation 8: 496–501, 1969.*

191. Epstein, R.B., Storb, R., and Thomas, E.D.: Relation of canine histocompatibility testing to marrow grafting. *Transplantation 3: 161–164, 1971.*

192. Epstein, R.J., McDonald, G.B., Sale, G.E., Shulman, H.M., and Thomas, E.D.: The diagnostic accuracy of the rectal biopsy in acute graft-versus-host disease: A prospective study of 13 patients. *Gastroenterology 78: 764–771, 1980.*

193. Eras, P., Goldstein, M.J., and Sherlock, P.: Candida infection of the gastrointestinal tract. *Medicine 51: 367–379, 1972.*

194. Fajardo, L.F., and Berthrong, M.: Radiation injury in surgical pathology. Part I. *Am J Surg Pathol 2: 159–199, 1978.*

195. Fajardo, L.F., and Colby, T.V.: Pathogenesis of veno-occlusive liver disease after radiation. *Arch Pathol Lab Med 104: 584–588, 1980.*

196. Fang, M.H., Ginsberg, A.L., and Dobbins, W.O., 3rd: Marked elevation in serum alkaline phosphatase activity as a manifestation of systemic infection. *Gastroenterology 78: 592–597, 1980.*

197. Fass, L., Ochs, H.D., Thomas, E.D., Mickelson, E., Storb, R., and Fefer, A.: Studies of immunological reactivity following syngeneic or allogeneic marrow grafts in man. *Transplantation 16: 630–640, 1973.*

198. Fefer, A., Einstein, A.B., Thomas, E.D., Buckner, C.D., Clift, R.A., Glucksberg, H., Neiman, P.E., and Storb, R.: Bone marrow transplantation for hematologic neoplasia in 16 patients with identical twins. *N Engl J Med 290: 1389–1393, 1974.*

199. Fefer, A., Buckner, C.D., Thomas, E.D., Cheever, M.A., Clift, R.A., Glucksberg, H., Neiman, P.E., and Storb, R.: Cure of hematologic neoplasia with transplantation of marrow from identical twins. *N Engl J Med 297: 146–148, 1977.*

200. Fefer, A., Cheever, M.A., Thomas, E.D., Appelbaum, F.R., Buckner, C.D., Clift, R.A., Glucksberg, H., Greenberg, P.D., Johnson, F.L., Kaplan, H.G., Sanders, J.E., Storb, R., and Weiden, P.L.: Bone marrow transplantation for refractory acute leukemia in 34 patients with identical twins. *Blood 57: 421–430, 1981.*

201. Fefer, A., Cheever, M.A., Greenberg, P.D., Appelbaum, F.R., Boyd, C.N., Buckner, C.D., Kaplan, H.G., Ramberg, R., Sanders, J.E., Storb, R., and Thomas, E.D.: Treatment of chronic granulocytic leukemia with chemoradiotherapy and transplantation of marrow from identical twins. *N Engl J Med 306: 63–68, 1982.*

202. Fennel, R.H., Jr.: Ductular damage in liver transplant rejection: Its similarity to that of primary biliary cirrhosis and graft-versus-host disease. *Pathol Annu 16: 289–294, 1981.*

203. Fenyk, J.R., Jr., Smith, C.M., Warkentin, P.I., Krivit, W., Goltz, R.W., Neely, J.E., Nesbit, M.E., Ramsay, N.K.C., Coccia, P.F., and Kersey, J.H.: Sclerodermatous graft-versus-host disease limited to an area of measles exanthem. *Lancet 1: 472–473, 1978.*

204. Ferguson, A., and Parrott, DMV: Histopathology and time course of rejection of allografts of mouse small intestine. *Transplantation 15: 546–554, 1973.*

205. Ferguson, A., and Jarrett, E.E.: Hypersensitivity reactions in the small intestine: I. Thymus dependence of experimental "partial villous atrophy." *Gut 16: 114–117, 1975.*

206. Ferguson, A.: Intraepithelial lymphocytes of the small intestine. *Gut 18: 921–937, 1977.*

207. Feron, V.J., and Mullink, J.W.M.A.: Mucosal cysts in the gastrointestinal tract of beagle dogs. *Lab Anim 5: 193–201, 1971.*

208. Ferrebee, J.W., and Thomas, E.D.: Radiation injury and marrow replacement: Factors affecting survival of the host and the homograft. *Ann Intern Med 49: 987–1003, 1958.*

209. Ferrebee, J.W., and Thomas, E.D.: Some experiences with irradiation injury. *Radiology 75: 1–5, 1960.*

210. Finegold, M.J., and Carpenter, R.J.: Obliterative cholangitis due to cytomegalovirus: A possible precursor of paucity of intrahepatic bile ducts. *Hum Pathol 13: 662–665, 1982.*

211. Fisk, J.D., Shulman, H.M., Greening, R.R., McDonald, G.B., Sale, G.E. and Thomas, E.D.: Gastrointestinal radiographic features of human graft-versus-host disease. *AJR 136: 329–336, 1981.*

212. Fleischmajer, R., Damiano, V., and Nedwich, A.: Scleroderma and the subcutaneous tissue (Abstract). *Science 171: 1019–1021, 1971.*

213. Fleischmajer, R., Perlish, J.S., and West, W.P.: Ultrastructure of cutaneous cellular infiltrates in scleroderma. *Arch Dermatol 113: 1661–1666, 1977.*

214. Fleischmajer, R., Perlish, J.S., and Reeves, J.R.T.: Cellular "infiltrates" in scleroderma skin. *Arthritis Rheum 20: 975–984, 1977.*

215. Fleischmajer, R., Gay, S., Meigel, W.N., and Perlish, J.S.: Collagen in the cellular and fibrotic stages of

scleroderma. *Arthritis Rheum 21: 418–428, 1978.*

216. Fleischmajer, R., Perlish, J.S., Krieg, T., and Timpl, R.: Variability in collagen and fibronectin synthesis by scleroderma fibroblasts in primary culture. *J Invest Dermatol 76: 400–403, 1981.*

217. Foster, J.H., Donohue, T.A., and Berman, M.M.: Familial liver cell adenomas in diabetes mellitus. *N Engl J Med 299: 239–241, 1978.*

218. Freeman, H.J., Schnitka, T.K., Piercey, J.R, and Weinstein, W.M.: Cytomegalovirus infection of the gastrointestinal tract in a patient with late onset immunodeficiency syndrome. *Gastroenterology 73: 1397–1403, 1977.*

219. Freeman, H.J., Rabeneck, L., and Owen, D.: Survival after necrotizing enterocolitis of leukemia treated with oral vancomycin. *Gastroenterology 81: 791–794, 1981.*

220. French, S.W., Burbige, E.J., Tarder, G., Bourke, E., Harkin, C.G., and Denton, T.: Lymphocyte sequestration by the liver in alcoholic hepatitis. *Arch Pathol Lab Med 103: 146–152, 1979.*

221. Friedrich, W., O'Reilly, R.J., Koziner, B., Gebhard, D.F., Jr., Good, R.A., and Evans, R.L.: T-lymphocyte reconstitution in recipients of bone marrow transplants with and without GVHD: Imbalances of T-cell subpopulations having unique regulatory and cognitive functions. *Blood 59: 696–701, 1982.*

222. Frizzera, G., Hanto, D.W., Gajl-Peczalska, K.J., Rosai, J., McKenna, R.W., Sibley, R.K., Holahan, K.P., and Lindquist, L.L.: Polymorphic diffuse B-cell hyperplasia and lymphomas in renal transplant recipients. *Cancer Res 41: 4262–4271, 1981.*

223. Fuks, Z., Strober, S., Bobrove, A.M., Sasazuki, T., McMichael, A., and Kaplan, H.S.: Long-term effects of radiation on T- and B-lymphocytes in the peripheral blood of patients with Hodgkin's disease. *J Clin Invest 58: 803–814, 1976.*

224. Fung, K.Y., and Sabbadini, E.: Cytotoxicity in graft-versus-host reaction. II. Lysis of target cells of parental genotype by $F_1$ hybrid macrophages. *Transplantation 22: 449–454, 1976.*

225. Gale, R.P., Opelz, G., Mickey, M.R., Graze, P.R., and Saxon, A. for the UCLA Bone Marrow Transplant Team: Immunodeficiency following allogeneic bone marrow transplantation. *Transplant Proc 10: 223–227, 1978.*

226. Gale, R.P., and Fox, C.F., Eds.: *Biology of Bone Marrow Transplantation*, Vol. 17, ICN-UCLA Symposia on Molecular and Cellular Biology. Academic Press, New York, 1980.

227. Gale, R.P.: Clinical trials of bone marrow transplantation in leukemia. In Gale and Fox, *op cit*, pp. 11–28.

228. Gale, R.P., Foon, K., Cline, M.J., Zighelboim, J., and UCLA Acute Leukemia Study Group: Intensive chemotherapy for acute myelogenous leukemia. *Ann Intern Med 94: 753–757, 1981.*

229. Gallucci, B.B., Shulman, H.M., Sale, G.E., Lerner, K.G., Caldwell, L.E., and Thomas, E.D.: The ultrastructure of the human epidermis in chronic graft-versus-host disease. *Am J Pathol 95: 643–662, 1979.*

230. Gallucci, B.B., Sale, G.E., McDonald, G.B., Epstein, R., Shulman, H.M., and Thomas, E.D.: The fine structure of human rectal epithelium in acute graft-versus-host disease. *Am J Surg Pathol 6: 293–305, 1982.*

231. Gatti, R.A., and Good, R.A.: Occurrence of malignancy in immunodeficiency disease. *Cancer 28: 89–98, 1971.*

232. Gauvreau, J.M., Lenssen, P., Cheney, C.L., Aker, S.N., Hutchinson, M.L., and Barale, K.V.: Nutritional management of patients with intestinal graft-versus-host disease. *J Am Diet Assoc 79: 673–677, 1981.*

233. Georgitis, J., Eigen, H., Provisor, D., and Baehner, R.L.: Isolated pulmonary leukemic relapse following successful bone marrow transplant in a child with acute lymphoblastic leukemia. *Pediatrics 64: 913–917, 1979.*

234. Gérard, H., and Kohler, F.: Modifications des espaces porto-biliaires au cours de la réaction du greffan contre l'hote chez l'embryon de Poulet et de foetus de at. *C R Soc Biol (Paris) 173: 758–766, 1979.*

235. Gerber, M.A.: Binding of antibody to hepatocytes: cause or effect of chronic active hepatitis? (Editorial). *Gastroenterology 77: 389–390, 1979.*

236. Ginsberg, S.J., and Comis, R.L.: The pulmonary toxicity of antineoplastic agents. *Semin Oncol 9: 34–51, 1982.*

237. Glasier, C.M., Siegel, M.J., McAllister, W.H., and Shackelford, G.D.: Henoch-Schonlein syndrome in children: Gastrointestinal manifestations. *AJR 136: 1081–1085, 1981.*

238. Gleichmann, H., Gleichmann, E., Andre-Schwartz, J., and Schwartz, R.S.: Chronic allogeneic disease: III. Genetic requirements for the induction of glomerulonephritis. *J Exp Med 135: 516–532, 1972.*

239. Gleichmann, E., and Gleichmann, H.: Graft-versus-host reaction: A pathogenetic principle for the development of drug allergy, autoimmunity, and malignant lymphoma in non-chimeric individuals. Hypothesis. *Z Krebsforsch 85: 91–109, 1976.*

240. Gleichmann, E., van Elven, F., and Gleichmann, H.: Immunoblastic lymphadenopathy, systemic lupus erythematosus, and related disorders. Possible pathogenetic pathways. *Am J Clin Pathol 72: 708–723, 1979.*

241. Gleichmann, E., and Gleichmann, H.: Spectrum of disease caused by autoreactive T-cells, mode of sensitization to the drug diphenylhydantain, and possible role of SLE-typical self antigens in B-cell triggering. In *Immunoregulation and Autoimmunity*, R.S. Krakauer and M.K. Cathcart, Eds., Elsevier/North-Holland, New York, 1980, pp. 73–83.

242. Gluckman, E., Andersen, E., Lepage, V., and Dausset, J.: Non-HLA lymphocytotoxic antibodies during GVHD after bone marrow transplantation (BMT). *Transplant Proc 9: 761–763, 1977.*

243. Gluckman, E., Devergie, A., Sohier, J., and Saurat, J.H.: Graft versus host disease in recipients of syngeneic bone marrow (Letter). *Lancet 1: 253–254, 1980.*

244. Gluckman, E., Gluckman, J.C., Andersen, E., Guillet, J., Devergie, A., and Daussat, J.: Lymphocytotoxic antibodies after bone marrow transplantation in aplastic anemia. II. Non-HLA antibodies. *Transplantation 29: 471–476, 1980.*

245. Glucksberg, H., Storb, R., Fefer, A., Buckner, C.D., Neiman, P.E., Clift, R.A., Lerner, K.G., and Thomas, E.D.: Clinical manifestations of graft-versus-host disease in human recipients of marrow from HL-A-matched sibling donors. *Transplantation 18: 295–304, 1974.*

246. Glucksberg, H., Cheever, M.A., Farewell, V.T., Fefer, A., Sale, G.E., and Thomas, E.D.: High-dose combination chemotherapy for acute nonlymphoblastic leukemia in adults. *Cancer 48: 1073–1081, 1981.*

247. Glucksmann, A.: Radiation histology. II. The response

of human tissues to radiation with special reference to differentiation. *Br J Radiol* 25: 38–43, 1952.

248. Glucksmann, A., and Cherry, C.P.: The induction of adenomas by the irradiation of salivary glands of rats. *Radiat Res* 17: 186–202, 1962.

249. Gold, J.A., Kosek, J., and Wanek, N.: Duodenal immunoglobulin deficiency graft-versus-host disease (GVHD) in mice. *J Immunol* 117: 471–476, 1976.

250. Goldberg, I.D., Bloomer, W.D., and Dawson, D.M.: Nervous system toxic effects of cancer therapy (Special Communications). *JAMA* 247: 1437–1441, 1982.

251. Goldstein, L.C., McDougall, J., Hackman, R., Meyers, J.D., Thomas, E.D., and Nowinski, R.C.: Monoclonal antibodies to cytomegalovirus: Rapid identification of clinical isolates and preliminary use in diagnosis of cytomegalovirus pneumonia. *Infect Immun* 38: 273–281, 1982.

252. Goldstein, L.C., Corey, L., McDougall, J.K., Tolentino, E., and Nowinski, R.C.: Monoclonal antibodies to herpes simplex viruses: Use in antigenic typing and rapid diagnosis. *J Infect Dis* 147: 829–837, 1983.

253. Gonzalez-Licea, A., and Yardley, J.H.: A comparative ultrastructural study of the mucosa in idiopathic ulcerative colitis, shigellosis, and other human colonic diseases. *Bull Hopkins Hosp* 118: 444–461, 166.

254. Gonzalez-Licea, A., and Yardley, J.H.: Nature of the tissue reaction in ulcerative colitis: Light and electron microscopic findings. *Gastroenterology* 51: 825–840, 1966.

255. Goodman, Z.D., Boitnott, J.K., and Yardley, J.H.: Perforation of the colon associated with cytomegalovirus infection. *Dig Dis Sci* 24: 376–380, 1979.

256. Gorer, P.A., and Boyse, E.A.: Pathological changes in $F_1$ hybrid mice following transplantation of spleen cells from donors of the parental strain. *Immunology* 2: 182–193, 1959.

257. Gorin, N.C., David, R., Stachowiak, J., Salmon, C., Petit, J.C., Parlier, Y., Najman, A., and Duhamel, G.: High-dose chemotherapy and autologous bone marrow transplantation in acute leukemias, malignant lymphomas, and solid tumors. A study of 23 patients. *Eur J Cancer* 17: 557–568, 1981.

258. Gosink, B.B., Friedman, P.J., and Liebow, A.A.: Bronchiolitis obliterans: Roentgenologic–pathologic correlations. *AJR* 117: 816–832, 1973.

259. Gossett, T.C., Gale, R.P., Fleischman, H., Austin, G.E., Sparkes, R.S., and Taylor, C.R.: Immunoblastic sarcoma in donor cells after bone-marrow transplantation. *N Engl J Med* 300: 904–907, 1979.

260. Gottfried, M.R., and Sudilovsky, O.: Hepatic veno-occlusive disease after high-dose mitomycin C and autologous bone marrow transplantation therapy. *Hum Pathol* 13: 646–650, 1982.

261. Gould, V.E., and Miller, B.S.: Sclerosing alveolitis produced by cyclophosphamide. Ultrastructural observations on alveolar injury and repair. *Am J Pathol* 81: 513–529, 1975.

262. Gratwohl, A.A., Moutsopoulos, H.M., Chused, T.M., Akizuki, M., Wolf, R.O., Sweet, J.B., and Deisseroth, A.B.: Sjögren-type syndrome after allogeneic bone-marrow transplantation. *Ann Intern Med* 87: 703–706, 1977.

263. Graze, P.R., and Gale, R.P.: Chronic graft-versus-host disease: A syndrome of disordered immunity. *Am J Med* 66: 611–620, 1979.

264. Grebe, S.C., and Streilein, J.W.: Graft-versus-host reactions: A review. *Adv Immunol* 22: 119–221, 1976.

265. Greco, F.A., Brereton, H.D., Kent, H., Zimbler, H., Merrill, J., and Johnson, R.E.: Adriamycin and enhanced radiation reaction in normal esophagus and skin. *Ann Intern Med* 85: 294–298, 1976.

266. Gregson, R.L., Davey, M.J., and Prentice, D.E.: The response of rat bronchus-associated lymphoid tissue to local antigenic challenge. *Br J Exp Pathol* 60: 471–482, 1979.

267. Griffin, W.S.T., Eriksson, M.A.E., Crom, E.N., and Head, J.R.: Malformation of Purkinje cell dendrites induced by graft-versus-host disease. *Brain Res Bull* 5: 673–678, 1980.

268. Griffin, W.S.T., Cron, E.N., and Head, J.R.: Alterations in cerebellar germinal cell division induced by graft-versus-host disease. *J Comp Neurol* 203: 91–101, 1981.

269. Grogan, T.M., Odom, R.B., and Burgess, J.H.: Graft-vs-host reaction. *Arch Dermatol* 113: 806–812, 1977.

270. Gross, N.J.: Pulmonary effects of radiation therapy. *Ann Intern Med* 86: 81–92, 1977.

271. Gumucio, J.J., and Miller, D.L.: Functional implications of liver cell heterogeneity. *Gastroenterology* 80: 393–403, 1981.

272. Hackman, R.C., and Sale, G.E.: Large airway inflammation as a possible manifestation of a pulmonary graft-versus-host reaction (Abstract). *Lab Invest* 44: 26A, 1981.

273. Hackman, R.C., Schubach, W.H., Neiman, P.E., Miller, G., and Thomas, E.D.: Development of non-Hodgkin's lymphoma subsequent to marrow transplantation (Abstract). *Lab Invest* 46: 32A–33A, 1982.

274. Hackman, R.C., Meyers, J.D., Springmeyer, S.C., and Seattle Bone Marrow Transplant Team: Application of a monoclonal antibody to the diagnosis of cytomegalovirus pneumonia (Abstract). *Lab Invest* 48: 31A, 1983.

275. Hackman, R.C., Meyers, J.D., Springmeyer, S.S., Myerson, D., and the Seattle Bone Marrow Transplant Team: Identification of a CMV antigen and CMV nucleic acid in studies of pneumonitis and hepatitis in marrow transplant recipients (Abstract). *J Cell Biochem Suppl* 7A: 56, #134, 1983.

276. Hager, E.B., Ferrebee, J.W., and Thomas, E.D.: Damage and repair of the gastrointestinal tract after supralethal radiation. Experience with dogs receiving 1800 to 2400 roentgens of whole-body gamma radiation. *Radiobiol Radiother (Ber)* 4: 1–12, 1963.

277. Halterman, R.H., Graw, R.G., Jr., Fuccillo, D.A., and Leventhal, B.G.: Immunocompetence following allogeneic bone marrow transplantation in man. *Transplantation* 14: 689–697, 1972.

278. Hamilton, B.L., Bevan, M.J., and Parkman, R.: Anti-recipient cytotoxic T-lymphocyte precursors are present in the spleens of mice with acute graft-versus-host disease due to minor histocompatibility antigens. *J Immunol* 126: 621–625, 1981.

279. Hansen, J.A., Clift, R.A., Thomas, E.D., Buckner, C.D., Storb, R., and Giblett, E.R.: Transplantation of marrow from an unrelated donor to a patient with acute leukemia. *N Engl J Med* 303: 565–567, 1980.

280. Hansen, J.A., Woodruff, J.M., and Good, R.A.: The graft-vs.-host reaction in man: Genetics, clinical features, and immunopathology. In *Immunodermatology*

(Comprehensive Immunology Series, Vol 7), B. Safai and R.A. Good, Eds., Plenum Publishing, New York, 1981, pp. 229–257.

280a. Harmon, J.B., Sibley, R.K., Peterson, P., and Ferguson, R.: Cytomegalovirus viremia and renal allograft morphology: are there distinct pathologic features? (Abstract) *Lab Invest 46: 35A, 1982.*

281. Harrison, D.T., Flournoy, N., Ramberg, R., Boyd, C., Erne, K., Buckner, C.D., Fefer, A., Sanders, J.E., Storb, R., and Thomas, E.D.: Relapse following marrow transplantation for acute leukemia. *Am J Hematol 5: 191–202, 1978.*

282. Haschek, W.M., Meyer, K.R., Ullrich, R.L., and Witschi, H.P.: Potentiation of chemically induced lung fibrosis by thorax irradiation. *Int J Radiat Oncol Biol Phys 6: 449–455, 1980.*

283. Heard, B.E., and Cooke, R.A.: Busulphan lung. *Thorax 23: 187–193, 1968.*

284. Hebard, D.W., Jackson, K.L., and Christensen, G.M.: The chronological development of late radiation injury in the liver of the rat. *Radiat Res 81: 441–454, 1980.*

285. Hedberg, C.A., Reiser, S., and Reilly, R.W.: Intestinal phase of the runting syndrome in mice. II. Observations on nutrient absorption and certain disaccharidase abnormalities. *Transplantation 6: 104–110, 1968.*

286. Heflin, A.C., Jr., and Brigham, K.L.: Prevention by granulocyte depletion of increased vascular permeability of sheep lung following endotoxemia. *J Clin Invest 68: 1253–1260, 1981.*

287. Heit, H., Wilson, R., Fliedner, T.M., and Kohne, E.: Mortality of secondary disease in antibiotic-treated mouse radiation chimeras. In *Germfree Research: Biological Effects of Gnotobiotic Environments*, J.B. Heneghan, Ed., Academic Press, New York, 1973, pp. 477–483.

288. Henson, D.: Cytomegalovirus hepatitis in an adult. An autopsy report. *Arch Pathol 88: 199–203, 1969.*

289. Hersh, E.M., Wong, V.G., Henderson, E.S., and Freireich, E.J.: Hepatotoxic effects of methotrexate. *Cancer 19: 600–606, 1966.*

289a. Hersman, J., Meyers, J.D., Thomas, E.D., Buckner, C.D., and Clift, R.: The effect of granulocyte transfusions on the incidence of cytomegalovirus infection after allogeneic marrow transplantation. *Ann Intern Med 96: 149–152, 1982.*

290. Herzenberg, L.A., Black, S.J., and Herzenberg, L.A.: Regulatory circuits and antibody responses. *Eur J Immunol 10: 1–11, 1980.*

291. Hill, Donald L.: *A Review of Cyclophosphamide.* C.C. Thomas, Springfield, Illinois, 1975, pp. 118–137.

292. Hirt, A., and Wagner, H.P.: Characterization of lymphoid cells in the blood of healthy adults: Sequential immunological, cytochemical, and cytokinetic studies. *Am J Hematol 9: 301–309, 1980.*

293. Hobbs, J.R.: Bone marrow transplantation for inborn errors. *Lancet 2: 735–739, 1981.*

294. Hochberg, F.H., Parker, L.M., Takvorian, T., Canellos, G.P., and Zervas, N.T.: High-dose BCNU with autologous bone marrow rescue for recurrent glioblastoma multiforme. *J Neurosurg 54: 455–460, 1981.*

295. Holland, P.V., and Alter, H.J.: Non-A, non-B viral hepatitis. *Hum Pathol 12: 1114–1122, 1981.*

296. Hong, R., Schulte-Wissermann, H., Jarred-Toth, E., Horowitz, S.D., and Manning, D.D.: Transplantation

of cultured thymic fragments. II. Results in nude mice. *J Exp Med 149: 398–415, 1979.*

297. Hoofnagle, J.H., Dusheiko, G.M., Schafer, D.F., Jones, A., Micetich, K.C., Young, R.C., and Costa, J.: Reactivation of chronic hepatitis B virus infection by cancer chemotherapy. *Ann Intern Med 96: 447–449, 1982.*

298. Hopf, U, zum Buschenfelde, K-H.M., and Arnold, W.: Detection of a liver-membrane autoantibody in HB$_s$ Ag-negative chronic active hepatitis. *N Engl J Med 294: 578–582, 1976.*

299. Howard, J.G.: Changes in the activity of reticulo-endothelial system (RES) following the injection of parental spleen cells into F$_1$ hybrid mice. *Br J Exp Pathol 42: 72–82, 1961.*

300. Hughes, W.T., Kuhn, S., Chaudhary, S., Feldman, S., Verzosa, M., Aur, R.J.A., Pratt, C., and George, S.L.: Successful chemoprophylaxis for *Pneumocystis carinii* pneumonitis. *N Engl J Med 297: 1419–1426, 1977.*

301. Hutton, S.W., Snoker, D.C., and Bloomer, J.R.: The role of liver tissue in evaluating patients with cytomegalovirus infection (Abstract). *Gastroenterology 82: 1088, 1982.*

302. Ishak, K.G.: Light microscopic morphology of viral hepatitis. *Am J Clin Pathol 65: 787–827, 1976.*

303. Ivanyi, J.: Prevention of graft-versus-host reactions and conditioning of recipients for bone marrow transplantation in chickens. In Thierfelder, Rodt, and Kolb, *op cit*, pp. 219–237.

304. Izutsu, K., Oberg, S., Shulman, H., Schubert, M., Sullivan, K., Morton, T., Sale, G., and Truelove, E.: Depressed salivary IgA and sodium flow changes in C-GVHD patients (Abstract). *J Supramol Struct (Suppl 4): 24, #50, 1980.*

305. Izutsu, K.T., Truelove, E.L., Shulman, H.M., Schubert, M.M., Sale, G.E., Oberg, S.G., Ensign, W.Y., and Thomas, E.D.: The predictive value of elevated labial saliva sodium concentration. Its relation to labial gland pathology in bone marrow transplant recipients. *Hum Pathol 13: 29–35, 1983.*

306. Izutsu, K.T., Sullivan, K.M., Schubert, M.M., Truelove, E.L., Shulman, H.M., Sale, G.E., Morton, G.H., Rice, J.C., Witherspoon, R.P., Storb, R., and Thomas, E.D.: Disordered salivary immunoglobulin secretions and sodium transport in human chronic graft-versus-host disease. *Transplantation 35: 441–446, 1983.*

307. Jack, M.K., Jack, G.M., Sale, G.E., Shulman, H.M., and Sullivan, K.M.: Ocular manifestations of graft-versus-host disease. *Arch Ophthalmol 101: 1080–1084, 1983.*

308. Jack, M.K., and Hicks, J.D.: Ocular complications in high-dose chemoradiotherapy and marrow transplantation. *Arch Ophthalmol 13: 709–711, 1981.*

309. Jacobs, P., Miller, J.L., Uys, C.J., and Dietrich, B.E.: Fatal veno-occlusive disease of the liver after chemotherapy, whole-body irradiation, and bone marrow transplantation for refractory acute leukemia. *S Afr Med J 55: 5–10, 1979.*

310. Jaffe, C.J., Vierling, J.M., Jones, E.A., Lawly, T.J., and Frank, M.M.: Receptor specific clearance by the reticuloendothelial system in chronic liver diseases. Demonstration of defective C3b-specific clearance in primary biliary cirrhosis. *J Clin Invest 62: 1069–1077, 1978.*

311. Jaffe, J.P., and Maki, D.G.: Lung biopsy in immunocompromised patients: One institution's experience and an approach to management of pulmonary disease in the compromised host. *Cancer 48: 1144–1153, 1981.*

312. James, S.P., Vierling, J.M., and Strober, W.: The role of the immune response in the pathogenesis of primary biliary cirrhosis. *Semin Liver Dis 1: 322–337, 1981.*

313. Janin-Mercier, A., Saurat, J.H., Bourges, M., Sohier, J., Didierjean, L., and Gluckman, E.: The lichen planus-like and sclerotic phases of the graft-versus-host disease in man: An ultrastructural study of six cases. *Acta Derm Venereol (Stockh) 61: 187–193, 1981.*

314. Janossy, G., Thomas, J.A., Bollum, F.J., Granger, S., Pizzolo, G., Bradstock, K.F., Wong, L., McMichael, A., Ganeshaguru, K., and Hoffbrand, A.V.: The human thymic microenvironment: An immunohistologic study. *J Immunol 125: 202–212, 1980.*

315. Jeannet, M., Rubenstein, A., and Pelet, B.: Studies on non-HL-A cytotoxic and blocking factor in a patient with immunological deficiency successfully reconstituted by bone marrow transplantation. *Tissue Antigens 3: 411–416, 1973.*

316. Jeannet, M., Klouda, P.T., Vassalli, P., Ramirez, E., Legendre, C., and Speck, B.: Anomalous MLC and CML tests in human bone marrow transplantation. In *Histocompatibility Testing,* F. Kissmeyer-Neilsen, Ed., Munksgaard, Copenhagen, 1975, pp. 885–892.

317. Jeffrey, R.B., Jr., Moss, A.A., Quivey, J.M., Federle, M.P., and Wara, W.M.: CT of radiation-induced hepatic injury. *AJR 135: 445–448, 1980.*

318. Jiminez, S.A., McArthur, W., and Rosenbloom, J.: Inhibition of collagen synthesis by mononuclear cell supernates. *J Exp Med 150: 1421–1431, 1979.*

319. Jirtle, R.L., Michalopoulous, G., McLain, J.R., and Crowley, J.: Transplantation system for determining the clonogenic survival of parenchymal hepatocytes exposed to ionizing radiation. *Cancer Res 41: 3512–3518, 1981.*

320. Johnson, F.L., Thomas, E.D., Clark, B.S., Chard, R.L., Hartmann, J.R., and Storb, R.: A comparison of marrow transplantation with chemotherapy for children with acute lymphoblastic leukemia in second or subsequent remission. *N Engl J Med 305: 846–851, 1981.*

321. Johnson, K.J., and Ward, P.A.: Biology of disease. Newer concepts in the pathogenesis of immune complex-induced tissue injury. *Lab Invest 47: 218–226, 1982.*

322. Johnson, R.L., and Ziff, M.: Lymphokine stimulation of collagen accumulation. *J Clin Invest 58: 240–252, 1976.*

323. Jones, E.A., Frank, M.M., Jaffe, C.J., and Vierling, J.M.: Primary biliary cirrhosis and the complement system. *Ann Intern Med 90: 72–84, 1979.*

324. Jones, J.M., Wilson, R., and Bealmear, P.M.: Mortality and gross pathology of secondary disease in germfree mouse radiation chimeras. *Radiat Res 45: 577–588, 1971.*

325. Jones, J.M.: Necrotizing *Candida* esophagitis. Failure of symptoms and roentgenographic findings to reflect severity. *JAMA 244: 2190–2191, 1980.*

326. Jones, J.M.: Granulomatous hepatitis due to *Candida albicans* in patients with acute leukemia. *Ann Intern Med 94: 475–477, 1981.*

327. Jonsson, P.E., and Andersson, A.: Postoperative acute acalculous cholecystitis. *Arch Surg. 111: 1097–1101, 1976.*

328. Jordan, S.W., Yuhas, J.M., Key, C.R., Hogstrom, K.R., Butler, J.L.B., and Kligerman, M.M.: Comparative late effects of x-rays and negative pimesons on the mouse kidney. *Am J Pathol 97: 315–326, 1979.*

329. Joshi, S.N., Garvin, P.J., and Sunwoo, Y.C.: Candidiasis of the duodenum and jejunum. *Gastroenterology 80: 829–833, 1981.*

330. Julia, A., and Font, L.: Hepatitis and leukemia (Letter). *Ann Intern Med 93: 780, 1980.*

331. Kahaleh, M.B., Sherer, G.K., and LeRoy, E.C.: Endothelial injury in scleroderma. *J Exp Med 149: 1326–1335, 1979.*

332. Kane, J.G., Chretien, J.H., and Garagusi, V.F.: Diarrhoea caused by *Candida. Lancet 1: 335–336, 1976.*

333. Kao, Y.S.: A technic for bone marrow imprints from postmortem specimens. *Am J Clin Pathol 63: 832–835, 1975.*

334. Kaplan, R.S., and Wiernik, P.H.: Neurotoxicity of antineoplastic drugs. *Semin Oncol 9: 103–130, 1982.*

335. Katzenstein, A.L., Bloor, C.M., and Liebow, A.A.: Diffuse alveolar damage—The role of oxygen, shock, and related factors. *Am J Pathol 85: 210–228, 1976.*

336. Katzenstein, A.L., and Maksem, J.: Candidal infection of gastric ulcers. Histology, incidence, and clinical significance. *Am J Clin Pathol 71: 137–141, 1979.*

337. Katzenstein, A.L., and Askin, F.B.: Interpretation and significance of pathologic findings in transbronchial lung biopsy. *Am J Surg Pathol 4: 223–234, 1980.*

338. Katzenstein, A.L., and Askin, F.B.: *Surgical Pathology of Non-neoplastic Lung Disease, Vol 8, Major Problems in Pathology Series,* J.L. Bennington, Ed., W.B. Saunders, Philadelphia, 1982.

339. Kawanishi, H.: Morphologic association of lymphocytes with hepatocytes in chronic liver disease. *Arch Pathol Lab Med 101: 286–290, 1977.*

340. Kay, H.E.M., Powles, R.L., Sloane, J.P., and Farthing, M.G.: Cyclosporin A in human bone marrow grafts. *Haematol Bluttransfus 25: 255–260, 1981.*

341. Keane, T.J., Van Dyk, J., and Rider, W.D.: Idiopathic interstitial pneumonia following bone marrow transplantation: The relationship with total body irradiation. *Int J Rad Oncol Biol Phys 7: 1365–1370, 1981.*

342. Keane, W.F., Crosson, J.T., Staley, N.A., Anderson, W.R., and Shapiro, F.L.: Radiation-induced renal disease. A clinicopathologic study. *Am J Med 60: 127–137, 1976.*

343. Keating, M.J., Smith, T.L., McCredie, K.B., Bodey, G.P., Hersh, E.M., Gutterman, J.U., Gehan, E., and Freireich, E.J.: A 4-year experience with anthracycline, cytosine arabinoside, vincristine, and prednisone combination chemotherapy in 325 adults with acute leukemia. *Cancer 47: 2779–2788, 1981.*

344. Kennedy, B.J., Smith, L.R., and Goltz, R.W.: Skin changes secondary to hydroxyurea therapy. *Arch Dermatol 111: 183–187, 1975.*

345. Kerr, J.F.R., Wyllie, A.H., and Currie, A.R.: Apoptosis: A basic biological phenomenon with wide-ranging implications in tissue kinetics. *Br J Cancer 26: 239–257, 1972.*

346. Kersey, J.H., Meuwissen, H.J. and Good, R.A.: Graft-versus-host reactions following transplantation of

allogeneic hematopoietic cells. *Hum Pathol* 2: 389–402, 1971.

347. Klatskin, G., and Kantor, F.S.: Mitochondrial antibody in primary biliary cirrhosis and other diseases. *Ann Intern Med* 77: 533–541, 1972.

348. Klein, G., and Purtilo, D.: Summary—Symposium on Epstein-Barr virus-induced lymphoproliferative disease in immunodeficient patients. *Cancer Res* 41: 4302–4304, 1981.

349. Klintmalm, G.B.G., Iwatsuki, S., and Starzl, T.E.: Nephrotoxicity of Cyclosporin A in liver and kidney transplant patients. *Lancet* 1: 470–471, 1981.

350. Knowles, D.M., II, Hoffman, T., Ferrarini, M., and Kunkel, H.G.: The demonstration of acid alpha-naphtyl acetate esterase activity in human lymphocytes: usefulness as a T-cell marker. *Cell Immunol* 35: 112–123, 1978.

351. Kodsi, B.E., Wickremesinghe, P.C., Kozinn, P.J., Iswara, K., and Goldberg, P.K.: *Candida* esophagitis. A prospective study of 27 cases. *Gastroenterology* 71: 715–719, 1976.

352. Kolb, H., Sale, G.E., Lerner, K.G., Storb, R., and Thomas, E.D.: Pathology of acute graft-versus-host disease in the dog. An autopsy study of 95 dogs. *Am J Pathol* 96: 581–594, 1979.

353. Kolb, H., Freytag, G., Kiesel, U., and Kolb-Bachofen, V.: Cellular immune reactions against pancreatic islets as a consequence of graft-versus-host disease. *Clin Exp Immunol* 43: 121–127, 1981.

354. Kolbenstvedt, A., Kjolseth, I., Klepp, O., and Kolmannskog, F.: Post irradiation changes of the liver demonstrated by computer tomography. *Radiology* 135: 391, 1980.

355. Kondo, H., Rabin, B.S., and Rodnan, G.P.: Cutaneous antigen-stimulating lymphokine production by lymphocytes of patients with progressive systemic sclerosis (scleroderma). *J Clin Invest* 58: 1388–1394, 1976.

356. Koretz, R.L., Stone, O., and Gitnick, G.L.: The longterm course of non-A, non-B post-transfusion hepatitis. *Gastroenterology* 79: 893–898, 1980.

357. Korn, J.H., Halushka, P.V., and LeRoy, E.C.: Mononuclear cell modulation of connective tissue function. Suppression of fibroblast growth by stimulation of endogenous prostaglandid production. *J Clin Invest* 65: 543–554, 1980.

358. Korotzer, T.I., Page, R.C., Granger, G.A., and Rabinovitch, P.S.: Regulation of growth of human diploid fibroblasts by factors elaborated by activated lymphoid cells. *J Cell Physiol* 111: 247–254, 1982.

359. Korsmeyer, S.J., Elfenbein, G.J., Goldmann, C.K., Marshall, S.L., Santos, G.W., and Waldmann, T.A.: B-cell, helper T-cell, and suppressor T-cell abnormalities contribute to disordered immunoglobulin synthesis in patients following bone marrow transplantation. *Transplantation* 33: 184–190, 1982.

360. Koss, L.G., Melamed, M.R., and Mayer, K.: The effect of busulfan on human epithelia. *Am J Clin Pathol* 44: 385–397, 1965.

361. Koss, L.G.: A light and electron microscopic study of the effects of a single dose of cyclophosphamide on various organs in the rat. I. The urinary bladder. *Lab Invest* 16: 44–65, 1967.

362. Koss, L.G.: *Diagnostic Cytology and Its Histopathologic Bases*, (2nd ed.). J.P. Lippincott, Philadelphia, 1968, pp. 527–528.

363. Krause, W., Matheis, H., and Wulf, K.: Fungaemia and funguria after oral administration of *Candida albicans*. *Lancet* 1: 598–599, 1969.

364. Krieg, T., Luderschmidt, C., Weber, L., Muller, P.K., and Braun-Falco, O.: Scleroderma fibroblasts: Some aspects of *in vitro* assessment of collagen synthesis. *Arch Dermatol Res* 270: 263–272, 1981.

365. Krueger, G.R.F., Berard, C.W., DeLellis, R.A., Graw, R.G., Jr., Yankee, R.A., Leventhal, B.G., Rogentine, G.N., Herzig, G.P., Halterman, R.H., and Henderson, E.S.: Graft-versus-host disease. Morphologic variation and differential diagnosis in eight cases of HL-A matched bone marrow transplantation. *Am J Pathol* 63: 179–202, 1971.

366. Krueger, G.R.F., Graw, R.G., Jr., Rogentine, G.N., Darrow, C.C., II, Neefe, J.R., and Luetzeler, J.: Pathology of modified graft-versus-host disease in bone marrow allografted monkeys treated with anti-lymphocyte serum. *Blut* 30: 19–30, 1975.

367. Lafferty, K.J., Cooley, M.A., Woolnough, J., and Walker K.: Thyroid allograft immunogenicity is reduced after a period in organ culture. *Science* 188: 259–261, 1975.

368. Lampert, I.A., Suitters, A.J., Janossy, G., Thomas, J.A., Palmer, S., and Smith, E.G.: Lymphoid infiltrates in skin in graft-versus-host disease (Letter). *Lancet* 2: 1352, 1981.

369. Lamy, M., Fallat, R.J., Koeniger, E., Dietrich, H-P, Ratliff, J.L., Eberhart, R.C., Tucker, H.J., and Hill, D.: Pathologic features and mechanisms of hypoxemia in adult respiratory distress syndrome. *Am Rev Resp Dis* 114: 267–284, 1976.

370. Editorial: "Preventing graft-versus-host disease." *Lancet* 2: 1343–1344, 1980.

371. Lange, B., Henle, W., Meyers, J.D., Yang, L.C., August, C., Koch, P., Arbeter, A., and Henle, G.: Epstein-Barr virus-related serology in marrow transplant recipients. *Int J Cancer* 26: 151–157, 1980.

372. Lapp, W.S., Mendes, M., Kirchner, H., and Gemsa, D.: Prostaglandin synthesis by lymphoid tissue of mice experiencing a graft-versus-host reaction: Relationship to immunosuppression. *Cell Immunol* 50: 271–281, 1980.

373. Lautenschlager, I., and Hayry, P.: Expression of the major histocompatibility complex antigens on different liver cellular-components in rat and man. *Scand J Immunol* 14: 421–426, 1981.

374. Lawley, T.J., Peck, G.L., Moutsopoulos, H.M., Gratwohl, A.A., and Deisseroth, A.B.: Scleroderma, Sjögren-like syndrome, and chronic graft-versus-host disease. *Ann Inter Med* 87: 707–709, 1977.

375. Lawley, T.J., James, S.P., and Jones E.A.: Circulating immune complexes: Their detection and potential significance in some hepatobiliary and intestinal diseases. *Gastroenterology* 78: 626–641, 1980.

376. Lee, C.C., Castles, T.R., and Kintner, L.D.: Single-dose toxicity of cyclophosphamide (NSC-26271) in dogs and monkeys. *Cancer Chemother Rep (Part 3)* 4: 51–76, 1973.

377. Lefkowitz, J.H.: Bile ductular cholestasis: An ominous histopathologic sign related to sepsis and "cholangitis lenta." *Hum Pathol* 13: 19–24, 1982.

378. Leibovich, S.J., and Ross, R.: A macrophage-dependent factor that stimulates the proliferation of fibroblasts *in vitro*. *Am J Pathol* 84: 501–513, 1976.

379. Lerner, K.G., Kao, G.F., Storb, R., Buckner, C.D., Clift, R.A., and Thomas, E.D.: Histopathology of graft-vs.-host reaction (GvHR) in human recipients of marrow from HL-A matched sibling donors. *Transplant Proc* 6: 367–371, 1974.

380. Letendre, L., Kovach, J.S., Ludwig, J., Smithson, W.A., Hoagland, H.C., Gilchrist, G.S., and Burgert, E.O., Jr.: Hepatic veno-occlusive disease (VOD) in patients (PTS) with acute leukemia (AL) treated with indicine N-oxide (Abstract). In *Proceedings of 17th Annual Meeting, American Society Clinical Oncology*, Waverly Press, Baltimore, 1981, p. 488, #C-607.

381. Lewis, R.M., Armstrong, M.Y.K., André-Schwartz, J., Muftuoglu, A., Beldotti, L., and Schwartz, R.S.: Chronic allogeneic disease. I. Development of glomerulonephritis. *J Exp Med* 128: 653–679, 1968.

382. Liebow, A.A.: Definition and classification of interstitial pneumonias in human pathology. In *Progress in Respiration Research, Vol 8: Alveolar Interstitium of the Lung. Pathological and Physiological Aspects*, F. Basset and R. Georges, Eds., Karger, New York, 1975, pp. 1–33.

383. Liepins, A., Faanes, R.B., Lifter, J., Choi, Y.S., and deHarven, E.: Ultrastructural changes during T-lymphocyte-mediated cytolysis. *Cell Immunol* 28, 109–124, 1977.

384. Lightdale, C.J., Wasser, J., Coleman, M., Brower, M., Tefft, M., and Pasmantier, M.: Anticoagulation and high-dose liver radiation. A preliminary report. *Cancer* 43: 174–181, 1979.

385. Lin, C.S., Penha, P.D., Krishnan, M.N., and Zak, F.G.: Cytomegalic inclusion disease of the skin. *Arch Dermatol* 117: 282–284, 1981.

386. Lippmann, M.: Pulmonary reactions to drugs. *Med Clin North Am* 61: 1353–1367, 1977.

387. Livnat, S., and Cohen, I.R.: Recruitment of effector lymphocytes by initiator lymphocytes. Circulating lymphocytes are trapped in the reacting lymph node. *J Immunol* 117: 608–613, 1976.

388. Livnat, S., Seigneuret, M., Storb, R., and Prentice, R.L.: Analysis of cytotoxic effector cell function in patients with leukemia or aplastic anemia before and after marrow transplantation. *J Immunol* 124: 481–490, 1980.

389. Lopez, C., Kirkpatrick, D., Sorell, M., O'Reilly, R.J., Ching, C., and the Bone Marrow Transplant Unit: Association between pre-transplant natural kill and graft-versus-host disease after stem-cell transplantation. *Lancet* 2: 1103–1107, 1979.

389a. Lopez, C., Kirkpatrick, D., Livnat, S., and Storb, R.: Natural killer cells in bone marrow transplantation (Letter). *Lancet* 2: 1025, 1980.

390. Loutit, J.F., and Micklem, H.S.: "Secondary disease" among lethally irradiated mice restored with haematopoietic tissues from normal or iso-immunized foreign mice. *Br J Exp Pathol* 43: 77–87, 1962.

391. Loutit, J.F.: Immunological and trophic functions of lymphocytes. *Lancet* 2: 1106–1108, 1962.

392. Loveland, B.E., and McKenzie, I.F.C.: Which T-cells cause graft rejection? *Transplantation* 33: 217–221, 1982.

393. Lowenberg, B.: *Fetal Liver Cell Transplantation. Role and Nature of the Fetal Haematopoietic Stem Cell*. Organization for Health Research TNO, Radiobiological Institute, Rijswijk, The Netherlands, 1975.

394. Ludwig, J.: Drug effects on the liver: A tabular compilation of drugs and drug-related hepatic diseases. *Dig Dis Sci* 24: 785–796, 1979.

395. Lum, L.G., Seigneuret, M.C., Storb, R., Witherspoon, R.P., and Thomas, E.D.: T- and B-cell deficiencies in patient with chronic graft-versus-host disease after HLA-identical marrow transplantation. *Transplant Proc* 13: 1231–1232, 1981.

396. Lum, L.G., Seigneuret, M.C., Storb, R.F., Witherspoon, R.P., and Thomas E.D.: *In vitro* regulation of immunoglobulin synthesis after marrow transplantation. I. T-cell and B-cell deficiences in patients with and without chronic graft-versus-host disease. *Blood* 58: 431–439, 1981.

397. Lum, L.G., Seigneuret, M.C., Orcutt-Thordarson, N., Ostenson, R.C., and Storb, R.: Immunoglobulin production after marrow transplantation. III. The functional heterogeneity of FC-IgG receptor positive and negative T-cell subpopulations. *Clin Exp Immunol* 48: 675–684, 1982.

398. Lum, L.G., Orcutt-Thordarson, N., Seigneuret, M.C., and Storb, R.: The regulation of Ig synthesis after marrow transplantation. IV. T4 and T8 subset function in patients with chronic graft-versus-host disease. *J Immunol* 129: 113–119, 1982.

399. Lusch, C.J., Ramsey, H.E., Smith, B., and Sweet, W.: Hemorrhagic ulcerative colitis after cyclophosphamide therapy: Report of a case (Wadley Institute of Molecular Medicine Quarterly) *J Clin Hematol Oncol* 8: 32–37, 1978.

400. MacDonald, T.T., and Ferguson, A.: Hypersensitivity reactions in the small intestine: II. Effects of allograft rejection on mucosal architecture and lymphoid cell infiltrate. *Gut* 17: 81–91, 1976.

401. MacDonald, T.T., and Ferguson, A.: Hypersensitivity reactions in the small intestine: III. The effects of allograft rejection and of graft-versus-host disease on epithelial cell kinetics. *Cell Tissue Kinet* 10: 301–312, 1977.

402. MacFarlane, I.G., Wojcicka, B.M., Tsantoulous, D.M., Portmann, B.C., Eddleston, A.L., and Williams, R.: Leukocyte migration inhibition in response to biliary antigens in primary biliary cirrhosis, sclerosing cholangitis, and other chronic liver diseases. *Gastroenterology* 76: 1333–1340, 1979.

403. MacSween, R.N.M., and Sumithran, E.: Histopathology of primary biliary cirrhosis. *Semin Liver Dis 1*: 282–292, 1981.

404. Magnussen, C.R., Olson, J.P., Ona, F.V., and Graziani, A.J.: *Candida* fungus balls in common bile duct. Unusual manifestations of disseminated candidiasis. *Arch Intern Med* 139: 821–822, 1979.

405. Mahan, C.T., and Sale, G.E.: Rapid methenamine silver stain for *Pneumocystis* and fungi. *Arch Pathol Lab Med* 102: 351–352, 1978.

406. Malmström, P., Jönsson, A., and Sjögren, H.O.: ANAE staining pattern of rat lymphocytes: Lack of correlation with lymphocyte subclasses. *Scand J Immunol* 14: 523–527, 1981.

407. Mandel, I.D., and Baurmash, H.: Sialochemistry in Sjögren's syndrome. *Oral Surg* 41: 182–187, 1976.

408. Mannick, J.A., Lochte, H.L., Jr., Ashley, C.A., Thomas, E.D., and Ferrebee, J.W.: Autografts of bone marrow in dogs after lethal total-body radiation. *Blood* 15: 255–266, 1960.

409. Marcus, J.N., Hurtubise, P.E., and Quiroga, L.E.: The T-gall granule has acid esterase-activity and marks T-helper lymphocytes (Abstract). *Lab Invest 44: A41, 1981.*

410. Marmary, Y., Glaiss, R., and Pisanty, S.: Scleroderma: Oral manifestations. *Oral Surg 52: 32–37, 1981.*

411. Martin, D.H., Counts, G., and Thomas, E.D.: Fungal infections in human bone marrow transplant recipients. In *Program and Abstracts of the Seventeenth Interscience Conference on Antimicrobial Agents and Chemotherapy.* American Society for Microbiology, Washington, D.C., 1977, P. 406.

412. Marubbio, A.T., and Danielson, B.: Hepatic veno-occlusive disease in a renal transplant patient receiving azathioprine. *Gastroenterology 69: 739–743, 1975.*

413. Mathé, G., Bernard, J., deVries, M.J., Schwarzenberg, L., Larrieu, M.J., Lalanne, C.M., Dutreix, A., Amiel, J.L., and Surmont, J.: Nouveaux assais de graffe de moelle osseuse homologue après irradiation totale chez des enfants attents de laucémias aigu en rémission. Le syndrome secondaire chez l'homme. *Rev Hemat (Par) 15: 115–161, 1960.*

414. Mathé, G., and Amiel, J.L.: Aspects histologiques des lésions induites dans les organes hematopoietiques par l'injection à des hybridés F₁ irradiés de cellules ganglionaires d'une des lignes parentales. *Rev Franc Etudes Clin Biol 5: 20–30, 1960.*

415. McClelland, D.B.L.: Bacterial and viral infections of the gastrointestinal tract. In *Immunology of the Gastrointestinal Tract,* P. Asquith, Ed., Churchill Livingstone, Edinburgh, 1979, pp. 214–245.

416. McDonald, G.B., Sullivan, K.M., Schuffler, M.D., Shulman, H.M., and Thomas, E.D.: Esophageal abnormalities in chronic graft-versus-host disease in humans. *Gastroenterology 80: 914–921, 1981.*

417. McDonald, G.B., and Sullivan, K.M.: Endoscopic and radiologic features of esophageal graft-vs.-host disease (GVHD) (Abstract). *Gastrointest Endosc 27: 137, 1981.*

418. McDonald, G.B., Sharma, P., and Shulman, H.M.: Pre-marrow transplant hepatitis is a risk factor for hepatic VOD (Abstract). *Gastroenterology 80: 1227, 1981.*

419. McDonald, G.B., Sharma, P., Sale, G.E., Shulman, H.M., Hackman, R.C., and Meyers, J.D.: Infectious esophagitis in immunosuppressed patients after marrow transplantation (Abstract). *Gastroenterology 82: 1127, 1982.*

420. McDonald, G.B., Sharma, P., Shulman, H.M., and Thomas, E.D.: Venocclusive disease of the liver after marrow transplant. Clinical course of 53 patients (Abstract). *Gastroenterology 82: 1237, 1982.*

421. McElwain, T.J., Hedley, D.W., Burton, G., Clink, H.M., Gordon, M.Y., Jarman, M., Juttner, C.A., Miller, J.L., Milsted, R.A., Prentice, G., Smith, I.E., Spence, D., and Woods, M.: Marrow autotransplantation accelerates haemotological recovery in patients with malignant melanoma treated with high-dose melphalan. *Br J Cancer 40: 72–80, 1979.*

422. McGuire, T.C., and Poppie, M.J.: Hypogammaglobulinemia and thymic hypoplasia in horses: A primary combined immunodeficiency disorder. *Infect Immun 8: 272–277, 1973.*

423. McIntyre, R.E., Magidson, J.G., Austin, G.G., and Gale, R.P.: Fatal veno-occlusive disease of the liver following high-dose 1,3 *bis* (2-chloroethyl)-1-nitro-sourea (BCNU) and autologous bone marrow transplantation. *Am J Clin Pathol 75: 614–617, 1981.*

424. McLean, E.K.: The toxic actions of pyrrolizidine (senecio) alkaloids. *Pharmacol Rev 22: 429–483, 1970.*

425. McLean, E.K., and Mattocks, A.R.: Environmental liver injury. Plant toxins. In *Toxic Injury of the Liver, Part B, Liver: Normal Function and Disease, Vol. 2,* E. Farber and M.M. Fisher Eds., Marcel Dekker, New York, 1979, pp. 517–540.

426. Mehrotra, T.N.: Hemorrhagic colitis after cyclophosphamide (Letter). *Lancet 2: 345, 1966.*

427. Meisel, J.L., Perera, D.R., Meligro, C., and Rubin, CE.: Overwhelming watery diarrhea associated with a cryptosporidium in an immunosuppressed patient. *Gastroenterology 70: 1157–1160, 1976.*

428. Menard, D.B., Gisselbrecht, C., Marty, M., Reyes, F., and Dhumeaux, D.: Antineoplastic agents and the liver. *Gastroenterology 78: 142–164, 1980.*

429. Mennie, A.T., and Dalley, V.M.: Treatment of radiation-induced gastrointestinal distress with acetylsalicylate. *Lancet 2: 942–943, 1975.*

430. Merritt, C.B., Mann, D.L., and Rogentine, G.N., Jr.: Cytotoxic antibody for epithelial cells in human graft-versus-host disease. *Nature 232: 638–639, 1971.*

431. Merritt, C.B., Darrow, C.C., II, Vaal, L., and Rogentine, G.N., Jr.: Bone marrow transplantation in rhesus moneys following irradiation. Modification of acute graft-versus-host disease with antilymphocyte serum. *Transplantation 14: 9–20, 1972.*

432. Meuwissen, H.J., Rodey, G., McArthur, J., Pabst, H., Gatti, R., Chilgren, R., Hong, R., Frommel, D., Coifman, R., and Good, R.A.: Bone marrow transplantation. Therapeutic usefulness and complications. *Am J Med 51: 513–532, 1971.*

433. Meyer zum Büschenfelde, K.H., Manns, M., Hütteroth, T.H., Hopf, U., and Arnold, W.: LM-Ag and LSP—Two different target antigens involved in the immunopathogenesis of chronic active hepatitis? *Clin Exp Immunol 37: 205–212, 1979.*

434. Meyers, J.D., Pifer, L.L., Sale, G.E., and Thomas, E.D.: The value of *Pneumocystis carinii* antibody and antigen detection for diagnosis of *Pneumocystis carinii* pneumonia after marrow transplantation. *Am Rev Respir Dis 120: 1283–1287, 1979.*

435. Meyers, J.D., Flournoy, N., and Thomas, E.D.: Infection with herpes simplex virus and cell-mediated immunity after marrow transplant. *J Infect Dis 142: 338–346, 1980.*

436. Meyers, J.D., Flournoy, N., and Thomas, E.D.: Cytomegalovirus infection and specific cell-mediated immunity after marrow transplant. *J Infect Dis 142: 816–824, 1980.*

437. Meyers, J.D., Hackman, R.C., and Stamm, W.E.: *Chlamydia trachomatis* infection as a cause of pneumonia after human marrow transplantation. *Transplantation* (in press).

438. Meyers, J.D., Wade, J.C., Mitchell, C.D., Saral, R., Lietman, P.S., Durack, D.I., Levin, M.J., Segreti, A.C., and Balfour, H.H., Jr.: Multicenter collaborative trial of intravenous acyclovir for treatment of mucocutaneous herpes simplex virus infection in the immunocompromised host. *Am J Med 73: 229–235, 1982.*

439. Meyers, J.D., Flournoy, N., and Thomas, E.D.: Nonbacterial pneumonia after allogeneic marrow transplantation: A review of 10 years' experience. *Rev Infect Dis* 4: 1119–1132, 1982.

440. Meyers, J.D., and Thomas, E.D. Infection complicating bone marrow transplantation. In *Clinical Approach to Infection in the Compromised Host*, R.H. Rubin and L.S. Young, Eds., Plenum Publishers, New York, 1981, pp. 507–551.

441. Mickelson, E.M., Fefer, A., Storb, R., and Thomas, E.D.: Correlation of the relative response index with marrow graft rejection in patients with aplastic anemia. *Transplantation* 22: 294–300, 1976.

442. Mickelson, E.M., Clift, R.A., Fefer, A., Storb, R., Thomas, E.D., Warren, R.P., and Hansen, J.A.: Studies of the responses in mixed leukocyte culture of cells from patients with aplastic anemia to cells from HLA-identical siblings. *Transplantation* 32: 90–95, 1981.

443. Miller, F., Lane, B., Soterakis, J., and D'Angelo, W.A.: Primary biliary cirrhosis and scleroderma. The possibility of a common pathogenetic mechanism. *Arch Pathol Lab Med* 103: 505–509, 1979.

444. Miller, G.G., Witwer, M.W., Braude, A.I., and Davis, C.E.: Rapid identification of *Candida albicans* septicemia by gas–liquid chromatography. *J Clin Invest* 54: 1235–1240, 1974.

445. Mitchell, J.R., and Jollow, D.J.: Progress in hepatology. Metabolic activation of drugs to toxic substances. *Gastroenterology* 68: 392–410, 1975.

446. Moraes, J.R., and Stastny, P.: A new antigen system expressed in human endothelial cells. *J Clin Invest* 60: 449–454, 1977.

447. Morecki, R., Glaser, J.H., Cho, S., Balistreri, W.F., and Horwitz, M.S.: Biliary atresia and reovirus type 3 infection. *N Engl J Med* 307: 481–484, 1982.

448. Morgan, W.S., and Castleman, B.: A clinicopathologic study of "Mikulicz's disease." *Am J Pathol* 29: 471–503, 1953.

449. Mori, T., Tsoi, M-S., Gillis, S., Santos, E., Thomas, E.D., and Storb, R.: Cellular interaction in marrow-grafted patients. I. Impairment of cell-mediated lympholysis associated with graft-vs.-host disease and the effect of interleukin 2. *J Immunol* 130: 712–716, 1983.

450. Morris, P.J.: Overview. Cyclosporin A. *Transplantation* 32: 349–354, 1981.

451. Morton, J.I., Siegel, B.V., and Moore, R.D.: Transplantation of autoimmune potential. II. Glomerulonephritis in lethally irradiated DBA/2 recipients of NZB bone marrow cells. *Transplantation* 19: 464–469, 1975.

452. Motta, P., Muto, M., and Fujita, T.: In *The Liver: An Atlas of Scanning Electron Microscopy*, Igaku-Shoin, Tokyo, 1978, pp. 92–95.

453. Mowat, A.M., and Ferguson, A.: Hypersensitivity reactions in the small intestine. 6. Pathogenesis of the graft-versus-host reaction in the small intestinal mucosa of the mouse. *Transplantation* 32: 238–243, 1981.

454. Mueller, J., Brun del Re, G., Buerki, H., Keller, H.U., Hess, M.W., and Cottier, H.: Nonspecific acid esterase activity: A criterion for differentiation of T- and B-lymphocytes in mouse lymph nodes. *Eur J Immunol* 5: 270–274, 1975.

455. Müller-Ruchholtz, W., Wottge, H.U, and Müller-Hermelink, H.K.: Restitution potentials of allogeneically or xenogeneically grafted lymphocyte-free hemopoietic stem cells. In Thierfelder, Rodt and Kolb, *op cit*, pp. 153–177.

456. Murphy, J.B.: The effect of adult chicken grafts on the chick embryo. *J Exp Med* 24: 1–5, 1916.

457. Myerowitz, R.L., Pazin, G.J., and Allen, C.M.: Disseminated candidiasis. Changes in incidence, underlying disease, and pathology. *Am J Clin Pathol* 68: 29–38, 1977.

458. Nagington, J., Cossart, Y.E., and Cohen, B.J.: Reactivation of hepatitis B after transplantation operations. *Lancet* 1: 558–560, 1977.

459. Nagington, J., and Gray, J.: Cyclosporin A immunosuppression, Epstein-Barr antibody, and lymphoma (Letter). *Lancet* 1: 536–537, 1980.

459a. Naeim, F., Smith, G.S., Gale, R.P., and the UCLA Bone Marrow Transplant Team: Morphologic aspects of bone marrow transplantation in patients with aplastic anemia. *Hum Pathol* 9: 295–308, 1978.

460. Nakanuma, Y., and Ohta, G.: Histometric and serial section observations of the intrahepatic bile ducts in primary biliary cirrhosis. *Gastroenterology* 76: 1326–1332, 1979.

461. Nash, G., and Ross, J.S.: Herpetic esophagitis: A common cause of esophageal ulceration. *Hum Pathol* 5: 339–345, 1974.

462. Neely, J.E., Neely, A.N., and Kersey, J.H.: Immunodeficiency following human marrow transplantation: *in vitro* studies. *Transplant Proc* 10: 229–231, 1978.

463. Neilson, E.G., Jimenez, S.A., and Phillips, S.M.: Cell-mediated immunity in interstitial nephritis. III. T-lymphocyte-mediated fibroblast proliferation and collagen synthesis: An immune mechanism for renal fibrogenesis. *J Immunol* 125: 1708–1714, 1980.

464. Neiman, P., Thomas, E.D., Buckner, C.D., Storb, R., Fefer, A., Glucksberg, H., and Lerner, K.G.: Marrow transplantation for aplastic anemia and acute leukemia. *Annu Rev Med* 25: 179–198, 1974.

465. Neiman, P.E., Thomas, E.D., Reeves, W.C., Ray, C.G., Sale, G., Lerner, K.G., Buckner, C.D., Clift, R.A., Storb, R., Weiden, P.L., and Fefer, A.: Opportunistic infection and interstitial pneumonia following marrow transplantation for aplastic anemia and hematologic malignancy. *Transplant Proc* 8: 663–667, 1976.

466. Neiman, P.E., Reeves, W., Ray, C.G., Flournoy, N., Lerner, K.G., Sale, G.E., and Thomas, E.D.: A prospective analysis of interstitial pneumonia and opportunistic viral infection among recipients of allogeneic bone marrow grafts. *J Infect Dis* 136: 754–767, 1977.

467. Neiman, P.E., Meyers, J.D., Medeiros, E., McDougall, J.K., and Thomas, E.D.: Interstitial pneumonia following marrow transplantation for leukemia and aplastic anemia. In Gale and Fox, *op cit*, pp. 75–82.

468. Nesbit, M., Krivit, W., Heyn, R., and Sharp, H.: Acute and chronic effects of methotrexate on hepatic, pulmonary, and skeletal systems. *Cancer* 37: 1048–1054, 1976.

469. Newburger, P.E., Cassady, J.R., and Jaffe, N.: Esophagitis due to adriamycin and radiation therapy for childhood malignancy. *Cancer* 42: 417–423, 1978.

470. Nime, F.A., Burek, J.D., Page, D.L., Holscher, M.A., and Yardley, J.H.: Acute enterocolitis in a human being infected with the protozoan Cryptosporidium. *Gastroenterology* 70: 592–598, 1976.

471. Nisbet, N.W., and Simonsen, M.: Primary immune response in grafted cells. Dissociation between the proliferation of activity and proliferation of cells. *J Exp Med* 125: 967–981, 1967.

472. Noel, D.R., Witherspoon, R.P., Storb, R., Atkinson, K., Doney, K., Mickelson, E.M., Ochs, H.D., Warren, R.P., Weiden, P.L., and Thomas, E.D.: Does graft-versus-host disease influence the tempo of immunologic recovery after allogeneic human marrow transplantation? An observation on 56 long-term survivors. *Blood* 51: 1087–1105, 1978.

473. Northway, M.G., Libshitz, H.I., Osborne, B.M., Feldman, M.S., Mamel, J.J., West, J.H., and Szwarc, I.A.: Radiation esophagitis in the opossum: Radioprotection with indomethacin. *Gastroenterology* 78: 883–892, 1980.

474. Novack, R., Wilimas, J., and Johnson, W.: Hypertrophy and hyperplasia of islets of Langerhans associated with androgen therapy. *Arch Pathol Lab Med* 103: 483–485, 1979.

475. Nyfors, A.: Liver biopsies from psoriatics related to methotrexate therapy. 3. Findings in post-methotrexate liver biopsies from 160 psoriatics. *Acta Pathol Microbiol Scand* 85: 511–518, 1977.

476. O'Brien, K.D., Hackman, R.C., Sale, G.E., Prentice, R., Deeg, J., Thomas, E.D., and Storb, R.: Lymphocytic bronchitis in canine marrow graft recipients. *Transplantation, March 1984.*

477. Ochs, H.D., Storb, R., Thomas, E.D., Kolb, H.J., Graham, T.C., Mickelson, E.M., Parr, M., and Rudolph, R.H.: Immunologic reactivity in canine marrow graft recipients. *J Immunol* 113: 1039–1057, 1974.

478. O'Connor, R.E., Ramsay, N.K.C., McGlave, P., Snover, D.C., Kersey, J.H., and Burke, B.A.: Pulmonary pathology in bone marrow transplant recipients (Abstract). *Lab Invest* 46: 3P, 1982.

479. Okada, M., Klimpel, G.R., Kuppers, R.C., and Henney, C.S.: The differentiation of cytotoxic T-cells *in vitro.* I. Amplifying factor(s) in the primary response is Lyt 1+ cell dependent. *J Immunol* 122: 2527–2533, 1979.

480. Opelz, G., Gale, R.P., and the UCLA Bone Marrow Transplant Team: Absence of specific mixed leukocyte culture reactivity during graft-versus-host disease and following bone marrow transplant rejection. *Transplantation* 22: 474–477, 1976.

481. Opelz, G., Walker, J., and Gale, R.P.: Detection of non-HLA antibodies in bone marrow transplant recipients. *Transplant Proc* 10: 963–964, 1978.

482. Opelz, G., Mickey, M.R., and Terasaki, P.I.: Blood transfusions and kidney transplants: Remaining controversies. *Transplant Proc* 13: 136–141, 1981.

483. O'Reilly, R.J., Lee, F.K., Grossbard, E., Kapoor, N., Kirkpatrick, D., Dinsmore, D., Stutzer, C., Shah, K.V., and Nahmias, A.J.: Papovirus excretion following marrow transplantation: Incidence and association with hepatic dysfunction. *Transplant Proc* 13: 262–266, 1981.

484. Otto, H.F.: The interepithelial lymphocytes of the intestinum. Morphological observations and immunological aspects of intestinal enteropathy. In *Current Topics in Pathology,* Vol. 57, K.W. Altmann et al., Eds. Springer-Verlag, Berlin, 1973, pp. 81–121.

485. Pahwa, S.G., Pahwa, R.N., Friedrich, W., O'Reilly, R.J., and Good, R.A.: Abnormal humoral immune responses in peripheral blood lymphocyte cultures of bone marrow transplant recipients. *Proc Natl Acad Sci USA* 79: 2663–2667, 1982.

486. Palacios, R., Möller, G.: Cyclosporin A blocks receptors for HLA-DR antigens on T-cells. *Nature* 290: 792–794, 1981.

487. Palmer, R.H., and Reilly, R.W.: Bile salt depletion in the runting syndrome. *Transplantation* 12: 479–483, 1971.

488. Pang, K.S., and Terrell, J.A.: Retrograde perfusion to prove the heterogeneous distribution of hepatic drug metabolizing enzymes in rats. *J Pharmacol Exp Ther* 216: 339–346, 1981.

489. Paradinas, F.J., Bull, T.B., Westaby, D., and Murray-Lyon, I.M.: Hyperplasia and prolapse of hepatocytes into hepatic veins during long-term methyltestosterone therapy: Possible relationships of these changes to the development of peliosis hepatis and liver tumours. *Histopathology* 1: 225–246, 1977.

490. Parkman, R., Rappeport, J., Geha, R., Belli, J., Cassaday, R., Levey, R., Nathan, D.G., and Rosen, F.S.: Complete correction of the Wiskott-Aldrich syndrome by allogeneic bone marrow transplantation. *N Engl J Med* 298: 921–927, 1978.

491. Parkman, R., Rappeport, J., and Rosen, F.: Human graft versus host disease. *J Invest Dermatol* 74: 276–279, 1980.

492. Paronetto, F., and Popper, H.: Hetero-iso- and autoimmune phenomena in the liver. In *Textbook of Immunopathology,* Vol. 2, 2nd ed., P.A. Miescher and H.J. Muller-Eberhard, Eds., Grune & Stratton, New York, 1976, pp. 789—817.

493. Paul, L.C., Claas, F.H.J., van Es, L.A, Kalff, M.W., and de Graeff, J.: Accelerated rejection of a renal allograft associated with pretransplantation antibodies directed against donor antigens on endothelium and monocytes. *N Engl J Med* 300: 1258–1260, 1979.

494. Perrault, J.: Paucity of interlobular bile ducts: Getting to know it better (Editorial). *Dig Dis Sci* 26: 481–484, 1981.

495. Perry, M.C.: Hepatotoxicity of chemotherapeutic agents. *Semin Oncol* 9: 65–74, 1982.

496. Perryman, L.E., Buening, G.M., McGuire, T.C., Torbeck, R.L., Poppie, M.J., and Sale, G.E.: Fetal tissue transplantation for immunotherapy of combined immunodeficiency in horses. *Clin Immunol Immunopathol* 12: 238–251, 1979.

497. Perryman, L.E., and Liu, I.K.: Graft versus host reactions in foals with combined immunodeficiency. *Am J Vet Res* 41: 187–192, 1980.

498. Peters, M., Weiner, J., and Whelan, G.P.: Fungal infection associated with gastroduodenal ulceration: Endoscopic and pathologic appearances. *Gastroenterology* 78: 350–354, 1980.

499. Peterson, P.K., Balfour, H.H., Marker, S.C., Fryd, D.S., Howard, R.J., and Simmons, R.L.: Cytomegalovirus disease in renal allograft recipients: A prospective study of the clinical features, risk factors, and impact on renal transplantation. *Medicine* 59: 283–300, 1980.

500. Phillips, M.J., and Poucell, S.: Modern aspects of the morphology of viral hepatitis. *Hum Pathol* 12: 1060–1084, 1981.

501. Phillips, R.K.S., Glazer, G., and Borriello, S.P.: Non-*Clostridium difficile* pseudomembranous colitis

responding to both vancomycin and metronidazole. *Br Med J* 283: 823, 1981.

502. Phillips, T.L., Wharam, M.D., and Margolis, L.W.: Modification of radiation injury to normal tissues by chemotherapeutic agents. *Cancer* 35: 1678–1684, 1975.

503. Pino, Y., Torres, J.L., Bross, D.S., Lam, W.C., Wharam, M.D., Santos, G.W., and Order, S.E.: Risk factors in interstitial pneumonitis following allogeneic bone marrow transplantation. *Int J Radiat Oncol Biol Phys* 8: 1301–1307, 1982.

504. Pitt, H.A., King, W., III, Mann, L.L., Roslyn, J.J., Berquist, W.E., Ament, M.E., and Den-Besten, L.: Increased risk of cholithiases with prolonged total parenteral nutrition. *Am J Surg* 145: 106–112, 1983.

505. Platt, J.L., LeBien, T.W., and Michael, A.F.: Interstitial mononuclear cell populations in renal graft rejection. Identification by monoclonal antibodies in tissue sections. *J Exp Med* 155: 17–30, 1982.

506. Podurgiel, B.J., McGill, D.B., Ludwig, J., Taylor, W.F., and Muller, S.A.: Liver injury associated with methotrexate therapy for psoriasis. *Mayo Clin Proc* 48: 787–792, 1973.

507. Porter, K.A.: Graft-versus-host reactions in the rabbit. *Br J Cancer* 14: 66–76, 1960.

508. Porter, K.A.: Immune haemolysis in rabbit radiation-chimeras. *Br J Exp Pathol* 41: 72–80, 1960.

509. Poulsen, H., and Christoffersen, P.: Abnormal bile duct epithelium in chronic aggressive hepatitis and cirrhosis. *Hum Pathol* 3: 217–225, 1972.

510. Powell, R.D., Larson, A.L., and Henkin, R.I.: Nasal mucous membrane biopsy in Sjögren's syndrome. *Ann Intern Med* 81: 25–31, 1974.

511. Powles, R.L., Barrett, A., Clink, H.M., Kay, H.E.M., Sloane, J., and McElwain, T.J.: Cyclosporin A for the treatment of graft-versus-host disease in man. *Lancet* 2: 1327–1331, 1978.

512. Powles, R.L., Morgenstern, G., Clink, H.M., Hedley, D., Bandini, G., Lumley, H., Watson, J.G., Lawson, D., Spence, D., Barrett, A., Jameson, B., Lawler, S., Kay, H.E.M., and McElwain, T.J.: The place of bone-marrow transplantation in acute myelogenous leukemia. *Lancet* 1: 1047–1050, 1980.

513. Powles, R.L., Clink, H.M., Spence, D., Morgenstern, G., Watson, J.G., Selby, P.J., Woods, M., Barrett, A., Jameson, B., Sloane, J., Lawler, S.D., Kay, H.E.M., Lawson, D., McElwain, T.J., and Alexander, P.: Cyclosporin A to prevent graft-versus-host disease in man after allogeneic bone-marrow transplantation. *Lancet* 1: 327–329, 1980.

514. Price, R.A., and Johnson, W.W.: The central nervous system in childhood leukemia. I. The arachnoid. *Cancer* 31: 520–533, 1975.

515. Quinnan, G.V., Jr., Kirmani, N., Esber, E., Saral, R., Manischewitz, J.F., Robers, J.L., Rook, A.H., Santos, G.W., and Burns, W.H.: HLA-restricted cytotoxic T-lymphocyte and nonthymic cytotoxic lymphocyte responses to cytomegalovirus infection of bone marrow transplant recipients. *J Immunol* 126: 2036–2041, 1981.

516. Ragaz, A., and Ackerman, A.B.: Evolution, maturation, and regression of lesions of lichen planus. New observations and correlations of clinical and histologic findings. *Am J Dermatopathol* 3: 5–25, 1981.

517. Rai, K.R., Holland, J.F., Glidewell, O.J., Weinberg, V., Brunner, K., Obrecht, J.P., Preisler, H.D.,

Nawabi, I.W., Prager, D., and Carey, R.W.: Treatment of acute myelocytic leukemia: A study of Cancer and Leukemia Group B. *Blood* 58: 1203–1212, 1981.

518. Ramsey, P.G., Fife, K.H., Hackman, R.C., Meyers, J.D., and Corey, L.: Herpes simplex virus pneumonia. Clinical, virologic, and pathologic features in 20 patients. *Ann Intern Med* 97: 813–820, 1982.

519. Rappaport, H., Khalil, A., Halle-Pannenko, O., Pritchard, L., Dantchev, D., and Mathé, G.: Histopathologic sequence of events in adult mice undergoing lethal graft-versus-host reaction developed across H-2 and/or non-H-2 histocompatibility barriers. *Am J Pathol* 96: 121–142, 1979.

520. Rappeport, J., Mihm, M., Reinherz, E., Lopansri, S., and Parkman, R.: Acute graft-versus-host disease in recipients of bone-marrow transplants from identical twin donors. *Lancet* 2: 717–720, 1979.

521. Reece, E.R., Gartner, J.G., Seemayer, T.A., Joncas, J.H., and Pagano, J.S.: Epstein-Barr virus in a malignant lymphoproliferative disorder of B-cells occurring after thymic epithelial transplantation for combined immunodeficiency. *Cancer Res* 41: 4243–4247, 1981.

522. Reed, R.J., Clark, W.H., and Mihm., M.C.: The cutaneous collagenoses. *Hum Pathol* 4: 165–186, 1973.

523. Reed, R.J., and Ackerman, A.B.: Pathology of the adventitial dermis: Anatomic observations and biologic speculations. *Hum Pathol* 4: 207–217, 1973.

524. Reinherz, E.L., Parkman, R., Rappeport, J., Rosen, F.S., and Schlossman, S.: Aberrations of suppressor T-cells in human graft-versus-host disease. *N Engl J Med* 300: 1061–1068, 1979.

525. Reinherz, E.L., and Schlossman, S.F.: Current concepts in immunology. Regulation of the immune response—Inducer and suppressor T-lymphocyte subsets in human beings. *N Engl J Med* 303: 370–373, 1980.

526. Reller, L.B.: Granulomatous hepatitis associated with acute cytomegalovirus infection. *Lancet* 1: 20–22, 1973.

526a. Richardson, W.P., Colvin, R.B., Cheeseman, S.H., Tolkoff-Rubin, N.E., Herrin, J.T., Cosimi, A.B., Collins, A.B., Hirsch, M.S., McCluskey, R.T., Russell, P.S., and Rubin, R.H.: Glomerulopathy associated with cytomegalovirus viremia in renal allografts. *N Engl J Med* 305: 57–63, 1981.

527. Richens, E.R., Thorp, C.M., Bland, P.W., and Hall, N.D.: Circulating immune complexes in Crohn's disease. Their characterization and interrelationship with components of the complement system. *Dig Dis Sci* 27: 129–138, 1982.

528. Riede, U.N., Mittermayer, C.H., Friedburg, H., Wybitul, K., and Sandritter, W.: Morphologic development of human shock lung. *Pathol Res Pract* 165: 269–286, 1979.

529. Rinaldo, J.E., and Rogers, R.M.: Adult respiratory-distress syndrome. Changing concepts of lung injury and repair. *N Engl J Med* 306: 900–909, 1982.

530. Ringden, O., Witherspoon, R.P., Storb, R., and Thomas, E.D.: The use of hemolysis-in-gel assays to study polyclonal antibody secretion in bone marrow transplant recipients. *Blut* 42: 221–226, 1981.

331. Rizzetto, M.: Biology and characterization of the delta agent. In *Viral Hepatitis: 1981 International Symposium*, W. Szmuness, H.J. Alter, and J.E. Maynard, Eds., Franklin Institute, Philadelphia, 1982, pp. 355–360.

532. Roca, J., Graňeña, A., Rodriguez-Roisin, R., Alvarez, P., Agusti-Vidal, A., and Rozman, C.: Fatal airway disease in an adult with chronic graft-versus-host disease. *Thorax 37: 77–78, 1982.*

533. Rodnan, G.P., Myerowitz, R.L., and Justh, G.O.: Morphologic changes in the digital arteries of patients with progressive systemic sclerosis (scleroderma) and Raynaud pnenomenon. *Medicine 59: 393–408, 1980.*

534. Rogers, L.F., and Goldstein, H.M.: Roentgen manifestations of radiation injury to the gastrointestinal tract. *Gastrointest Radiol 2: 281–291, 1977.*

535. Rosen, P.R., and Hajdu, S.I.: Visceral herpesvirus infections in patients with cancer. *Am J Clin Pathol 56: 459–465, 1971.*

536. Rosen, P., Armstrong, D., and Rice, N.: Gastrointestinal cytomegalovirus infection. *Arch Intern Med 132: 274–276, 1973.*

537. Rosenberg, H.K., Serota, F.T., Koch, P., Borden, S., IV, and August, C.S.: Radiographic features of gastrointestinal graft-vs.-host disease. *Radiology 138: 371–374, 1981.*

538. Rosenberg, J.L., Wall, A.J., Scanu, A.M., and Reilly, R.W.: Fat malabsorption in the immunologically runted mouse (Abstract). *Gastroenterology 64: A109, 1973.*

539. Roswit, B., and White, D.C.: Severe radiation injuries of the lung. *AJR 129: 127–136, 1977.*

540. Rouse, R.V., van Ewijk, W., Jones, P.P., and Weissman, I.L.: Expression of MHC antigens by mouse thymic dendritic cells. *J Immunol 122: 2508–2515, 1979.*

541. Rubinstein, L.J., Herman, M.M., Long, T.F., and Wilbur, J.R.: Disseminated necrotizing leukoencephalopathy: A complication of treated central nervous system leukemia and lymphoma. *Cancer 35: 291–305, 1975.*

542. Rudolph, R., Stein, R.S., and Pattillo, R.A.: Skin ulcers due to adriamycin. *Cancer 38: 1087–1094, 1976.*

543. Rudolph, R.H., Hered, B., Epstein, R.B., and Thomas, E.D.: Canine mixed leukocyte reactivity and transplantation antigens. *Transplantation 8: 141–146, 1969.*

544. Sale, G.E., and Lerner, K.G.: Multiple tumors after androgen therapy. *Arch Pathol Lab Med 101: 600–603, 1977.*

545. Sale, G.E., Lerner, K.G., Barker, E.A., Shulman, H.M., and Thomas, E.D.: The skin biopsy in the diagnosis of acute graft-versus-host disease in man. *Am J Pathol 89: 621–635, 1977.*

546. Sale, G.E., Storb, R., and Kolb, H.: Histopathology of hepatic acute graft-versus-host disease in the dog. A double-blind study confirms the specificity of small bile duct lesions. *Transplantation 26: 103–106, 1978.*

547. Sale, G.E., Shulman, H.M., McDonald, G.B., and Thomas, E.D.: Gastrointestinal graft-versus-host disease in man. A clinicopathologic study of the rectal biopsy. *Am J Surg Pathol 3: 291–299, 1979.*

548. Sale, G.E., Shulman, H.M., Schubert, M.M., Sullivan, K.M., Kopecky, K.J., Hackman, R.C., Morton, T.H., Storb, R., and Thomas, E.D.: Oral and ophthalmic pathology of graft-versus-host disease in man: Predictive value of the lip biopsy. *Hum Pathol 12: 1022–1030, 1981.*

549. Sale, G.E., and Marmont, P.: Marrow mast cell counts do not predict bone marrow graft rejection. *Hum Pathol 12: 605–608, 1981.*

550. Sale, G.E.: Histochemical demonstration of T lymphocytes in the lesions of human graft-versus-host disease (Abstract). *Am J Clin Pathol 77: 247–248, 1982.*

551. Sale, G.E., Shulman, H.M., Hackman, R.C., and Meyers, J.D.: Frozen-section diagnosis of cytomegalovirus infections: Sensitivity in lung biopsy after marrow transplant. A model for possible use in other tissue sites. *Diagn Gynecol Obstet 4: 389–396, 1982.*

552. Sandberg, J.S., Owens, A.H., and Santos, G.W.: Clinical and pathologic characteristics of graft-versus-host disease produced in cyclophosphamide-treated adult mice. *J Natl Cancer Inst 46: 151–160, 1971.*

553. Sanders, J., Sale, G.E., Ramberg, R., Clift, R., Buckner, C.D., and Thomas, E.D.: Glioblastoma multiforme in a patient with acute lymphoblastic leukemia who received a marrow transplant. *Transplant Proc 14: 770–774, 1982.*

554. Sanderson, C.J., and Glauert, A.M.: The mechanism of T-cell-mediated cytotoxicity. V. Morphological studies by electron microscopy. *Proc R Soc Lond (Biol) 198: 315–323, 1977.*

555. Sanderson, C.J., and Glauert, A.M.: The mechanism of T-cell-mediated cytotoxicity. VI. T-cell projections and their role in target cell killing. *Immunol 36: 119–129, 1979.*

556. Saulsbury, F.T., Winkelstein, J.A., and Yolken, R.H.: Chronic rotavirus infection in immunodeficiency. *J Pediatr 97: 61–65, 1980.*

557. Saurat, J.H., Didierjean, L., Gluckman, E., and Bussel, A.: Graft-versus-host reaction and lichen planus-like eruption in man. *Br J Dermatol 92: 591–592, 1975.*

558. Saurat, J.H., Gluckman, E., Didierjean, L., Sockeel, F., Bonnetblanc, J.M., and Puissant, A.: Anticorps anticytoplasme des cellules de l'épiderme humain. *Ann Dermatol Venereol 104: 121–126, 1977.*

559. Saurat, J.H., Didierjean, L., Beucher, F., and Gluckman, E.: Immunofluoroescent tracing of cytoplasmic components involved in keratinocyte differentiation. *Br J Dermatol 98: 155–163, 1978.*

560. Saurat, J.H., Gluckman, E., Bonnetblanc, J-M., Didierjean, L., Bussel, A., and Puissant, A.: Caractères cliniques et biologiques des éruptions lichéniennes après graffe de moelle osseuse. *Ann Dermatol Syphiligr (Paris) 102: 521–525, 1975.*

561. Saurat, J.H.: Cutaneous manifestations of graft-versus-host disease. *Int J Dermatol 20: 249–256, 1981.*

562. Saxon, A., McIntyre, R.E., Stevens, R.H., and Gale, R.P.: Lymphocyte dysfunction in chronic graft-versus-host disease. *Blood 58: 746–751, 1981.*

563. Schatz, M., Patterson, R., and Fink, J.: Immunologic lung disease. *N Engl J Med 300: 1310–1320, 1979.*

563a. Schilsky, R.L.: Renal and metabolic toxicities of cancer chemotherapy. *Semin Oncol 9: 75–83, 1982.*

564. Schimmelpenninck, M., and Zwaan, F.: Radiographic features of small intestinal injury in human graft-versus-host disease. *Gastrointest Radiol 7: 29–33, 1982.*

565. Schimpff, S.C.: Infection prevention during profound granulocytopenia. New approaches to alimentary canal microbial suppression. *Ann Intern Med 93: 358–361, 1980.*

566. Schimpff, S.C.: Surveillance cultures. *J Infect Dis 144: 81–84, 1981.*

567. Schlesinger, M., and Essner, E.: Histochemical and electron microscopic studies of the liver in runt disease.

*Am J Pathol 47: 371–401, 1965.*

568. Schlossberg, D., Devig, P.M., Travers, H., Kovalcik, P.J., and Mullen, J.T.: Bowel perforation with candidiasis. *JAMA 238: 2520–2521, 1977.*

569. Schubach, W.H., Hackman, R., Neiman, P.E., Miller, G., and Thomas, E.D.: A monoclonal immunoblastic sarcoma in donor cells bearing Epstein-Barr virus genomes following allogeneic marrow grafting for acute lymphoblastic leukemia. *Blood 60: 180–187, 1982.*

570. Scowden, E.B., Schaffner, W., and Stone, W.J.: Overwhelming strongyloidiasis: An unappreciated opportunistic infection. *Medicine 57: 527–544, 1978.*

571. Searle, J., Kerr, J.F.R., Battersby, C., Egerton, W.S., Balderson, G., and Burnett, W.: An electron microscopic study of the mode of donor cell death in unmodified rejection of pig liver allografts. *Aust J Exp Biol Med Sci 55: 401–406, 1977.*

572. Seddik, M.H., Seemayer, T.A., and Lapp, W.S.: T-cell functional defect associated with thymic epithelial cell injury induced by a graft-versus-host reaction. *Transplantation 29: 61–66, 1980.*

573. Seemayer, T.A., Lapp, W.S., and Bolande, R.P.: Thymic involution in murine graft-versus-host reaction. Epithelial injury mimicking human thymic dysplasia. *Am J Pathol 88: 119–133, 1977.*

574. Seemayer, T.A., Lapp, W.S., and Bolande, R.P.: Thymic epithelial injury in graft-versus-host reactions following adrenalectomy. *Am J Pathol 93: 325–338, 1978.*

575. Seemayer, T.A.: The GVHR: a pathogenetic mechanism of experimental and human disease. In *Perspectives in Pediatric Pathology*, Vol. 5, H.S. Rosenberg and R.P. Bolande, Eds., Masson Publishing, USA, New York, 1979, pp. 93–136.

576. Seemayer, T.A., Gartner, J.G., Colle, E., and Lapp, W.S.: Acute graft-versus-host disease in the pancreas. *Transplantation 36: 72–77, 1983.*

577. Serota, F.T., Rosenberg, H.K., Rosen, J., Koch, P.A., and August, C.S.: Delayed onset of gastrointestinal disease in the recipients of bone marrow transplants. A variant graft-versus-host reaction. *Transplantation 34: 60–64, 1982.*

578. Sharma, P., McDonald, G.B., and Banaji, M.: The risk of bleeding after percutaneous liver biopsy: Relation to platelet count. *J Clin Gastroenterol 4: 451–453, 1982.*

579. Shearer, G.M., and Schmitt-Verhulst, A.M.: Major histocompatibility complex restricted cell-mediated immunity. *Adv Immunol 25: 55–91, 1977.*

580. Shimkin, P.M., DeLellis, R.A., Carolla, R.L., and Weinstein, M.A.: Graft-versus-host disease. Radiographic findings in a patient with severe intestinal involvement. *Radiology 102: 623–624, 1972.*

581. Shouval, D., Eliakim, M., and Levij, I.S.: Chronic active hepatitis with cholestatic features. II. A histopathological study. *Am J Gastroenterol 72: 551–555, 1979.*

582. Shulman, H.M., Sale, G.E., Lerner, K.G., Barker, E.A., Weiden, P.L., Sullivan, K., Gallucci, B., Thomas, E.D., and Storb, R.: Chronic cutaneous graft-versus-host disease in man. *Am J Pathol 91: 545–570, 1978.*

583. Shulman, H.M., McDonald, G.B., Matthews, D., Doney, K.C., Kopecky, K.J., Gauvreau, J.M., and Thomas, E.D.: An analysis of hepatic venocclusive disease and centrilobular hepatocyte degeneration following bone marrow transplantation. *Gastroenterology 79: 1178–1191, 1980.*

584. Shulman, H.M., Sullivan, K.M., Weiden, P.L., McDonald, G.B., Striker, G.E., Sale, G.E., Hackman, R.C., Tsoi, M.S., Storb, R., and Thomas, E.D.: Chronic graft-versus-host syndrome in man. A long-term clinicopathologic study of 20 Seattle patients. *Am J Med 69: 204–217, 1980.*

585. Shulman, H., Striker, G., Deeg, H.J., Kennedy, M., Storb, R., and Thomas, E.D.: Nephrotoxicity of cyclosporin A after allogeneic marrow transplantation. *N Engl J Med 305: 1391–1394, 1981.*

585a. Shulman, H.M., Hackman, R.C., Sale, G.E., and Meyers, J.D.: Rapid cytologic diagnosis of cytomegalovirus interstitial pneumonia on touch imprints from open-lung biopsy. *Am J Clin Pathol 77: 90–94, 1982.*

586. Shusterman, N.H., Frauenhoffer, C., and Kinsey, M.D.: Fatal massive hepatic necrosis in cytomegalovirus mononucleosis. *Ann Intern Med 88: 810–812, 1978.*

587. Simonsen, M.: Graft-versus-host reactions. Their natural history and applicability as tools of research. *Prog Allergy 6: 349–467, 1962.*

588. Singer, C., Armstrong, D., Rosen, P.P., Walzer, P.D., and Yu, B.: Diffuse pulmonary infiltrates in immunosuppressed patients. Prospective study of 80 cases. *Am J Med 66: 110–120, 1979.*

589. Singer, J.B., Spiro, H.M., and Thayer, W.R.: Colonic manifestations of runt disease. *Yale J Biol Med 39: 106–112, 1966.*

590. Singer, R.M., and Gelfant, S.: Continuous inhibition of DNA synthesis in mouse ear epidermis using hydroxyurea. *Exp Cell Res 73: 270–271, 1972.*

591. Slavin, R.E., and Santos, G.W.: The graft-versus-host reaction in man after bone marrow transplantation: Pathology, pathogenesis, clinical features, and implication. *Clin Immunol Immunopathol 1: 472–498, 1973.*

592. Slavin, R.E., and Woodruff, J.M.: The pathology of bone marrow transplantation. *Pathol Annu 9: 291–344, 1974.*

593. Slavin, R.E., Millan, J.C., and Mullins, G.M.: Pathology of high-dose intermittent cyclophosphamide therapy. *Hum Pathol 6: 693–709, 1975.*

594. Slavin, R.E., Dias, M.A., and Saral, R.: Cytosine arabinoside-induced gastrointestinal toxic alterations in sequential chemotherapeutic protocols: A clinico-pathologic study of 33 patients. *Cancer 42: 1747–1759, 1978.*

595. Slavin, S., and Strober, S.: Mechanisms of transplantation tolerance to allogeneic bone marrow cells following total lymphoid irradiation (TLI). In Thierfelder, Rodt, and Kolb, *op cit*, pp. 323–332.

596. Sloane, J.P., Farthing, M.J., and Powles, R.L.: Histopathological changes in the liver after allogeneic bone marrow transplantation. *J Clin Pathol 33: 344–350, 1980.*

597. Sloane, J.P., and Powles, R.L.: Graft-versus-host disease in recipients of syngeneic bone marrow (Letter). *Lancet 1: 253, 1980.*

598. Smedile, A., Dentico, P., Zanetti, A., Sagnexlli, E., Nordenfelt, E., Actis, G.C., and Rizzetto, M.: Infection with the delta agent in chronic HB$_s$Ag carriers. *Gastroenterology 81: 992–997, 1981.*

599. Smith, C., and Gelfant, S.: Effects of methotrexate and hydroxyurea on psoriatic epidermis. Preferential

cytotoxic effects on psoriatic epidermis. *Arch Dermatol* 110: 70–72, 1974.

600. Smith, K.C., and Hanawalt, P.C.: Recovery from photochemical damage. In *Molecular Photobiology. Inactivation and Recovery.* Academic Press, New York, 1969, pp. 131–164.

601. Snell, G.D., Dausset, J., and Nathenson, S.: *Histocompatibility.* Academic Press, New York, 1976.

602. Soligner, A.M., Bhatnagar, R., and Stobo, J.D.: Cellular, molecular, and genetic characteristics of T-cell reactivity to collagen in man. *Proc Natl Acad Sci USA* 78: 3877–3881, 1981.

603. Soligner, A.M., and Stobo, J.D.: Immune response gene control of collagen reactivity in man: Collagen unresponsiveness in HLA-DR4 negative nonresponders is due to the presence of T-dependent suppressive influences. *J Immunol* 129: 1916–1920, 1982.

604. Sopko, J., and Anuras, S.: Liver disease in renal transplant recipients. *Am J Med* 64: 139–146, 1978.

605. Sosa, R., Weiden, P.L., Storb, R., Syrotuck, J., and Thomas, E.D.: Granulocyte function in human allogeneic marrow graft recipients. *Exp Hematol* 8: 1183–1189, 1980.

606. Sparberg, M., Simon, N., and Del Greco, F.: Intrahepatic cholestasis due to azathioprine. *Gastroenterology* 57: 439–441, 1969.

607. Spector, J.I., Zimbler, H., and Ross, J.S.: Early-onset cyclophosphamide-induced interstitial pneumonitis. *JAMA* 242: 2852–2854, 1979.

608. Spencer, H.: *Pathology of the Lung (Excluding Pulmonary Tuberculosis).* WB Saunders, Philadelphia, 1977.

609. Spielvogel, R.L., Ullman, S., and Goltz, R.W.: Skin changes in graft-vs.-host disease. *South Med J* 69: 1277–1281, 1976.

610. Spitzer, G., Dicke, K.A., Litam, J., Verma, D.S., Zander, A., Lanzotti, V., Valdivieso, M., McCredie, K.B., and Samuels, M.L.: High-dose combination chemotherapy with autologous bone marrow transplantation in adult solid tumors. *Cancer* 45: 3075–3085, 1980.

611. Springmeyer, S.C., Silvestri, R.C., Sale, G.E., Peterson, D.L., Weems, C.E., Huseby, J.S., Hudson, L.D., and Thomas, E.D.: The role of transbronchial biopsy for the diagnosis of pneumonias in immunocompromised marrow transplant recipients. *Am Rev Respir Dis* 126: 763–765, 1982.

612. Spruce, W.E., Forman, S.J., Blume, K.G., Bearman, R.M., Bixby, H., Ching, A., Drinkard, J., and San Marco, A.: Hemolytic uremic syndrome after bone marrow transplantation. *Acta Haematol (Basel)* 67: 206–210, 1982.

613. Starzl, T.E., Penn, I., Putnam, C.W., Groth, C.G., and Halgrimson, C.G.: Iatrogenic alterations of immunologic surveillance in man and their influence on malignancy. *Transplant Rev* 7: 112–145, 1971.

614. Starzl, T.E., Klintmalm, G.B., Porter, K.A., Iwatsuki, S., and Shröter, G.P.J.: Liver transplantation with use of cyclosporin A and prednisone. *N Engl J Med* 305: 266–269, 1981.

615. Stastny, P., Stembridge, V.A., and Ziff, M.: Homologous disease in the adult rat: a model for autoimmune disease. I. General features and cutaneous lesions. *J Exp Med* 118: 635–647, 1963.

616. Stastny, P., Stembridge, V.A., and Vischer, T., and Ziff, M.: Homologous disease in the adult rat: A model for autoimmune disease. II. Findings in the joints, heart, and other tissues. *J Exp Med* 122: 681–709, 1965.

617. Steinmuller, D., and Motulsky, A.G.: Treatment of hereditary spherocytosis in Peromyscus by radiation and allogeneic bone marrow transplantation. *Blood* 29: 320–330, 1967.

618. Steinmuller, D.: Allograft immunity produced with skin isografts from immunologically tolerant mice. *Transplant Proc* 1: 593–596, 1969.

619. Steinmuller, D., and Rogers, R.S.: Lymphokine production in the human autologous mixed lymphocyte epidermal cell reaction (MLECR) (Abstract). *Clin Res* 29: 615A, 1981.

620. Steinmuller, D., Tyler, J.D., and David, C.S.: Cell-mediated cytotoxicity to non-MHC alloantigens on mouse epidermal cells. I. H-2 restricted reactions *J Immunol* 126: 1747–1753, 1981.

621. Steinmuller, D., Tyler, J.D., and David, C.S.: Cell-mediated cytotoxicity to non-MHC alloantigens on mouse epidermal cells. II. Genetic basis of the response of C3H mice. *J Immunol* 126: 1754–1758, 1981.

622. Stein-Streilein, J., Lipscomb, M.F., Hart, D.A., and Darden, A.: Graft-versus-host reaction in the lung. *Transplantation* 32: 38–44, 1981.

623. Stephens, R.S., Tam, M.R., Kuo, C-C., and Nowinski, R.C.: Monoclonal antibodies to *Chlamydia trachomatis:* Antibody specificities and antigen characterization. *J Immunol* 128: 1083–1089, 1982.

624. Stockman, G.D., Heim, L.R., South, M.A., and Trentin, J.J.: Differential effects of cytophosphamide on the B- and T-cell compartments of adult mice. *J Immunol* 110: 277–282, 1973.

625. Stone, H.H., Kolb, L.D., Currie, C.A., Geheber, C.E., and Cuzzell, J.Z.: *Candida* sepsis: Pathogenesis and principles of treatment. *Ann Surg* 179: 697–711, 1974.

626. Storb, R., Epstein, R.B., Ragde, H., Bryant, J., and Thomas, E.D.: Marrow engraftment by allogeneic leukocytes in lethally irradiated dogs. *Blood* 30: 805–811, 1967.

627. Storb, R., Epstein, R.B., Bryant, J., Ragde, H., and Thomas, E.D.: Marrow grafts by combined marrow and leukocyte infusions in unrelated dogs selected by histocompatibility typing. *Transplantation* 6: 587–593, 1968.

628. Storb, R., Graham, T.C., Shiurba, R., and Thomas, E.D.: Treatment of canine graft-versus-host disease with methotrexate and cyclophosphamide following bone marrow transplantation from histoincompatible donors. *Transplantation* 10: 165–172, 1970.

629. Storb, R., Epstein, R.B., Graham, T.C., and Thomas, E.D.: Methotrexate regimens for control of graft-versus-host disease in dogs with allogeneic marrow grafts. *Transplantation* 9: 240–246, 1970.

630. Storb, R., Epstein, R.B., Rudolph, R.H., and Thomas, E.D.: The effect of prior transfusion on marrow grafts between histocompatible canine siblings. *J Immunol* 105: 627–633, 1970.

631. Storb, R., Rudolph, R.H., and Thomas, E.D.: Marrow grafts between canine siblings matched by serotyping and mixed leukocyte culture. *J Clin Invest* 50: 1272–1275, 1971.

632. Storb, R., Kolb, H.J., Graham, T.C., LeBlond, G.R.,

Kolb, H., Lerner, K.G., and Thomas, E.D.: Marrow grafts between histoincompatible canine family members. *Eur J Clin Biol Res 17: 680–685, 1972.*

633. Storb, R., Rudolph, R.H., Kolb, H.J., Graham, T.C., Mickelson, E., Erickson, V., Lerner, K.G., Kolb, H., and Thomas, E.D.: Marrow grafts between DL-A-matched canine littermates. *Transplantation 15, 92–100, 1973.*

634. Storb, R., Thomas, E.D., Buckner, C.D., Clift, R.A., Johnson, F.L., Fefer, A., Glucksberg, E.R., Giblett, E.R., Lerner, K.G., and Neiman, P.: Allogeneic marrow grafting for treatment of aplastic anemia. *Blood 43: 157–180, 1974.*

635. Storb, R., Gluckman, E., Thomas, E.D., Buckner, C.D., Clift, R.A., Fefer, A., Glucksberg, H., Graham, T.C., Johnson, F.L., Lerner, K.G., Neiman, P.E., and Ochs, H.D.: Treatment of established human graft-versus-host disease by antithymocyte globulin. *Blood 44: 57–75, 1974.*

636. Storb, R., Ochs, H.D., Weiden, P.L., and Thomas, E.D.: Immunologic reactivity in marrow graft recipients. *Transplant Proc 8: 637–639, 1976.*

637. Storb, R., Thomas, E.D., Weiden, P.L., Buckner, C.D., Clift, R.A., Fefer, A., Fernando, L.P., Giblett, E.R., Goodell, B.W., Johnson, F.L., Lerner, K.G., Neiman, P.E., and Sanders, J.E.: Aplastic anemia treated by allogeneic bone marrow transplantation: A report on 49 new cases from Seattle. *Blood 48: 817–841, 1976.*

638. Storb, R., Graham, T.C., Epstein, R.B., Sale, G.E., and Thomas, E.D.: Demonstration of hematopoietic stem cells in the peripheral blood of baboons by cross circulation. *Blood 50: 537–542, 1977.*

639. Storb, R., Prentice, R.L., and Thomas, E.D.: Marrow transplantation for treatment of aplastic anemia. An analysis of factors associated with graft rejection. *N Engl J Med 296: 61–66, 1977.*

640. Storb, R. for the Seattle Marrow Transplant Team: Decrease in the graft rejection rate and improvement in survival after marrow transplantation for severe aplastic anemia. *Transplant Proc 11: 196–198, 1979.*

641. Storb, R. for the Seattle Marrow Transplant Team: Current status of marrow transplantation for the treatment of aplastic anemia. In Gale and Fox, *op cit,* pp. 1–10.

642. Storb, R., Thomas, E.D., Buckner, C.D., Clift, R.A., Deeg, H.J., Fefer, A., Goodell, B.W., Sale, G.E., Sanders, J.E., Singer, J., Stewart, P., and Weiden, P.L.: Marrow transplantation in thirty "untransfused" patients with severe aplastic anemia. *Ann Intern Med 92: 30–36, 1980.*

643. Storb, R., and Weiden, P.L.: Transfusion problems associated with transplantation. *Semin Hematol 18: 163–176, 1981.*

644. Storb, R., Doney, K.C., Thomas, E.D., Appelbaum, F., Buckner, C.D., Clift, R.A., Deeg, H.J., Goodell, B.W., Hackman, R.C., Hansen, J.A., Sanders, J., Sullivan, K., Weiden, P.L., and Witherspoon, R.P.: Marrow transplantation with or without donor buffy coat cells for 65 transfused aplastic anemia patients. *Blood 59: 236–246, 1982.*

645. Storb, R., Prentice, R.L., Buckner, C.D., Clift, R.A., Appelbaum, F., Deeg, J., Doney, K., Hansen, J.A., Mason, M., Sanders, J.E., Singer, J., Sullivan, K.M., Witherspoon, R.P., and Thomas, E.D.: Graft-versus-host disease and survival in patients with aplastic ane-

mia treated by marrow grafts from HLA-identical siblings. Beneficial effect of a protected environment. *N Engl J Med 308: 302–307, 1983.*

646. Straus, S.E., Smith, H.A., Brickman, C., de Miranda, P., McLaren, C., and Keeney, R.E.: Acyclovir for chronic mucocutaneous herpes simplex virus infection in immunosuppressed patients. *Ann Intern Med 96: 270–277, 1982.*

647. Streilein, J.W., and Billingham, R.E.: An analysis of graft-versus-host disease in Syrian hamsters. I. The epidermolytic syndrome: Description and studies on its procurement. *J Exp Med 132: 163–180, 1970.*

648. Streilein, J.W., and Billingham, R.E.: An analysis of graft-versus-host disease in Syrian hamsters. II. The epidermolytic syndrome: Studies on its pathogenesis. *J Exp Med 132: 181–197, 1970.*

649. Streilein, J.W.: An analysis of epidermolysis in hamsters suffering from homologous disease. In *Advances in Biology of Skin, Vol 11: Immunology and the Skin,* W. Montagna and R.E. Billingham, Eds., Appleton-Century-Crofts, New York, 1971.

650. Strober, W., Krakauer, R., Klaeveman, H.L., Reynolds, H.Y., and Nelson, D.L.: Secretory component deficiency. A disorder of the IgA immune system. *N Engl J Med 294: 351–356, 1976.*

651. Su, W.P.D., and Person, J.R.: Morphea profunda. A new concept and a histopathologic study of 23 cases. *Am J Dermatopathol 3: 251–260, 1981.*

652. Sullivan, J.L., Wallen, W.C., and Johnson, F.L.: Epstein-Barr virus infection following bone-marrow transplantation. *Int J Cancer 22: 132–135, 1978.*

653. Sullivan, K.M., Shulman, H.M., Storb, R., Weiden, P.L., Witherspoon, R.P., McDonald, G.B., Schubert, M.M., Atkinson, K., and Thomas, E.D.: Chronic graft-versus-host disease in 52 patients: Adverse natural course and successful treatment with combination immunosuppression. *Blood 57: 267–276, 1981.*

654. Sullivan, K.M., Storb, R., Flournoy, N., Shulman, H.M., Weiden, P.L., and Thomas, E.D.: Day 100 screening studies predict development of chronic graft-vs.-host disease (GVHD) (Abstract). *Blood 58 (Suppl 1): 176a, #615, 1981.*

655. Sullivan, K.M., Storb, R., Shulman, H.M., Shaw, C.M., Spence, A., Beckham, C., Clift, R.A., Buckner, C.D., Stewart, P., and Thomas, E.D.: Immediate and delayed neurotoxicity after mechlorethamine preparation for bone marrow transplantation. *Ann Intern Med 97: 182–189, 1982.*

656. Sullivan, K.M., Dahlberg, S., Storb, R., Shulman, H., and Thomas, E.D.: Chronic graft-versus-host disease (GVHD): Risk factor analysis in patients surviving > 70 days after marrow transplantation (Abstract). *Exp Hematol 10: (Suppl) 7, #9 1982.*

657. Sumner, H.W., and Tedesco, F.J.: Rectal biopsy in clindamycin-associated colitis: An analysis of 23 cases. *Arch Pathol 99: 237–241, 1975.*

658. Sutherland, D.E.R., Chan, F.Y., Foucar, E., Simmons, P.L., Howard, R.J., and Najarian, J.S.: The bleeding cecal ulcer in transplant patients. *Surgery 86: 386–398, 1979.*

659. Sweny, P., Hopper, J., Gross, M., and Varghese, Z.: Nephrotoxicity of cyclosporin A (Letter). *Lancet 1: 663, 1981.*

660. Swisher, S.N., and Young, L.E.: The blood grouping systems of dogs. *Physiol Rev 41: 495–520, 1961.*

661. Tamerius, J.D., Garrigues, H.J., Hellström, I., and Hellström, K.E.: An isotope release assay and terminal-labeling assay for measuring cell-mediated allograft and tumor immunity to small numbers of adherent target cells. *J Immunol Meth* 22: 1–22, 1978.

662. Tan, E.M.: Immunopathology and pathogenesis of cutaneous involvement in systemic lupus erythematosus. *J Invest Dermatol* 67: 360–365, 1976.

663. Tarpila, S.: Morphologic and functional response of human small intestine to ionizing radiation. *Scand J Gastroenterol (Suppl)* 6: 9–48, 1971.

664. Thein, S.L., Goldman, J.M., and Galton, D.A.G.: Acute "graft-versus-host disease" after autografting for chronic granulocytic leukemia in transformation. *Ann Intern Med* 94: 210–211, 1981.

665. Thierfelder, S., Rodt, H., and Kolb, H.J., (Eds.): *Immunobiology of Bone Marrow Transplantation, Vol 25: Haemotology and Blood Transfusion.* Springer-Verlag, New York, 1980.

666. Thomas, E.D., Ashley, C.A., Lochte, H.L., Jaretzki, A. III, Sahler, O.D., and Ferrebee, J.W.: Homografts of bone marrow in dogs after lethal total-body radiation. *Blood* 14: 720–736, 1959.

667. Thomas, E.D., LeBlond, R., Graham, T.C., and Storb, R.: Marrow infusions in dogs given midlethal or lethal irradiation. *Radiat Res* 41: 113–124, 1970.

668. Thomas, E.D., and Storb, R.: Technique for human marrow grafting. *Blood* 36: 507–515, 1970.

669. Thomas, E.D., Storb, R., Clift, R.A., Fefer, A., Johnson, F.L., Neiman, P.E., Lerner, K.G., Glucksberg, H., and Buckner, C.D.: Bone-marrow transplantation. *N Engl J Med* 292: 832–843; 895–902, 1975.

670. Thomas, E.D., Storb, R., Giblett, E.R., Longpre, B., Weiden, P.L., Fefer, A., Witherspoon, R., Clift, R.A., and Buckner, C.D.: Recovery from aplastic anemia following attempted marrow transplantation. *Exp Hematol* 4: 97–102, 1976.

671. Thomas, E.D., Buckner, C.D., Banaji, M., Clift, R.A., Fefer, A., Flournoy, N., Goodell, B.W., Hickman, R.O., Lerner, K.G., Neiman, P.E., Sale, G.E., Sanders, J.E., Singer, J., Stevens, M., Storb, R., and Weiden, P.L.: One hundred patients with acute leukemia treated by chemotherapy, total body irradiation, and allogeneic marrow transplantation. *Blood* 49: 511–533, 1977.

672. Thomas, E.D., Buckner, C.D., Clift, R.A., Fefer, A., Johnson, F.L., Neiman, P.E., Sale, G.E., Sanders, J.E., Singer, J.W., Shulman, H., Storb, R., and Weiden, P.L.: Marrow transplantation for acute nonlymphoblastic leukemia in first remission. *N Engl J Med* 301: 597–599, 1979.

673. Thomas, E.D., Sanders, J.E., Flournoy, N., Johnson, F.L., Buckner, C.D., Clift, R.A., Fefer, A., Goodell, B.W., Storb, R., and Weiden, P.L.: Marrow transplantation for patients with acute lymphoblastic leukemia in remission. *Blood* 54: 468–476, 1979.

674. Thomas, E.D.: Bone marrow transplantation. *Univ Wash Med* 8: 17–22, 1981.

675. Thomas, E.D.: Clinical bone marrow transplantation. Proceedings of the Cancer 1981/Cancer 1001 International Colloquium, Houston, Texas, 1981. *Cancer Bull* 34: 268–270, 1982.

675a. Thomas, E.D., Buckner, C.D., Sanders, J., Papayannopoulou, T., Borgna-Pignatti, C., De Stefano, P., Sullivan, K.M., Clift, R.A., and Storb, R.: Marrow transplantation for thalassemia. *Lancet* 2: 227–229, 1982.

676. Thorsby, E., and Helgesen, A.: Possible detection of sensitization against non-HL-A histocompatibility antigens "in vitro." In *Series Immunobiology Standard, Vol. 18,* International Symposium on Standardization of HL-A Reagents, 1972. Karger, Basel, 1973, pp. 141–148.

677. Thung, S.N., Gerber, M.A., and Bodenheimer, H.C., Jr.: Nodular regenerative hyperplasia of the liver in a patient with diabetes mellitus. *Cancer* 49: 543–546, 1982.

678. Tobias, H., and Auerbach, R.: Hepatotoxicity of long-term methotrexate therapy for psoriasis. *Arch Intern Med* 132: 391–396, 1973.

679. Toner, P.G., and Ferguson, A.: Intraepithelial cells in the human intestinal mucosa. *J Ultrastruc Res* 34: 329–344, 1971.

680. Touraine, R., Revuz, J., Dreyfus, B., Rochant, H., and Mannoni, P.: Graft-versus-host-reaction and lichen planus. *Br J Dermatol* 92: 589, 1975.

681. Townsend, T.R., Bolyard, E.A., Yolken, R.H., Beschorner, W.E., Bishop, C.A., Burns, W.H., Santos, G.W., and Saral, R.: Outbreak of Coxsackie A1 gastroenteritis: A complication of bone-marrow transplantation. *Lancet* 1: 820–823, 1982.

682. Travis, E.L., Harley, R.A., Fenn, J.O., Klobukowski, C.J., and Hargrove, H.B.: Pathologic changes in the lung following single and multi-fraction irradiation. *Int J Radiat Oncol Biol Phys* 2: 475–490, 1977.

683. Trier, J.S.: Morphologic alterations induced by methotrexate in the mucosa of human proximal intestine. II. Electron microscopic observations. *Gastroenterology* 43: 407–424, 1962.

684. Trier, J.S., and Browning, T.H.: Morphologic response of the mucosa of human small intestine to x-ray exposure. *J Clin Invest* 45: 194–204, 1966.

685. Trier, J.S., and Rubin, C.E.: Electron microscopy of the small intestine: A review. *Gastroenterology* 49: 574–603, 1965.

686. Tsoi, M.S., Storb, R., Weiden, P.L., Graham, T.C., Schroeder, M.L., and Thomas, E.D.: Canine marrow transplantation: Are serum blocking factors necessary to maintain the stable chimeric state? *J Immunol* 114: 531–539, 1975.

687. Tsoi, M.S., Storb, R., Weiden, P.L., and Thomas, E.D.: Studies on cellular inhibition and serum-blocking factors in 28 human patients given marrow grafts from HLA identical siblings. *J Immunol* 118: 1799–1805, 1977.

688. Tsoi, M.S., Storb, R., Jones, E., Weiden, P.L., Shulman, H., Witherspoon, R., Atkinson, K., and Thomas, E.D.: Deposition of IgM and complement at the dermo-epidermal junction in acute and chronic graft-vs.-host disease in man. *J Immunol* 120: 1485–1492, 1978.

689. Tsoi, M.S., Storb, R., Dobbs, S., Kopecky, K.J., Santos, E., Weiden, P.L., and Thomas, E.D.: Nonspecific suppressor cells in patients with chronic graft-vs.-host disease after marrow grafting. *J Immunol* 123: 1970–1976, 1979.

690. Tsoi, M.S., Storb, R., Dobbs, S., Medill, L., and Thomas, E.D.: Cell-mediated immunity to non-HLA antigens of the host by donor lymphocytes in patients with chronic graft-vs.-host disease. *J Immunol* 125:

2258–2262, 1980.

691. Tsoi, M.S., Storb, R., Dobbs, S., Sullivan, K.M., and Thomas, E.D.: Suppressor cells in patients with HLA identical marrow grafts. In Gale and Fox, *op cit*, pp. 119–125.

692. Tsoi, M.S., Storb, R., Dobbs, S., Santos, E., and Thomas, E.D.: Specific suppressor cells and immune response to host antigens in long-term human allogeneic marrow recipients. Implications for the mechanisms of graft–host tolerance and chronic graft-versus-host disease. *Transplant Proc 13*: 237–240, 1981.

693. Tsoi, M.S., Storb, R., Dobbs, S., and Thomas, E.D.: Specific suppressor cells in graft–host tolerance of HLA-identical marrow transplantation. *Nature 292*: 355–357, 1981.

694. Tsoi, M.S., Storb, R., Weiden, P., Santos, E., Kopecky, K.J., and Thomas, E.D.: Sequential studies of cell inhibition of host fibroblasts in 51 patients given HLA-identical marrow grafts. *J Immunol 128*: 239–242, 1982.

695. Tsoi, M.S.: Overview. Immunological mechanisms of graft-versus-host disease in man. *Transplantation 33*: 459–464, 1982.

695a. Tsoi, M.S., Storb, R., Santos, E., and Thomas, E.D.: Antihost cytotoxicity in patients with acute graft-versus-host disease after HLA-identical marrow grafting. *Transplant Proc 15*: 1484–1486, 1983.

696. Tutschka, P.: *Experimental chemotherapy of graft versus host disease.* (Workshop Summary). In Gale and Fox, *op cit*, pp. 291–295.

697. Tutschka, P.J., Körbling, M., Hess, A.D., Beschorner, W.E., and Santos, G.W.: Graft-vs.-host reactions: Prevention of graft-versus-host disease (GVHD) by chemoseparation of marrow cells. *Transplant Proc 13*: 1202–1206, 1981.

698. Tyler, J.D., and Steinmuller, D.: Cell-mediated cytotoxicity to non-MHC alloantigens on mouse epidermal cells. III. Epidermal cell-specific cytotoxic T-lymphocytes. *J Immunol 126*: 1759–1763, 1981.

699. Tytgat, G.N., Huibregtse, K., Schellekens, P.T., and Feltkamp-Vroom, T.H.: Clinical and immunologic observations in a patient with late onset immunodeficiency. *Gastroenterology 76*: 1458–1465, 1979.

700. Tzipori, S., Angus, K.W., Gray, E.W., and Campbell, I.: Vomiting and diarrhea associated with cryptosporidial infection (Letter). *N Engl J Med 303*: 818, 1980.

701. UCLA Bone Marrow Transplantation Group: Bone marrow transplantation with intensive combination chemotherapy/radiation therapy (SCARI) in acute leukemia. *Ann Intern Med 86*: 155–161, 1977.

702. UCLA Bone Marrow Transplant Team: Prevention of graft rejection following bone marrow transplantation. *Blood 57*: 9–12, 1981.

703. Uitto, J., Bauer, E.A., and Eisen, A.Z.: Scleroderma: Increased biosynthesis of triple-helical type I and type III procollagens associated with unaltered expression of collagenase by skin fibroblasts in culture. *J Clin Invest 64*: 921–930, 1979.

704. Ulbright, T.M., and Katzenstein, A.L.A.: Solitary necrotizing granulomas of the lung: Differentiating features and etiology. *Am J Surg Pathol 4*: 13–28, 1980.

705. Ullman, S., Spielvogel, R.L., Kersey, J.H., and Goltz, R.W.: Immunoglobulins and complement in skin in graft-versus-host disease (Letter). *Ann Intern Med 85*: 205, 1976.

706. Underwood, J.C.E., and Corbett, C.L.: Persistent diarrhoea and hypoalbuminaemia associated with cytomegalovirus enteritis. *Br Med J 1*: 1029–1030, 1978.

707. van Bekkum, D.W., and Vos, D.: Treatment of secondary disease in radiation chimeras. *Int J Radiat Biol 3*: 173–181, 1961.

708. van Bekkum, O., and deVries, H.: *Radiation Chimeras.* Academic Press, New York, 1967, pp. 138, 146–150.

709. van Bekkum, D.W., deVries, M.J., and van der Waaij, D.: Lesions characteristic of secondary disease in germfree heterologous radiation chimeras. *J Natl Cancer Inst 38*: 223–231, 1967.

710. van Bekkum, D.W., Roodenburg, J., Heidt, P.J., and van der Waaij, D.: Mitigation of secondary disease of allogeneic mouse radiation chimeras by modification of the intestinal microflora. *J Natl Cancer Inst 52*: 401–404, 1974.

711. van Bekkum, D.W., and Knaan, S.: Role of bacterial microflora in development of intestinal lesions from graft-versus-host reaction. *J Natl Cancer Inst 58*: 787–790, 1977.

712. van Bekkum, D.W., Knaan, S., and Zurcher, C.: Effects of cyclosporin A on experimental graft-versus-host disease in rodents. *Transplant Proc 12*: 278–282, 1980.

713. van Bekkum, D.W.: Immunological basis of graft-versus-host disease. In Gale and Fox, *op cit*, pp. 175–193.

714. van de Waaij, D., Berghuis, J.M., and Lekkerkerk, J.E.C.: Colonization resistance of the digestive tract of mice during systemic antibiotic treatment. *J Hyg (Camb) 70*: 605–610, 1972.

715. van Dongen, J.M., Kooyman, J., and Visser, W.J.: The influence of 400r x-irradiation on the number and the localization of mature and immature goblet cells and Paneth cells in intestinal crypt and villus. *Cell Tissue Kinet 9*: 66–75, 1976.

716. Van Dyk, J., Keane, T.J., Kan, S., Rider, W.D., and Fryer, C.J.H.: Radiation pneumonitis following large single-dose irradiation. A re-evaluation based on absolute dose to lung. *Int J Radiat Oncol Biol Phys 7*: 461–467, 1981.

717. Vergani, D., Locasciulli, A., Masera, G., Alberti, A., Moroni, G., Tee, D.E.H., Portmann, B., Vergani, G.M., and Eddleston, A.L.W.F.: Histological evidence of hepatitis-B-virus infection with negative serology in children with acute leukaemia who develop chronic liver disease. *Lancet 1*: 361–364, 1982.

718. Vos, O., deVries, M.J., Collenteur, J.C., and van Bekkum, D.W.: Transplantation of homologous and heterologous lymphoid cells in x-irradiated and nonirradiated mice. *J Natl Cancer Inst 23*: 53–73, 1959.

719. Vosak, E., Atkinson, K., Munro, V., and Biggs, J.: Lymphoid subpopulations in the skin after human marrow transplantation: Definition with monoclonal antibodies (Abstract). *Transplant Proc* (in press).

720. Vowels, M., Lam-Po-Tang, R., Zagars, G., et al.: Total body irradiation and Budd-Chiari syndrome. In *Abstracts of 1978 Annual Meeting of the Royal College of Pathologists of Australia*, 1979, p. 306.

721. Vriesendorp, H.M., Rothengatter, C., Bos, E., Westbroek, D.L., and van Rood, J.J.: The production and

evaluation of dog allolymphocytotoxins for donor selection in transplantation experiments. *Transplantation* 11: 440–445, 1971.

722. Vriesendorp, H.M., Gross-Wilde, H., and Dorf, M.E.: The major histocompatibility system of the dog. In *The Major Histocompatibility System in Man and Animals*, D. Götze, Ed., Springer-Verlag, New York, 1977, pp. 129–163.

723. Wade, J.C., Schimpf, S.C. Hargadon, M.T., Fortner, C.L., Young, V.M., and Wiernik, P.H.: A comparison of trimethoprim-sulfamethoxazole plus nystatin with gentamicin plus nystatin in the prevention of infections in acute leukemia. *N Engl J Med* 304: 1057–1062, 1981.

724. Wade, J., and Meyers, J.: Randomized trial of ketaconazole for mucocutaneous candidiasis in bone marrow transplant recipients (unpublished observation).

725. Wade, J.C., Newton, B., McLaren, C., Flournoy, N., Keeney, R.E., and Meyers, J.D.: Intravenous acyclovir to treat mucocutaneous herpes simplex virus infections after bone marrow transplantation. A double-blind trial. *Ann Intern Med* 96: 265–269, 1982.

726. Wagemaker, G., Vriesendorp, H.M., and van Bekkum, D.W.: Successful bone marrow transplantation across major histocompatibility barriers in rhesus monkeys. *Transplant Proc* 13: 875–880, 1981.

727. Wagman, L.D., Burt, M.E., and Brennan, M.F.: The impact of total parenteral nutrition on liver function tests in patients with cancer. *Cancer* 49: 1249–1257, 1982.

728. Wahl, S.M., Wahl, L.M., and McCarthy, J.B.: Lymphocyte-mediated activation of fibroblast proliferation and collagen production. *J Immunol* 121: 942–946, 1978.

729. Wands, J.R., Dienstag, J.L., Bhan, A.K., Feller, E.R., and Isselbacher, K.J.: Circulating immune complexes and complement activation in primary biliary cirrhosis. *N Engl J Med* 298: 233–237, 1978.

730. Ward, P.A.: Immune complex injury of the lung. *Am J Pathol* 97: 85–91, 1979.

731. Ware, C.F., and Granger, G.A.: Mechanisms of lymphocyte-mediated cytotoxicity. III. Characterization of the mechanism of inhibition of the human alloimmune lymphocyte-mediated cytotoxic reaction by polyspecific antilymphotoxin sera *in vitro*. *J Immunol* 126: 1934–1940, 1981.

732. Warren, R.P., Storb, R., Weiden, P.L., Su, P.J., and Thomas, E.D.: Immunologic monitoring of marrow graft recipients following transplantation from HLA-identical siblings. *Transplant Proc* 10: 535–536, 1978.

733. Weedon, D., Searle, J., and Kerr, J.F.R.: Apoptosis: Its nature and implications for dermatopathology. *Am J Dermatopathol* 1: 133–144, 1979.

734. Weiden, P.L., Storb, R., Slichter, S., Warren, R.P., and Sale, G.E.: Effect of six weekly transfusions on canine marrow grafts: Tests for sensitization and abrogation of sensitization by procarbazine and antithymocyte serum. *J Immunol* 117: 143–150, 1976.

735. Weiden, P.L., Storb, R., Tsoi, M-S., Graham, T.C., Lerner, K.G., and Thomas, E.D.: Infusion of donor lymphocytes into stable canine radiation chimeras. Implications for mechanism of transplantation tolerance. *J Immunol* 116: 1212–1219, 1976.

735a. Weiden, P.L., Hackman, R.C., Deeg, H.J., Graham, T.C., Thomas, E.D., and Storb, R.: Long-term survival and reversal of iron overload after marrow transplantation in dogs with congenital hemolytic anemia. *Blood* 57: 66–70, 1981.

736. Weiden, P.L., Doney, K., Storb, R., and Thomas, E.D.: Anti-human thymocyte globulin (ATG) for prophylaxis and treatment of graft-versus-host disease in recipients of allogeneic marrow grafts. *Transplant Proc* 10: 213–216, 1978.

737. Weiden, P.L., Flournoy, N., Thomas, E.D., Prentice, R., Fefer, A., Buckner, C.D., and Storb, R.: Antileukemic effects of graft-versus-host disease in human recipients of allogeneic-marrow grafts. *N Engl J Med* 300: 1068–1073, 1979.

738. Weiden, P.L., and the Seattle Marrow Transplant Team: Graft-vs.-host disease in allogeneic marrow transplantation. In Gale and Fox, *op cit*, pp. 37–48.

739. Weiden, P.L., Zuckerman, N., Hansen, J.A., Sale, G.E., Remlinger, K., Beck, T.M., and Buckner, C.D.: Fatal graft-versus-host disease in a patient with lymphoblastic leukemia following normal granulocyte transfusions. *Blood* 57: 328–332, 1981.

740. Weiden, P.L., Sullivan, K.M., Flournoy, N., Storb, R., Thomas, E.D., and the Seattle Marrow Transplant Team: Antileukemic effect of chronic graft-versus-host disease. *N Engl J Med* 304: 1529–1533, 1981.

741. Weinstein, G.D., and Velsaco, J.: Selective action of methotrexate on psoriatic epidermal cells. *J Invest Dermatol* 59: 121–127, 1972.

742. Weinstein, G., Roenigk, H., Maibach, H., Cosmides, J., Halprin, K., and Millard, M.: Psoriasis–liver–methotrexate interactions. *Arch Dermatol* 108: 36–42, 1973.

743. Weinstein, L., Edelstein, S.M., Madara, J.L., Falchuk, K.R., McManus, B.N., and Trier, J.S.: Intestinal cryptosporidiosis complicated by disseminated cytomegalovirus infection. *Gastroenterology* 81: 584–591, 1981.

744. Weisbrot, I.M., Liber, A.F., and Gordon, B.S.: The effects of therapeutic radiation on colonic mucosa. *Cancer* 36: 931–940, 1975.

745. Weisdorf, S.A., Longsdorf, J.A., Salati, L.M., Ramsay, N.K., and Sharp, H.L.: Intestinal graft-versus-host disease: A new protein losing enteropathy (Abstract). *Gastroenterology* 80: 1313, 1981.

746. Weiser, B., Lange, M., Fialk, M.A., Singer, C., Szatrowski, T.H., and Armstrong, D.: Prophylactic trimethoprim-sulfamethoxazole during consolidation chemotherapy for acute leukemia: A controlled trial. *Ann Intern Med* 95: 436–438, 1981.

747. Weiss, R.B., and Muggia, F.M.: Cytotoxic drug-induced pulmonary disease: Update 1980. *Am J Med* 68: 259–266, 1980.

748. West, J.C., Armitage, J.O., Mitros, R.A., Klassen, L.W., Corry, R.J., and Ray, T.: Cytomegalovirus cecal erosion causing massive hemorrhage in a bone marrow transplant recipient. *World J Surg* 6: 251–255, 1982.

749. Williams, R.C., Jr.: In *Immune Complexes in Clinical and Experimental Medicine*. Harvard University, Cambridge, 1980.

750. Willson, R.A., and Hart, J.R.: *In vivo* drug metabolism and liver lobule heterogeneity in the rat. *Gastroenterology* 81: 563–569, 1981.

751. Winston, D.J., Meyer, D.V., Gale, R.P., Young, L.S., and the UCLA Bone Marrow Transplant Team: Fur-

ther experience with infections in bone marrow transplant recipients. *Transplant Proc 10: 247–254, 1978.*

752. Winston, D.J., Schiffman, G., Wang, D.C., Feig, S.A., Lin, C.H., Marso, E.L., Ho, W.G., Young, L.S., and Gale, R.P.: Pneumococcal infections after human bone-marrow transplantation. *Ann Intern Med 91: 835–841, 1979.*

753. Winston, D.J., Gale, R.P., Meyer, D.V., Young, L.S., and the UCLA Bone Marrow Transplantation Group: Infectious complications of human bone marrow transplantation. *Medicine 58: 1–31, 1979.*

754. Winston, D.J., Ho, W.G., Young, L.S., and Gale, R.P.: Prophylactic granulocyte transfusions during human bone marrow transplantation. *Am J Med 68: 893–897, 1980.*

755. Winston, D.J., Ho, W.G., Howell, C.L., Miller, M.J., Mickey, R., Martin, W.J., Lin, C.H., and Gale, R.P.: Cytomegalovirus infections associated with leukocyte transfusions. *Ann Intern Med 93: 671–675, 1980.*

756. Withers, H.R.: The four R's of radiotherapy. *Adv Radiat Biol 5: 241–271, 1975.*

757. Witherspoon, R.P., Storb, R., Ochs, H.D., Flournoy, N., Kopecky, K.J., Sullivan, K.M., Deeg, H.J., Sosa, R., Noel, D.R., Atkinson, K., and Thomas, E.D.: Recovery of antibody production in human allogeneic marrow graft recipients. Influence of time post-transplantation, the presence or absence of chronic graft-versus-host disease, and antithymocyte globulin treatment. *Blood 58: 360–368, 1981.*

758. Wojcicka, B.: Separation and characterization of bile antigens. In *Immune Reactions in Liver Disease,* A.L.W.F. Eddleston, J.C.P. Weber and R. Williams, Eds., Pitman Medical, Tunbridge Wells, England, 1979.

759. Woodruff, J.M., Eltringham, J.R., and Casey, H.W.: Early secondary disease in the Rhesus monkey. I. A comparative histopathologic study. *Lab Invest 20: 499–511, 1969.*

760. Woodruff, J.M., Butcher, W.I., and Hellerstein, L.J.: Early secondary disease in the Rhesus monkey. II. Electron microscopy of changes in mucous membranes and external epithelia as demonstrated in the tongue and lip. *Lab Invest 27: 85–98, 1972.*

761. Woodruff, J.M., Hansen, J.A., Good, R.A., Santos, G.W., and Slavin, R.E.: The pathology of the graft-ver-

sus-host reaction (GVHR) in adults receiving bone marrow transplants. *Transplant Proc 8: 675–684, 1976.*

762. Woods, W.G., Dehner, L.P., Nesbit, M.E., Krivit, W., Coccia, P.F., Ramsay, N.K.C., Kim, T.H., and Kersey, J.H.: Fatal veno-occlusive disease of the liver following high-dose chemotherapy, irradiation, and bone marrow transplantation. *Am J Med 68: 285–290, 1980.*

763. Wulff, J., Sale, G.E., Deeg, H.J., and Storb, R.: Nonspecific acid esterase activity as a marker for canine T-lymphocytes. *Exp Hematol 9: 865–870, 1981.*

764. Yolken, R.H., Bishop, C.A., Townsend, T.R., Bolyard, E.A., Bartlett, J., Santos, G.W., and Saral, R.: Infectious gastroenteritis in bone-marrow transplant recipients. *N Engl J Med 306: 1009–1012, 1982.*

765. Zahradnik, J.M., Spencer, M.J., and Porter, D.D.: Adenovirus infection in the immunocompromised patient. *Am J Med 68: 725–732, 1980.*

766. Zachariae, H., Kragballe, K., and Søgaard, H.: Methotrexate induced liver cirrhosis. Studies including serial liver biopsies during continued treatment. *Br J Dermatol 102: 407–412, 1980.*

767. Zander, A.R., Vellekoop, L., Spitzer, G., Verma, D.S., Litam, J., McCredie, K.B., Keating, M., Hester, J.P., and Dicke, K.A.: Combination of high-dose cyclophosphamide, BCNU, and VP-16-213 followed by autologous marrow rescue in the treatment of relapsed leukemia. *Cancer Treat Rep 65: 377–381, 1981.*

768. Zimmerman, H.J., Fang, M., Utili, R., Seeff, L.B., and Hoofnagle, J.: Jaundice due to bacterial infection. *Gastroenterology 77: 362–374, 1979.*

769. Zimmerman, H.J.: Drug-induced liver injury: An overview. *Semin Liver Dis 1: 93–103, 1981.*

770. Zurcher, C., Van Kessel, A.C.M., and Vriesendorp, H.M.: Graft-versus-host reactions after total body irradiation and bone marrow transplantation. In *Annual Report, Radiobiologica Institute,* TNO, Rijswijk, The Netherlands, 1977, pp. 278–280.

771. Zwann, F.E., Jansen, J., and Noordijk, E.M.: Graft-versus-host disease limited to area of irradiated skin (Letter). *Lancet 1: 1081–1082, 1980.*

*Additional Reference:*
Gale, R.P. (ed.): *Recent Advances in Bone Marrow Transplantation.* Alan R. Liss Inc., New York, 1983.

# Glossary of abbreviations and terms

**Acidophilic body** Same as eosinophilic body: a shrunken, eosinophilic mass, usually anucleate, which represents a dead cell. In liver, same as Councilman body. In skin, same as "mummy" cell, apoptotic cell, individual cell necrosis.

**Aggressor lymphocyte lesion** Term coined by Woodruff to describe presumed attack upon epithelial cells by lymphocytes in target tissues of GVHD.[759]

**Allogeneic** Adjective defining the relationship between a donor and host who are of the same species but not genetically identical. Allografts may be matched at one or more MHC loci, or may be mismatched, as is the case in most random donors of blood products.

**Allograft** (= **Homograft**) A graft undertaken between genetically nonidentical individuals of the same species.

**ANA** Antinuclear antigen.

**ANAE** Acid naphthylacetate esterase. A "nonspecific" esterase present diffusely in the cytoplasm of the monocyte–macrophage series of cells and focally in some lymphocytes. The focal reaction is thought in mice and humans to characterize a T-cell subset, possibly helper cells.

**Apoptosis, apoptotic body** A form of individual cell death characterized by the formation of a membrane-bound cell fragment containing cytoplasm, intact organelles, and fragments of disrupted nucleus.[345]

**Ara-A** Adenine arabinoside: an antiviral and antineoplastic agent.

**Ara-C** Cytosine arabinoside: an antineoplastic drug.

**ATG** Antithymocyte globulin. Relatively crude xenogeneic antisera against T-cells used as immunosuppression.

**Autograft** A graft of an individual's own tissue.

**B-cell** "Bursal-derived" or "bursal-equivalent" lymphocyte. Refers to antibody-producing lymphocyte class which can differentiate into immunoglobulin-producing plasma cells. Originally discovered in the bursa of Fabricius of chickens.

**BMT** Bone marrow transplantation. The infusion of nucleated bone marrow cells from one individual to another.

**Chimera** An individual bearing cells of another individual, such as a stable bone marrow allograft recipient whose peripheral blood cells are all of donor genetic type.

**CY plus TBI** A frequently used "preconditioning" or "preparative" regimen to prepare a leukemia patient for bone marrow transplantation. A frequent combination is 60 mg/kg of cyclophosphamide (CY) on days −5, −3, and −1, followed by a single 1000r dose of total body irradiation (TBI). The marrow infusion is given later on the same day as the TBI in cases in which single TBI doses are given. More recently, fractioned radiation has been used in divided doses of 200–275r per day.

**"Day" convention** Throughout this book (and the publications of the Oncology Division, FHCRC) "day" refers to any day after bone marrow transplantation. Day of transplant is day zero, and those days prior to transplant, are indicated by a minus sign preceding the number: −1, −2, etc.

**DLA** Refers to the "dog leukocyte antigen" major histocompatibility complex.

**Eosinophilic body** Synonymous with apoptosis, acidophilic body, mummified cell.

**Exploding crypt** Term coined to describe gut crypt showing multiple necrotic epithelial cells, particularly in rectal histopathology of GVHD.[547]

**FTS** Factor thymic serique. A nonapeptide thymic epithelial product found in normal human serum.[24]

**GVH** Graft-vs.-host.

**GVHR** Graft-vs.-host reaction. Reaction of donor lymphoid cells against host tissue antigens. The reaction usually refers to the stimulation, recruitment, and cytotoxic phases in lymphoid tissues, whereas the "disease" is often considered the aftermath of the "reaction."

**GVHD** Graft-vs.-host disease.

**Acute** Syndrome of dermatitis, enteritis, and hepatitis occurring during the first 100 days after a bone marrow allograft in humans. In rodent models, acute GVHD is often used to refer to the disease occurring in $H_2$-mismatched donor–host pairs, whereas chronic GVHD is used to refer to that following more nearly matched transplantations.[519]

**Pseudo-GVHD** An autoimmune phenomenon occurring in syngeneic graft recipients resembling an alloimmune reaction (see Chapter 2).

**Chronic** Syndrome of lichenoid lesions, scleroderma, and immunodeficiency occurring more than 100 days after transplantation. In rodents, may refer to all GVHD after $H_2$-matched marrow allografting.

**Helper cell** A T-cell subset (equivalent to the OKT4 or Leu-2 marker-bearing cell in humans) which is capable of inducing (or helping) B-cells to synthesize immunoglobulin.

**HLA** Human leukocyte antigen.

**Homograft** (= **Isograft** = **Syngeneic graft**) A graft between genetically identical individuals of the same species.

**HSV** Herpes simplex virus.

**IgA, -G, -M, etc.** Immunoglobulin A, -G, -M, etc.

**IIP** Idiopathic interstitial pneumonia.

**Karyolytic body** Individual cell necrosis corresponding to the mummified or apoptotic cell.[192]

**Killer cell** Cell capable of cell-mediated cytotoxicity. T killer cells, macrophage killer cells, and null (natural) killer cells have been identified and characterized in several species.

**LAF** Laminar airflow.

**MHC** Major histocompatibility complex.

**MCTD** Mixed connective tissue disease.

**MLC** Mixed leukocyte culture.

**MTX** Methotrexate.

**Mummified cell** Necrotic individual cell with eosinophilic change found, for example, in basal layer of epidermis in GVHD of skin.

**Network theory** A system proposed by Jerne providing hypothetical servo-mechanisms by which circuits of T-lymphocytes might regulate cellular and humoral immune functions.[290]

**Nikolsky's sign** The ready desquamation of epidermis on gentle lateral digital pressure, associated with toxic epidermal necrolysis and with histological grade IV acute GVHD of the skin.

**NK cell** Natural killer cell. A null cell, identified by some with the "large granular lymphocyte" which may be related to a T-cell subset. These cells are efficient and highly specific cytotoxic cells under certain conditions and some have been grown in culture. They may relate to the phenomenon of natural (nonacquired) immunity. They have been implicated as mediators of "natural resistance" to marrow grafts and to tumors.

**OKT4 (or Leu-2)** Designation of a mouse monoclonal antibody against a cell surface phenotype of a lymphocyte T-cell subset, associated with "help."

**OKT8 (or Leu-3)** Cell surface phenotype of a suppressor/cytotoxic T-cell subset, identified by a monoclonal mouse antibody to human lymphocytes.

**Parabiosis intoxication** Refers to secondary disease (or GVHD) induced by connecting the peripheral blood circulations of donor and host animals.

**PBC** Primary biliary cirrhosis.

**rad (r)** Tissue unit dose of irradiation (100 ergs/g tissue).

**Gray (Gy)** = 100 rad.

**Roentgen (R)** Unit of x-irradiation. The amount of radiation which will produce in one cc of atmospheric air at zero degrees and 76 mm mercury pressure, a sufficient degree of conductivity so that one electrostatic unit of charge may be measured at saturation. Equivalent to $2.58 \times 10^{-4}$ coulomb/kg dry air.

**RA** Rheumatoid arthritis.

**RES** Reticuloendothelial system.

**SCID** Severe combined immunodeficiency.

**Secondary disease** General term for the sequelae of a GVHR which avoids the issue of the allogeneic specificity of the systemic syndrome. Includes both GVHR and GVHD with infectious and wasting sequelae.

**Simonson assay** Spleen weight assay for quantitative GVHR in animals.

**SLE** Systemic lupus erythematosus.

**SS** Systemic scleroderma.

**Syngeneic graft** (= **Isograft**) Graft between genetically identical individuals.

**TBB** Transbronchial biopsy.

**TBI** Total body irradiation.

**T-lymphocyte** (Thymus-derived lymphocyte) A lymphocyte influenced by the thymus to differentiate into a "T-cell" type, serving several functions, but lacking the secretion of circulating antibody.

**TNP** Trinitrophenol.

**TPN** Total parenteral nutrition.

**VOD** Venocclusive disease.

**VZV** Varicella zoster virus.

**Xenogeneic, xenograft** Graft between different species.

# Index